MAYO CLINIC

Heart Book

MAYO CLINIC

Heart Book

MICHAEL D. McGOON, M.D.
EDITOR-IN-CHIEF

William Morrow and Company, Inc.
New York

Mayo Clinic Heart Book provides comprehensive health information in a single, authoritative source. *Mayo Clinic Health Letter*, a monthly, eight-page newsletter offers the same kind of easy-to-understand, reliable information, with a special focus on timely topics. For information on how this award-winning newsletter can be delivered to your doorstep every month, call 1-800-333-9037.

Mayo Clinic Heart Book provides reliable, practical, comprehensive, easy-to-understand information on heart disease and heart health. Much of its information comes directly from the experience of Mayo's 1,300 physicians and medical scientists.

Mayo Clinic Heart Book supplements advice of your personal physician, whom you should consult for individual medical problems. No endorsement of any company or product is implied or intended.

The triple-shield Mayo logo and the words MAYO and MAYO CLINIC are registered marks of Mayo Foundation, and are used under license by Mayo Foundation for Medical Education and Research.

Library of Congress Cataloging-in-Publication Data

Mayo Clinic heart book : the ultimate guide to heart health.
p. cm.
Includes bibliographical references and index.
ISBN 0-688-09972-6
1. Heart—Diseases—Popular works. 2. Cardiology—Popular works. 3. Consumer education. I. Mayo Clinic.
RC672.M4 1993
616.1′2—dc20   93-25353
                                                CIP

Printed in the United States of America

First Edition

1 2 3 4 5 6 7 8 9 10

BOOK DESIGN BY MARSHA COHEN/PARALLELOGRAM

FOREWORD

Sharing ideas and information is a tradition at Mayo Clinic which is grounded in the philosophy of our institution's founders. This cooperative spirit guides our clinical practice, educational programs, and research efforts.

This book is a natural extension of the information that is available to patients and visitors who travel to Mayo facilities in Rochester, Minnesota; Jacksonville, Florida; and Scottsdale, Arizona. We recognize that preservation of health and the struggle against illness neither begin nor end with the clinic, the hospital, the physician, or the health care team. These are daily efforts that depend not only on the cooperation of the individual but also on his or her informed and active control of issues related to health and life.

On behalf of the physicians, medical support staff, editors, illustrators, and everyone who helped create *Mayo Clinic Heart Book*, we hope that this book will serve as a practical understandable guide to heart disease and heart health.

Robert R. Waller, M.D.
*President and Chief
Executive Officer
Mayo Foundation*

EDITORIAL STAFF AND CONTRIBUTORS

Editor-in-Chief Michael D. McGoon, M.D.
Managing Editor Sara C. Gilliland

Medical Illustrator John V. Hagen
Editorial Production LeAnn M. Stee

Reviewers and Contributors

Julie A. Abbott, M.D.
Susan L. Ahlquist, R.N.
Gerald M. Alborn, R. Tech., Radiology
Thomas G. Allison, Ph.D.
J. Michael Bacharach, M.D.
William T. Bardsley, M.D.
Malcolm R. Bell, M.D.
Peter B. Berger, M.D.
Sherri Schreifels Berning, R.N.
Jerome F. Breen, M.D.
Barbara K. Bruce, Ph.D.
W. Mark Brutinel, M.D.
Thomas F. Bugliosi, M.D.
Jean Buithieu, M.D.
Father James Buryska
John A. Callahan, M.D.
Mark J. Callahan, M.D.
Randi R. Campbell
J. William Charboneau, M.D.
Timothy F. Christian, M.D.
Roger L. Click, M.D., Ph.D.
Richard C. Daly, M.D.
Charles H. Dicken, M.D.
David J. Driscoll, M.D.
Brooks S. Edwards, M.D.
William D. Edwards, M.D.
Maurice Enriquez-Sarano, M.D.
Patricia J. Erwin
Titus C. Evans, Jr., M.D., Ph.D.
Glenn Forbes, M.D.
Robert P. Frantz, M.D.
William K. Freeman, M.D.
Robert L. Frye, M.D.
Kirk N. Garratt, M.D.
Gerald T. Gau, M.D.
Judith I. Giacabazi, R.N.
Raymond J. Gibbons, M.D.
John W. Hallett, M.D.
Stephen C. Hammill, M.D.
Thomas R. Harman, M.D.
Carlos E. Harrison, M.D.
David L. Hayes, M.D.
Sharonne N. Hayes, M.D.
Sharlene P. Hegland
John A. Heit, M.D.
Jane L. Heser

Stuart T. Higano, M.D.
Ann R. Hinikier, R.N.
Michael J. Hogan, M.D.
David R. Holmes, Jr., M.D.
Richard D. Hurt, M.D.
Robyn A. Hutchinson, R.N.
Michael D. Jensen, M.D.
Mary E. Johnson, Chaplain
Donald L. Johnston, M.D.
Paul R. Julsrud, M.D.
Barry L. Karon, M.D.
Frank P. Kennedy, M.D.
Bijoy K. Khandheria, M.D.
Stephen L. Kopecky, M.D.
Bruce A. Kottke, M.D., Ph.D.
Thomas E. Kottke, M.D.
Andre C. Lapeyre III, M.D.
Scott C. Litin, M.D.
Rick Madsen
Douglas D. Mair, M.D.
James K. Marttila, Pharm.D.
Craig N. Mattson, Registered Pharmacist
Dwight C. McGoon, M.D.
Bonnie K. McGoon
Christopher G.A. McGregor, M.D.
Kristina K. Menke
Peggy A. Menzel, Registered Dietitian
Virginia V. Michels, M.D.
John M. Miles, M.D.
Fletcher A. Miller, Jr., M.D.
Todd D. Miller, M.D.
Wayne L. Miller, M.D.
John C. Mitchell, M.D.
Michael B. Mock, M.D.
Pamela B. Morris, M.D.
Michael J. Muehlenbein, R.N.
Sharon L. Mulvagh, M.D.
Naomi E. Munene, R.N.
Joseph G. Murphy, M.D.
Jennifer K. Nelson, Registered Dietitian
Susan M. Nelson, L.P.N.
Barbara A. Nichols, R.N.
Rick A. Nishimura, M.D.
M. Kevin O'Connor, M.D.
Jae K. Oh, M.D.
Byron A. Olney, M.D.

Lyle J. Olson, M.D.
Thomas A. Orszulak, M.D.
Philip J. Osmundson, M.D.
Douglas L. Packer, M.D.
P.J. Palumbo, M.D.
Patricia A. Pellikka, M.D.
Co-burn J. Porter, M.D.
Stephanie M. Quigg
Mary Jane Rasmussen, R.N.
Guy S. Reeder, M.D.
Richard J. Rodeheffer, M.D.
Veronique L. Roger, M.D.
Jeffrey D. Rome, M.D.
Thom W. Rooke, M.D.
John A. Rumberger, M.D., Ph.D.
Michael G. Sarr, M.D.
Hartzell V. Schaff, M.D.
Thomas T. Schattenberg, M.D.
William A. Schnell, Jr.
Robert S. Schwartz, M.D.
Mary E. Seresse, R.N.
F. John Service, M.D.
James B. Seward, M.D.
Patrick F. Sheedy II, M.D.
Win-Kuang Shen, M.D.
Roger F.J. Shepherd, M.D.
Peg Sherman, R.N.
Clarence Shub, M.D.
Martha J. Siska, R.N.
John A. Spittell, Jr., M.D.
Peter C. Spittell, M.D.
Ray W. Squires, Ph.D.
Marshall S. Stanton, M.D.
Rich J. Streit, Registered Pharmacist
Lois A. Thorkelson, R.N.
Susan K. Tointon, R.N.
Gary J. Truex
Richard J. Vetter, Ph.D.
Roger A. Warndahl, Registered Pharmacist
Carole A. Warnes, M.D.
William H. Weidman, M.D.
Arnold M. Weissler, M.D.
Roger D. White, M.D.
Daniel J. Wilson, M.D.
Douglas L. Wood, M.D.
Vincent P. Zuck, M.D.

ACKNOWLEDGMENTS

People who come to the Mayo Clinic for medical care often remark about the efficient organization that greets nearly 380,000 patients a year and yet focuses on providing each individual with comprehensive and compassionate medical care of the highest quality. This is the result of teamwork among Mayo's 1,300 staff physicians and medical scientists and 17,000 administrative and allied health personnel.

Mayo Clinic Heart Book is the result of the same spirit of teamwork, focused on the goal of creating a comprehensive, reliable, user-friendly reference for anyone interested in heart disease. The content of the book is based on the collective knowledge of Mayo specialists in cardiology, in conjunction with colleagues in preventive medicine, surgery, endocrinology, dietetics, and other specialties. But the information is only one aspect of the book's contents. The accuracy, clarity, and dissemination of its message have required the dedication and skills of many other team members.

Medical illustrator John Hagen prepared all of the medical illustrations, including the elegant full-color section. John has the ability to turn an idea into a clear, beautifully rendered drawing that interprets complicated concepts and images into understandable, meaningful, and memorable images. His skills have been recognized with numerous professional awards.

Ms. Terry Jopke was instrumental in assimilating the contributions of numerous collaborators into a cohesive and readable document.

Joseph Kane, from our Visual Information Services, was principal photographer for the book. Assisted by George DeVinny, we obtained photographs in medical settings such as the Cardiac Laboratory at Saint Marys Hospital to demonstrate what you, the reader, might experience as you undergo certain tests and procedures. We are grateful to everyone who served as models. X-rays and imaging scans were provided by Mayo Clinic Department of Diagnostic Radiology, Cardiac Laboratory, Echocardiography Laboratory, Nuclear Cardiology Laboratory, and Gonda Vascular Center.

The highly capable staff of Mayo's Section of Publications provided complete manuscript services. Through numerous revisions, LeAnn Stee, editor, improved the readability and clarity of the material; Rose Ann Ptacek-Vitse and Mary Horsman typed the manuscript, Jen Schlotthauer coordinated the many stages of printer's proof, and Mary Schwager was responsible for proofreading and for incorporating the hundreds of cross-references. Roberta Schwartz supervised and tracked the various stages of manuscript production.

Many individuals in Mayo Medical Ventures had a hand in planning and supporting this project. Dr. Lynwood Smith, Rick Colvin, and Vicki Moore sought and gained institutional support for this project. Dr. David E. Larson, editor-in-chief of Mayo's first book for the public, *Mayo Clinic Family Health Book*, provided valuable advice and guidance. The work of Lindsay A. E. Dingle, Scott D. Olson, and Christie L. Herman will ultimately result in wider distribution of the book. Krista Clouse of our Division of Communications coordinated all Mayo publicity efforts. Joan Benjamin skillfully executed secretarial responsibilities while dealing with three different computer systems used by writers, physicians, and editors.

The insights, efforts, and enthusiasm of Adrian Zackheim, our editor at William Morrow and Company, provided the guidance and ideas that could come only from a skilled professional. Many thanks also go to Al Marchioni, Deborah Weiss-Geline, Ann Cahn, Harvey Hoffman, Suzanne Oaks, Susan Halligan, Caroline Sykes, Bob Aulicino, Scott Manning, Larry Norton, Lisa Queen, Skip Dye, and Nick Mazzella. Because of this supportive and experienced team at Morrow, we could focus on the all-important messages of the book, confident that the logistics of its production were in the best of hands. Marsha Cohen, Parallelogram Graphic Communications, designed and executed the layout with creativity and precision.

Special thanks go to Arthur M. Klebanoff, our literary agent, for his enthusiasm and good advice.

Our greatest debt of gratitude is to the thousands of patients who have asked their questions, raised their concerns, voiced their opinions, expressed their joys, and wept their tears with us, in short, those who have taken us into their confidence in the hope that we might help. It is they who have provided both the inspiration and the fundamental guidance for the creation of this book.

Michael D. McGoon, M.D.
Editor-in-Chief

Sara C. Gilliland
Managing Editor

CONTENTS

PART 5. WHAT CAN BE DONE TO TREAT HEART DISEASE?   237

PART 6. ISSUES IN CARDIOLOGY   321

PREFACE

At the risk of presumption, this book will attempt to take Leonardo da Vinci to task. In his notebooks he wrote: "How in words can you describe this heart without filling a whole book? Yet the more detail you write concerning it, the more you will confuse the mind of the hearer." Based on the cumulative expertise of the 97 cardiologists at the Mayo Clinic, this book is filled with information about the heart and circulation, their diseases, and means of diagnosis and treatment. This book is written to dispel confusion.

The contributors to this book are particularly well suited to the task of explaining all facets of cardiovascular medicine. The depth and breadth of their shared knowledge and experience are unsurpassed and widely recognized. Their enthusiasm is equally great. It comes from the perception that people who already have heart disease and those who are concerned about preventing it want fundamental information about the heart. Yet, straightforward, reliable information is sorely lacking.

A nation in which 70 million of its citizens have some form of cardiovascular disease might be expected to benefit from knowing as much as possible about the heart and the risks to its health. That is the philosophy behind this book. Whether you are interested in charting a course to a healthy life-style or in learning more about your mother's upcoming coronary artery bypass surgery, this book is intended to provide you with guidance and the tools of understanding.

INTRODUCTION

The heart has long been recognized as crucial to life. However, throughout history, the heart has acquired an almost sacred quality that transcends even its importance to the physical body.

Our language is filled with references to the heart, from "broken-hearted" to "the heart of the matter." Although we think with our brains, we "feel" with our hearts; opinions we hold most dear are "heartfelt." The heart is the repository of romantic love, most tangibly demonstrated by the classic valentine heart, despite its structural inaccuracy. Now, of course, we also comprehend the central role of the heart and blood vessels in our overall vitality: "cardiovascular fitness" has become virtually synonymous with good health.

The ancients were aware of the role of the heart and circulation in the normal functioning of the body. As long as 4,500 years ago, Huang Ti, the Yellow Emperor of China, wrote: "The heart influences the face and fills the pulse with blood" and "The blood current flows continuously in a circle and never stops." Early Egyptian writings from about 1550 B.C. referred to the heart as a "well" with vessels: "Everywhere he feels his Heart," it was observed in the Ebers papyrus, "because its vessels run to all his limbs." In 400 B.C., Greek writers noted that the heart is a muscle and is a part of the vascular system (although at least some writers seemed to think that the vessels contained air rather than blood); they described the pericardium, the heart valves, and the characteristics of the

pulse. Centuries later, many of their conclusions were proved incorrect, but the foundations of knowledge were slowly being laid.

It has been said that the extensive teachings of Galen, a physician in the Roman Empire who lived from A.D. 129 to 199, had "more influence on medical history than those of any other physician, before or since." Unfortunately, although he was considered the final word in medical matters for the next 1,400 years, much of what he wrote was erroneous. So highly regarded was Galen that even in the 1600s one French physician stated that if research disclosed differences from what Galen taught, then nature must have changed! This reverence for past teachings slowed progress in medical knowledge for many centuries. Among the isolated examples of forward steps was the observation of the Arabian physician Ibn al-Nafis (1210–1288) that the heart was nourished by its own vessels (later to be called the coronary arteries).

Finally, during the Renaissance, from about 1450 to 1600, substantial strides in knowledge began. They were largely a result of direct observation by dissection of cadavers, rather than speculation and theorizing. The greatest contributions to the understanding of the anatomy of the body and heart came from Vesalius (1514–1564) in Padua, Italy. Even before, Leonardo da Vinci (1452–1519) had done dissections and made elegant artistic renderings of his observations, but these were not published at the time and therefore had little influence. Examples of knowledge about the heart which emerged during the Renaissance include descriptions of the veins, the general structure of the heart and coronary vessels, aneurysms of the aorta, details of the heart valves, and the pulmonary (lung) circulation. Indeed, the term "circulation" was first used during this period.

If the advance of knowledge during the Renaissance about the heart and circulation could be considered the result of cumulative steps forward, then the 17th century was a time of leaps and bounds. It was then that the big picture of how the heart and circulation actually functioned came into focus, due mainly to the work of William Harvey (1578–1657). Harvey's discoveries were published in 1628 in the magnificent *De Motu Cordis* (*On the Motion of the Heart*). In it (and in subsequent writings), he accurately described, on the basis of observation and experimentation, the way the blood circulates throughout the body and lungs and returns to the heart.

Marcello Malpighi (1628–1694), using the newly invented microscope, discovered and made the initial descriptions of the "missing link" in Harvey's description of the circulation: the previously invisible small capillaries that connect the arteries and veins. Other scientists made the first conclusions that the purpose of the circulation through the lungs was to "aerate" the blood (oxygen was not yet discovered), a process that changed it from dark to bright red.

In the later part of the 18th century, knowledge about the heart and vessels continued to grow, especially as it applied to disease. Descriptions of heart failure, pericardial disease, disease of the heart valves, thickening of blood vessel walls, chest pain, palpitations and slow heartbeat, and the phenomenon of blood pressure all emerged during this time.

Not unexpectedly, as knowledge about diseased organs (the science of pathology) grew, the effort to diagnose the nature of the disease in ill patients began to take precedence. This attempt to correlate clinical conditions with pathologic states was the thrust of progress in the early 1800s. The first suggestions that angina pectoris is chest pain related to an inadequate supply of blood to the heart muscle were made at this time. Many of the basic aspects of the physical examination of the patient were developed, including methods of visual inspection, examination by touch (palpation), percussion (for example, tapping on the chest), and auscultation (listening, especially through a stethoscope).

The last part of the 1800s built in a logical fashion on the knowledge that had developed previously. Understanding of the general structure (anatomy), basic microscopic structure (histology), derangements caused by disease (pathology), and some relationships to medical illnesses (diagnosis) was well under way, and it continued to advance. Now inquiry began to emphasize how the parts of the body, including the heart, actually worked. A branch of science called physiology was developed, aided by new instruments and techniques. During this time, the areas of electrophysiology and electrocardiography began to reveal the electrical aspects of the heart.

All of these trends continued into the 20th century, right up to the present. The means of investigation have become more refined and new technological advances have allowed more detailed and accurate understanding of the body. X-rays, electrocardiography and electrophysiology, radioactive scanning, chemical analysis of the blood and tissues, ultrasound imaging of the heart, and analysis of blood flow all have been developed in this century. All these will be described as they apply to you.

The hallmark of the 20th century is that for the first time, medical science systematically developed effective treatments for illnesses. For heart disease, medications, devices, and surgical procedures evolved which are now capable of prolonging life, reducing symptoms, and eliminating the causes of many disease processes. There is still much progress to be made in the treatment of heart disease, and this will require further development in our understanding of its causes. Ironically, it is the capability of some treatments that has led to discussions about when the line is crossed between enough treatment to prolong life and too much.

What hallmark of the upcoming era will build on the progress of the past? Likely, we will focus on prevention of disease and on the wise distribution of resources for combating disease. These will be efforts not just for doctors and medical scientists but for everyone. Prevention involves more than being a "patient" whose concern with health develops only at the moment illness develops. Rather, it involves an ongoing, active interest in maintaining one's own health and the well-being of all of society's members. Developing and maintaining that interest require knowledge and understanding. The subsequent chapters of this book provide for you the foundations of that knowledge about cardiovascular health and disease.

ORGANIZATION OF THIS BOOK

In a sense, Leonardo da Vinci was right when he implied that the more you write about the heart, the more likely you are to confuse the reader. Therefore, this book conscientiously focuses on what is important in understanding the heart in health and disease. It is *not* a medical textbook or encyclopedia, nor is it isolated snippets of information about separate heart-related topics. It is *definitely not* another book preaching yet another way to change your life for the better in two easy steps. It *is* a broad, accessible reference that is useful in various contexts.

The sections of the book progress from understanding the normal heart to discussing what can go wrong and how it affects you. They are followed by an important review of how to minimize the chances of heart disease developing. Then there are detailed sections about what is done to evaluate and treat heart disease. Finally, there is a section about special issues in the area of heart health and disease.

Most of the sections are constructed to reflect the way the heart functions. The heart can be thought of as a mechanical pumping system with several components: the pump itself (the heart muscle), valves, fuel lines to the pump (the coronary arteries), electrical wiring (the conduction system), pipes (the blood vessels), and a container for the pump (the pericardium).

Page guides throughout the book direct you to further reading in subsequent portions of the book. The page guides are useful if you want to read as much as possible about one component of the heart, such as the normal heart valves, how the valves might become diseased, what tests are used to evaluate the valves, and what treatment options can be used for valve problems.

REASONS TO READ THIS BOOK

This book is intended for everyone with an interest in the heart: heart health, heart disease, or the care of the heart. It is organized to be useful to several types of readers; *how* you read it depends on your *reasons* for reading it.

General Knowledge

One reason to read this book is to obtain a general base of knowledge about the normal function of the heart, what can go wrong with the heart, how heart disease can be evaluated and treated, and how you can best maintain your own cardiovascular health. If that is your goal, then the best method is to approach the book very much like a novel, reading it from beginning to end. When read in this fashion, its organization systematically develops and increases your knowledge.

Learning About Symptoms

If your goal is to learn about the implications of your symptoms, refer to the *Symptoms Guide* starting on page 22. This will be a starting point for you to learn about the significance of heart and blood vessel symptoms and about what diagnoses may be suggested by them. Page guides refer you to other portions of the book, so you can be sure that you have been informed about every aspect of the particular problem you are having.

Please be careful, however. This book is not intended to take the place of a careful evaluation by your doctor. Similar symptoms may have substantially different meanings in different people, depending on circumstances. The *Symptoms Guide* cannot ask you pertinent questions about issues that have an important bearing on assessing your situation. It is a *"guide"* only, intended to assist your interaction with your doctor and perhaps dispel some of the mystery surrounding the symptoms you are having. *The Symptoms Guide should not cause you to delay or avoid consultation with your doctor.*

Learning About a Particular Condition

Your mother has been told that she has aortic regurgitation. What does this mean? The doctor may have explained things, but she did not understand everything and forgot some items, and you were not with her when she saw the doctor. Now you would like to know what her problem is, what the aortic valve is and what it does, whether there is a need for further evaluation, and what the options for treatment are. The logical starting point for you is Part 2, "What Is Heart Disease?", specifically the section "Defects of Valves" (page 57).

Most sections on specific diseases can be located through the Contents; occasionally the index may be handier. Once you read about the specific problem, you can follow the page guides, which refer you ahead to discussions about relevant testing procedures.

Learning About Tests or Treatments

It is natural to feel anxious as you await a procedure to evaluate or treat heart problems. Most of the anxiety is related to concern about the unknown— why is it being done, what exactly will happen, what will be accomplished, what will be the next step? Two parts of the book—"Tests to Diagnose Heart Disease" and "What Can Be Done to Treat Heart Disease?"—cover precisely these issues. If you are scheduled for some tests or treatment procedures, or if you are provided with

a new prescription, these sections will be useful.

Learning About Maintaining Your Cardiovascular Health

Fortunately, there is a great deal of interest in healthy living. This widespread interest has spawned a wealth of recommendations, advice, information, and sales pitches. What can you do that will actually be of benefit? What should you know to help sort through the barrage of information appearing on television, in newspapers and newsmagazines, in health publications, and in advertisements? Part 3, "Reducing Your Risk of Coronary Artery Disease," organizes this information for you. First, it provides background about *what* constitutes healthy (and unhealthy) living and why. Second, recommendations are made about how you can change from a higher-risk to a lower-risk life-style. These recommendations are practical, effective, and achievable; you will not find gimmicks, quick fixes, or promotions.

The Heart's Location

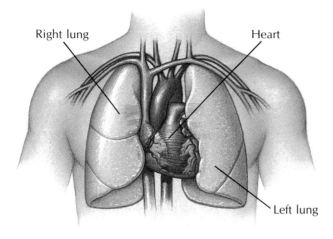

Right lung

Heart

Left lung

Figure 1

THE HEART

The heart is a muscular pump the size of your fist. Located to the left of the center of your chest between the lungs, its lower tip (apex) points toward the left.

The heart pumps blood into arteries. The major arteries that emerge from the heart are the aorta and the pulmonary arteries. The coronary arteries, which supply the heart muscle itself with nourishing blood, branch off directly from the aorta.

Veins return blood to the heart. The large veins that enter the heart are the superior vena cava, the inferior vena cava, and the pulmonary veins. In these illustrations, red blood vessels carry oxygen-rich blood and blue blood vessels contain blood with low oxygen levels.

Major Arteries and Veins

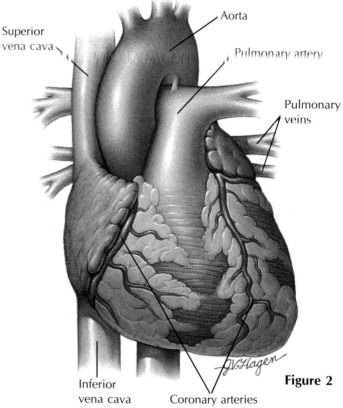

Superior vena cava

Aorta

Pulmonary artery

Pulmonary veins

Inferior vena cava

Coronary arteries

Figure 2

Chambers and Valves

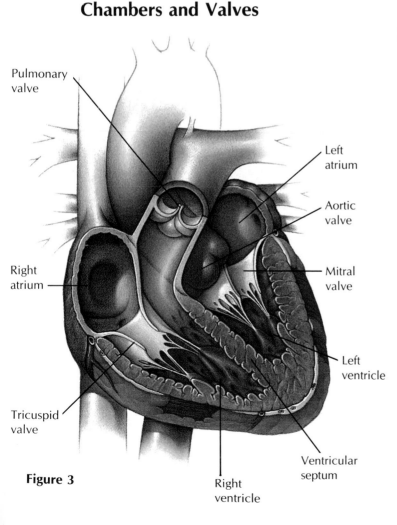

Pulmonary valve

Left atrium

Aortic valve

Mitral valve

Right atrium

Left ventricle

Tricuspid valve

Ventricular septum

Right ventricle

Figure 3

The heart consists of four chambers. Two atria on top are receiving chambers for blood returning from veins. Two ventricles beneath pump blood into the arteries. Valves allow the blood to move in only one direction. The mitral valve on the left side and the tricuspid valve on the right side control the flow of blood from the atria to the ventricles. The aortic valve (between the left ventricle and aorta) and the pulmonary valve (between the right ventricle and pulmonary artery) control the flow of blood out of the ventricles.

"Figure-Eight" Circulation

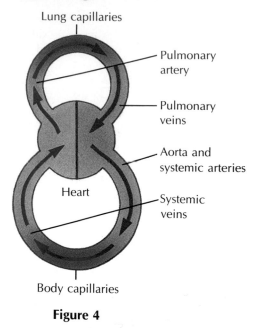

Figure 4

THE CIRCULATION

Circulating blood carries oxygen and nutrients to your body's organs and carries carbon dioxide and other waste products away from the organs to the sites of their elimination.

At its simplest, the circulation is like a figure-eight. One loop is the circulation to the lungs, in which blood is pumped through the pulmonary arteries, carbon dioxide is exchanged for oxygen in the capillaries, and the blood returns to the heart through the pulmonary veins. The other loop is the circulation to the body, in which blood is pumped through the arteries, oxygen and nutrients are exchanged for carbon dioxide and waste products in the capillaries, and the blood returns to the heart through the systemic veins.

In reality, the circulation is more complicated. Arteries branch repeatedly, transporting blood to all the cells of every organ. Veins join together, bringing blood back to the heart from every organ. The central focus is the heart: the right-sided chambers receive blood from the body and pump it into the pulmonary arteries. The left-sided chambers receive blood from the lungs and pump it into the aorta and systemic arteries.

Here is how a typical blood cell journeys through the circulatory system. It is pumped out of the left ventricle into the aorta, where it courses through smaller and smaller branches until it passes through a capillary in single file with other blood cells. Then it enters a tiny venule that joins up with others, like tributaries of a river, to form bigger veins until finally the blood cell passes through the vena cava (superior if it is returning from the head or arms, inferior if from the abdomen or legs) and into the right atrium. It passes into the right ventricle, which pumps it into the pulmonary artery. After going through a capillary in the lungs, it enters the pulmonary vein and is carried to the left atrium and then back to its starting point in the left ventricle.

The Circulatory System

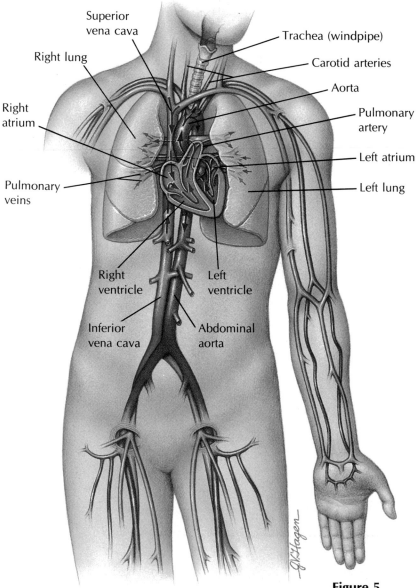

Figure 5

THE CAPILLARIES

Arteries branch until they become capillaries, so tiny that only one blood cell can pass through at a time and so numerous that there is a capillary near each cell of the body. The capillary walls are thin enough that nutrients, wastes, and gases pass freely between the blood inside the capillaries and the nearby cells. In the tissues of the body, such as the skin and muscles of the finger, oxygen passes from the blood to the cells, and carbon dioxide and other waste products pass into the blood.

In the lungs, carbon dioxide is released from the blood in the capillaries into the nearby alveoli (air sacs), and oxygen passes from the air in the alveoli into the blood. This oxygenated blood flows from the capillaries into the pulmonary veins to the left-sided chambers of the heart. Then it is pumped into the arteries to the capillaries of the body. This cycle repeats itself for a lifetime.

Capillaries in the General Circulation

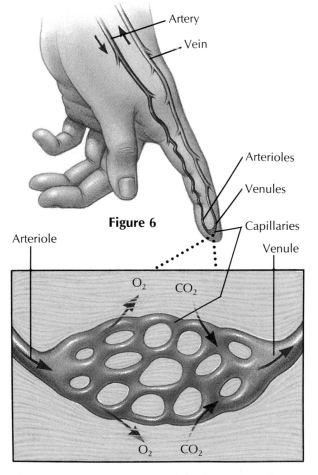

Figure 6

Figure 7: In most tissues of the body, capillaries release oxygen and nutrients in exchange for carbon dioxide and waste products.

Capillaries in the Lung Circulation

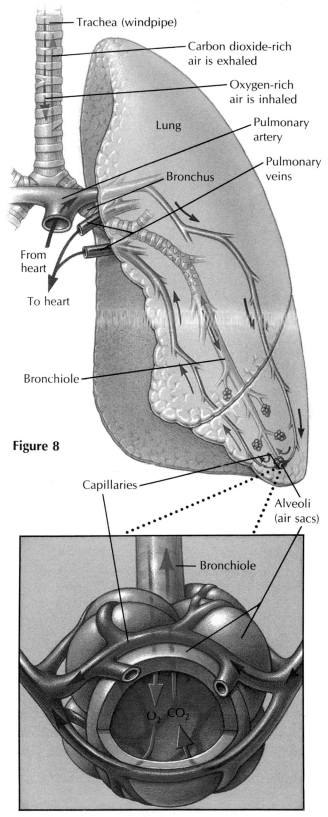

Figure 8

Figure 9: Lung capillaries release carbon dioxide into alveoli in exchange for oxygen.

THE HEART MUSCLE

The heart is a muscular pump that propels blood by squeezing it out of the powerful ventricles into the arteries. The muscular wall of the heart has three layers: a thin inner lining (endocardium), the bulk of working muscle (myocardium), and the outer surface (epicardium).

The squeezing action of the heart is produced by coordinated shortening of the muscle fibers that make up the walls of the heart. When the muscles shorten (contract), the ventricular chambers become smaller, forcing blood out. The valves ensure that the blood goes out the right direction. This phase of the heart action is *systole*. After contracting, the heart muscle relaxes, the muscle fibers lengthen, the ventricular chambers become more spacious, and blood flows into them from the atria. This phase is *diastole*.

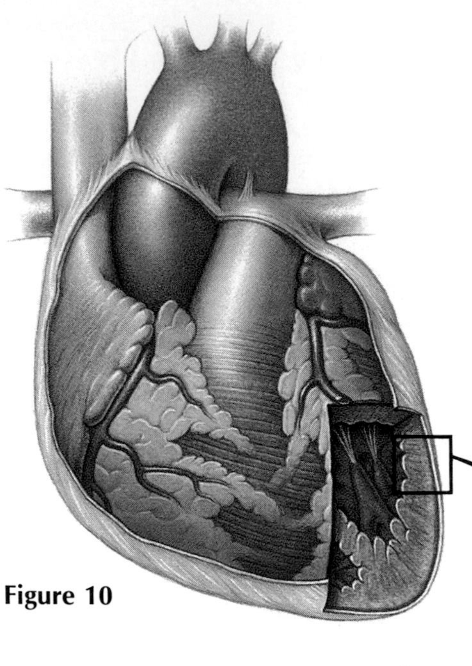

Figure 10

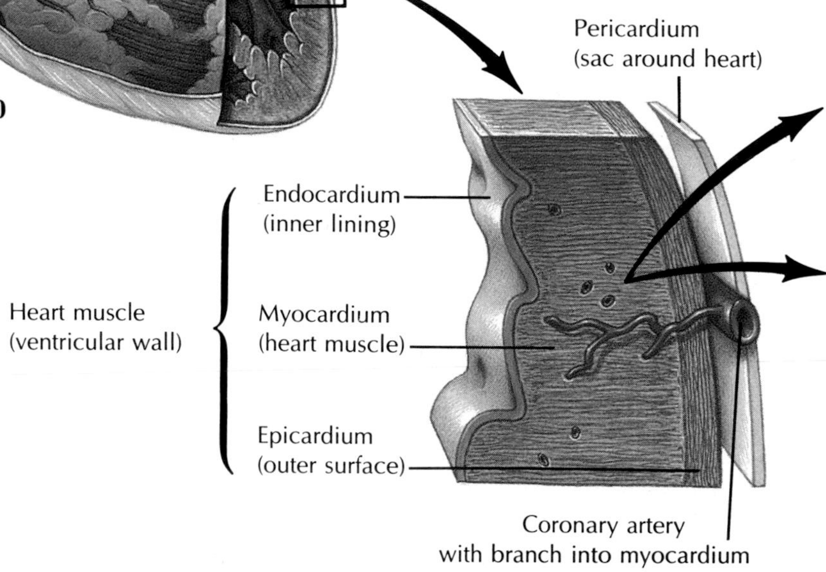

Pericardium (sac around heart)

Endocardium (inner lining)

Heart muscle (ventricular wall)

Myocardium (heart muscle)

Epicardium (outer surface)

Coronary artery with branch into myocardium

Figure 11

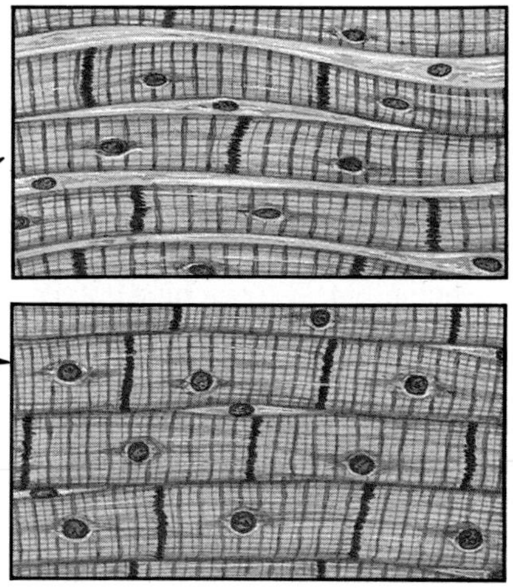

Figure 12: When microscopic muscle fibers relax, they are long and thin (top). When they contract, they become short and thick (bottom).

Normal

The nuclear "MUGA" scans (at right) show a normal heart. The orange ventricles (*arrow* points to left ventricle) are large during diastole and contracted during systole.

Dilated

The nuclear "MUGA" scans (at right) show a weakened heart. It cannot squeeze as hard. The size of the ventricles changes very little between diastole and systole.

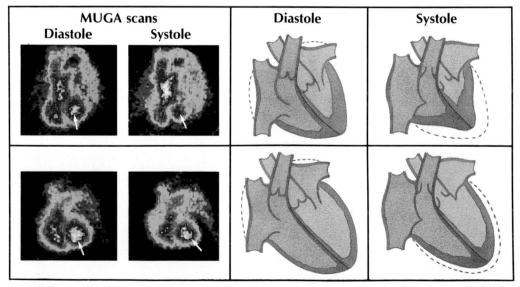

MUGA scans
Diastole   Systole

Diastole   Systole

Figure 13: If the heart muscle weakens, it cannot squeeze as hard. The heart gradually enlarges (dilates) to compensate for its inability to expel the normal amount of blood.

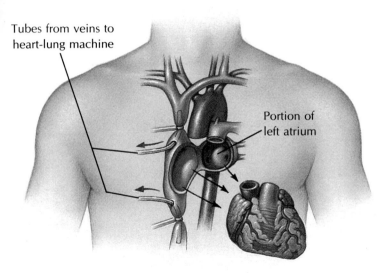

Tubes from veins to
heart-lung machine

Portion of
left atrium

HEART TRANSPLANTS

Transplantation of a weakened heart may be the
best solution when medications do not adequately
improve symptoms or when life expectancy is
short. The original heart is replaced with a normally
functioning heart donated by someone who has
died from causes unrelated to heart disease. The
ventricles and part of the atria, together with the
heart valves and coronary arteries, are transplanted
from the donor to the recipient. After the heart is
removed from the donor, it is cooled and stored in
special fluid. The time the heart is out of the body
must be kept short, generally less than 4 hours.

Figure 14: Before the weakened original
heart is removed, tubes must be positioned
to take blood from the body and transport it
to a cardiopulmonary bypass pump (heart-
lung machine). The machine puts oxygen
into the blood and then pumps the
blood back into an artery (not
shown). Because the machine
functions as the heart and
lungs, the weakened
heart can be removed.

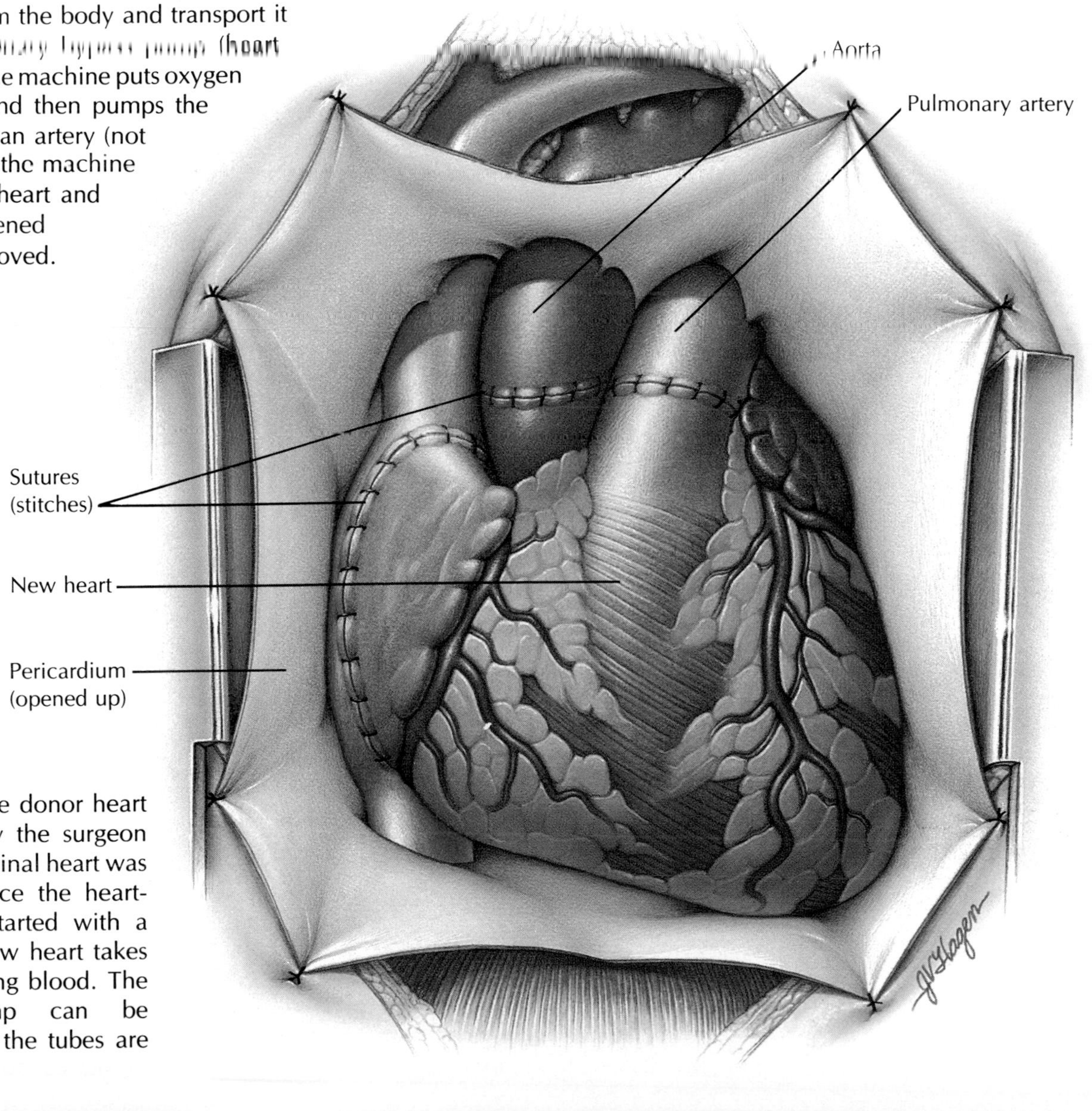

Aorta

Pulmonary artery

Sutures
(stitches)

New heart

Pericardium
(opened up)

Figure 15: The donor heart
is sewn in by the surgeon
where the original heart was
removed. Once the heart-
beats are restarted with a
shock, the new heart takes
over circulating blood. The
bypass pump can be
stopped, and the tubes are
removed.

HOW THE HEART'S VALVES WORK

Valves keep blood flowing in one direction through the heart. As the ventricles relax (*diastole*), the pressure within them decreases. The mitral and tricuspid valves are pushed open, allowing blood to flow from the atria to the ventricles. The aortic and pulmonary valves are pushed shut, preventing the return of blood that was pumped out on the preceding beat. During contraction (*systole*), the pressure pushes the aortic and pulmonary valves open, and the mitral and tricuspid valves are pushed shut and prevent back flow of blood.

Tricuspid valve
(open)

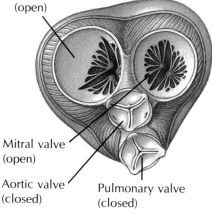

Mitral valve
(open)

Aortic valve
(closed)

Pulmonary valve
(closed)

Tricuspid valve
(open)

Pulmonary valve
(closed)

Figure 16: *Diastole.* A view of the heart from above, cut through the plane of the valves, during diastole. The mitral and tricuspid valves are open; the pulmonary and aortic valves are shut.

Figure 16A

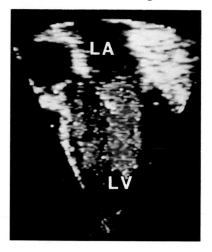

LA

LV

Figures 16A and 17A: Color Doppler echocardiograms. This study vividly demonstrates blood flow through the chambers on the left side of your heart. In *diastole* (above), blood flowing through the mitral valve from the left atrium (LA) to the left ventricle (LV) appears orange. In *systole* (below), blood is ejected through the aortic valve and appears blue on the echocardiograph monitor screen.

Tricuspid valve
(closed)

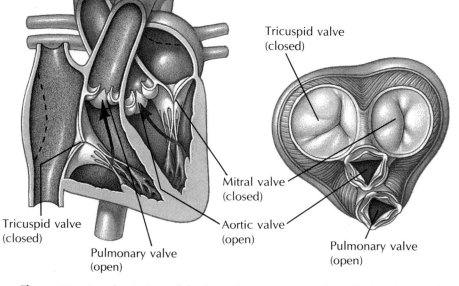

Mitral valve
(closed)

Aortic valve
(open)

Pulmonary valve
(open)

Tricuspid valve
(closed)

Pulmonary valve
(open)

Figure 17: *Systole.* A view of the heart from above, cut through the plane of the valves, during systole. The mitral and tricuspid valves are closed; the pulmonary and aortic valves are open.

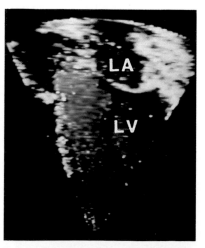

LA

LV

Figure 17A

DISEASES OF THE VALVES

Diseases of the valves may cause them to become too narrow, restricting blood flow (valve stenosis). They can also become "leaky," allowing blood to flow backward (valve regurgitation).

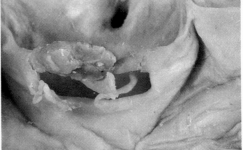

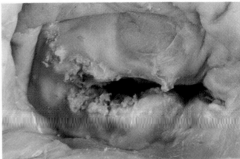

Figure 18A: Regurgitant aortic valve damaged by infection (infective endocarditis).

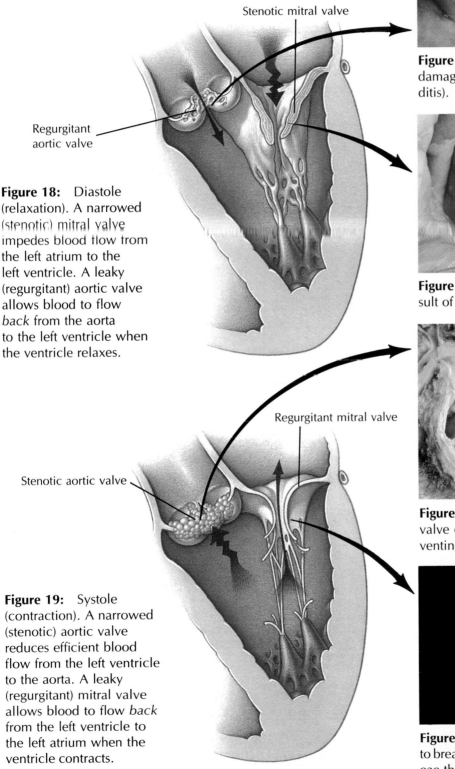

Stenotic mitral valve

Regurgitant aortic valve

Figure 18: Diastole (relaxation). A narrowed (stenotic) mitral valve impedes blood flow from the left atrium to the left ventricle. A leaky (regurgitant) aortic valve allows blood to flow *back* from the aorta to the left ventricle when the ventricle relaxes.

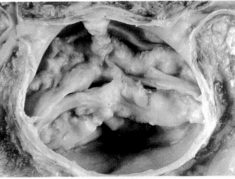

Figure 18B: Mitral valve stenosis as a result of rheumatic fever.

Figure 19A: Stenosis of a bicuspid aortic valve caused by deposits of calcium preventing adequate opening of the valve.

Regurgitant mitral valve

Stenotic aortic valve

Figure 19: Systole (contraction). A narrowed (stenotic) aortic valve reduces efficient blood flow from the left ventricle to the aorta. A leaky (regurgitant) mitral valve allows blood to flow *back* from the left ventricle to the left atrium when the ventricle contracts.

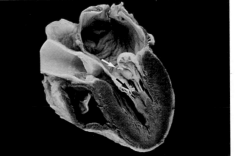

Figure 19B: Regurgitant mitral valve due to breakage (*arrows*) of the chordae tendineae that tether the valve leaflets.

A8

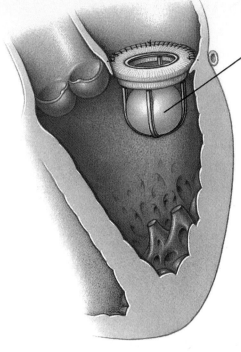

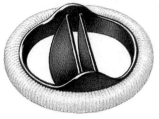

Caged ball valve (open)

Figure 21

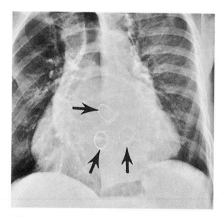

Bileaflet valve (open)

ARTIFICIAL VALVES

One means of correcting a defective heart valve is for a surgeon to remove it and replace it with an artificial valve. Various artificial (prosthetic) valves are available, each with its own advantages.

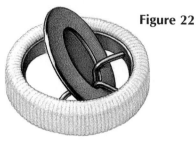

Figure 22

Tilting disk valve (open)

Figure 23

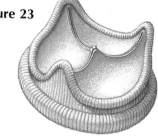

Tissue valve (closed)

Figure 20: An artificial valve is sewn in by the surgeon after the diseased valve is removed. It is positioned to allow the blood to flow freely in the correct direction and not leak back.

Figure 20A
X-ray of three artificial valves

BALLOON VALVULOPLASTY

Figure 24: Mitral stenosis can often be effectively treated by threading a catheter with an inflatable balloon through a vein and across the atrial septum (which is carefully punctured). It is positioned through the tight mitral opening. Then the balloon is inflated, pressing the valve leaflets apart, producing a wider opening.

Catheter crossing atrial septum

Catheter in left atrium

Balloon across mitral valve

Catheter in inferior vena cava

Figure 24

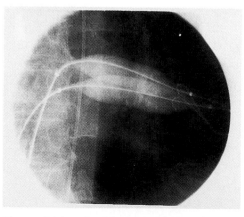

Figure 24A: In this X-ray, two inflated balloons extend across the mitral valve to produce a wider opening. The valve itself is not visible on an X-ray.

CORONARY ARTERIES

The coronary arteries emerge from the aorta and extend along the surface of the heart. Branches extend into the heart wall to supply the myocardial cells with oxygen and nourishment. The blood returns to the heart through coronary veins.

An arteriogram (photograph below) provides an image of the coronary arteries by showing contrast dye flowing within the arteries. This normal arteriogram reveals that the arteries are smooth and wide open.

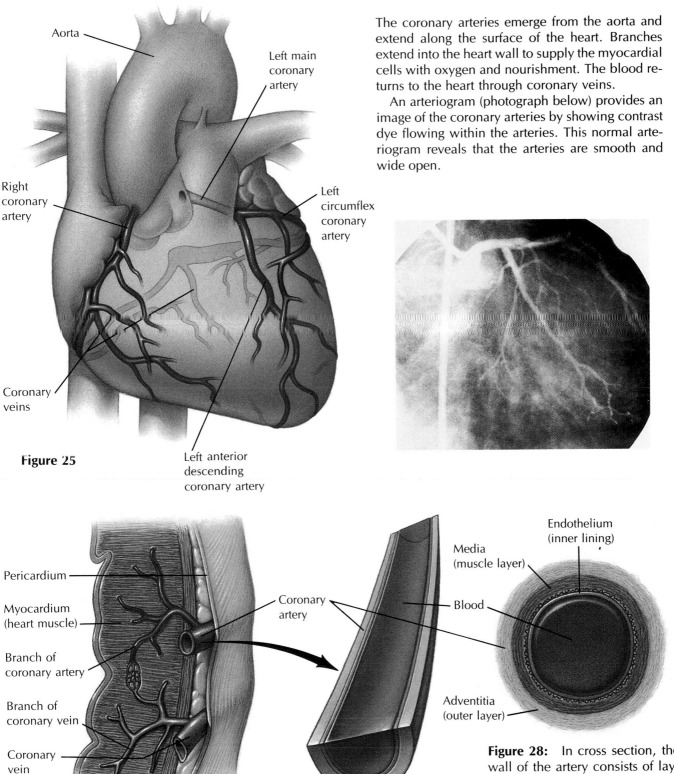

Figure 25

Labels in Figure 25:
- Aorta
- Left main coronary artery
- Right coronary artery
- Left circumflex coronary artery
- Coronary veins
- Left anterior descending coronary artery

Labels in Figure 26:
- Pericardium
- Myocardium (heart muscle)
- Branch of coronary artery
- Branch of coronary vein
- Coronary vein
- Coronary artery

Labels in Figure 27/28:
- Coronary artery
- Media (muscle layer)
- Endothelium (inner lining)
- Blood
- Adventitia (outer layer)

Figure 26: Cross section of a portion of heart wall. The coronary arteries send branches into the heart tissue.

Figure 27: The coronary artery is a conduit supplying blood to the heart. The inner lining is normally smooth.

Figure 28: In cross section, the wall of the artery consists of layers: the smooth inner endothelium, the middle layer of muscle that controls the width of the artery to regulate blood flow through it, and an outer surrounding layer.

DISEASED CORONARY ARTERIES

Blood flow through the coronary arteries can become obstructed by blood clot (thrombosis), causing total blockage that results in a heart attack (myocardial infarction); atherosclerosis, causing partial blockage leading to angina pectoris; or coronary spasm, which temporarily cuts off blood flow.

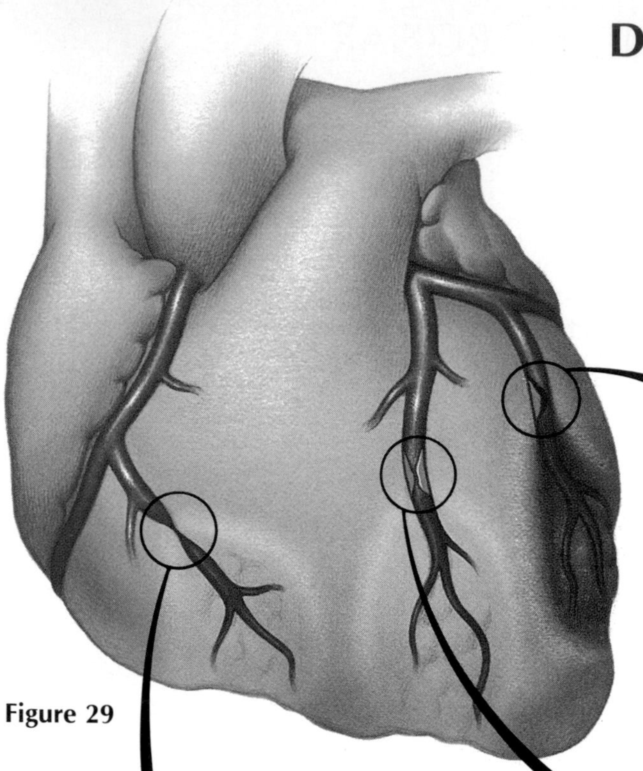

Figure 29

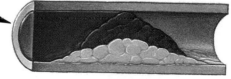

Figure 30:
Atherosclerosis with blood clot (lengthwise view)

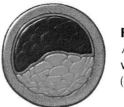

Figure 31:
Atherosclerosis with blood clot (cross section)

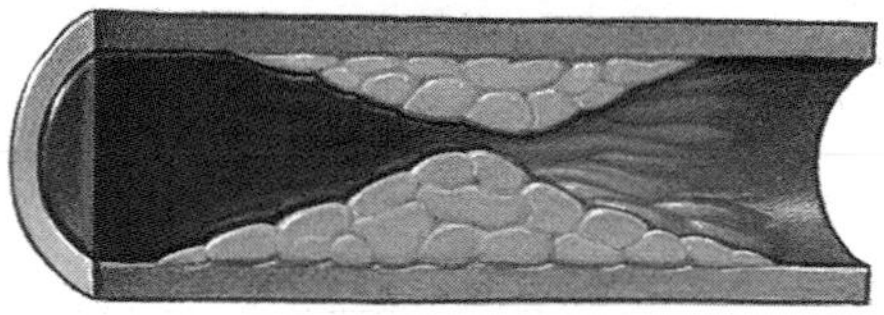

Figure 32:
Atherosclerosis (lengthwise view)

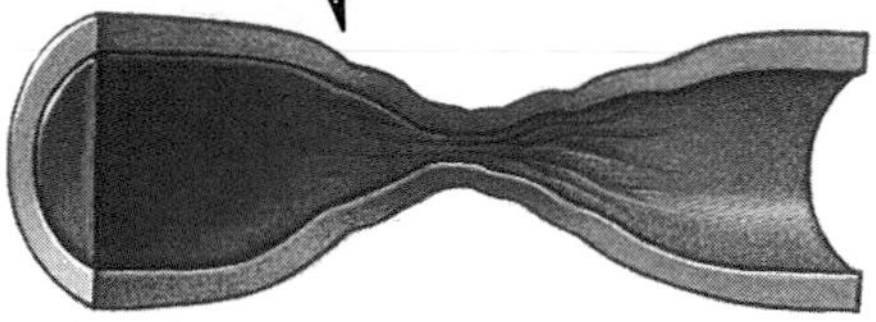

Figure 34:
Spasm (lengthwise view)

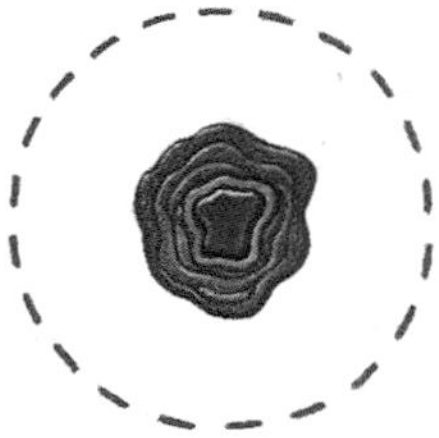

Figure 35:
Spasm (cross section)

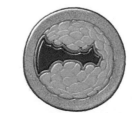

Figure 33:
Atherosclerosis (cross section)

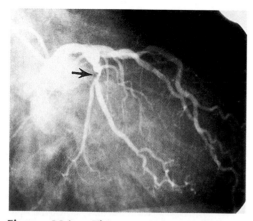

Figure 32A: This arteriogram shows a partial blockage in a coronary artery (*arrow*). Narrowing of the artery restricts the flow of blood to the heart muscle.

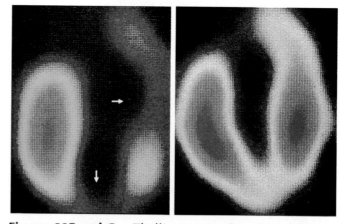

Figures 32B and C: Thallium scans show blood flow to the heart muscle. The "gaps" are areas that do not receive adequate blood flow during stress (*arrows*). During rest (right), blood flow is sufficient throughout.

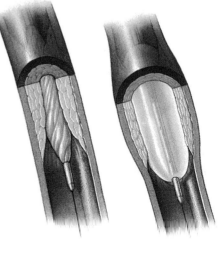

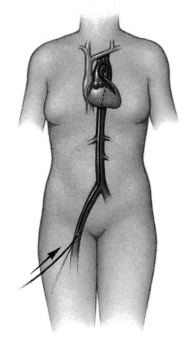

RESTORING CORONARY BLOOD FLOW

In some circumstances, coronary blockages can be reduced with specially designed catheters. Various methods and techniques are available.

Figure 37: Percutaneous transluminal coronary angioplasty (PTCA; balloon dilation). In this procedure, the cardiologist passes a catheter with a small balloon into the coronary artery. The deflated balloon is positioned at the site of the blockage.

Figure 38: The balloon is then inflated, pushing the atherosclerotic plaque aside and widening the artery.

Figure 37　　**Figure 38**

Figure 36. A large artery in the groin (or, in some cases, the arm) is the site where the angioplasty catheter is inserted. From there, it is threaded into the blocked coronary artery.

Figure 41

Saphenous vein bypass graft

Blockage in left anterior descending coronary artery

Right internal mammary artery

Blockage in right coronary artery

Figure 39: Atherectomy. A special device at the tip of the catheter actually shears the plaque off the artery wall. This material is compressed into a small compartment and removed when the catheter is pulled out.

Figure 40: Laser angioplasty. A laser beam emitted from the end of the catheter vaporizes the plaque or heats the tip of the catheter so that the plaque is "burned" or "melted" away.

Figure 39　　**Figure 40**

CORONARY ARTERY BYPASS SURGERY

Instead of trying to open a blocked artery, another approach is to bypass the artery. Bypasses around blockage sites can be surgically constructed out of veins taken from the leg (saphenous veins) or from arteries arising near the collarbone (internal mammary arteries).

THE CONDUCTION SYSTEM

The conduction system is like the "wiring" of the heart, designed to conduct electrical impulses throughout the heart muscle to make it beat. In actuality, the "wires" would not be visible, but follow the paths (shown in green) illustrated. The impulses begin in the sinus node, spread throughout the atria, pass through the atrioventricular node, and then are distributed throughout the ventricles.

During each heartbeat (a duration of about 1 second during a resting state), these stages can be seen on the electrocardiogram (ECG). The current flowing through the atria produces a small "blip" (the P wave). As the impulse crosses the atrioventricular node, the ECG line becomes level (the PR segment). When the impulse spreads throughout the muscular ventricles, a larger "blip" (the QRS complex) is produced on the ECG. Finally, the electrical system recovers in preparation for the next impulse. During this stage, the T wave appears on the ECG.

Figure 42

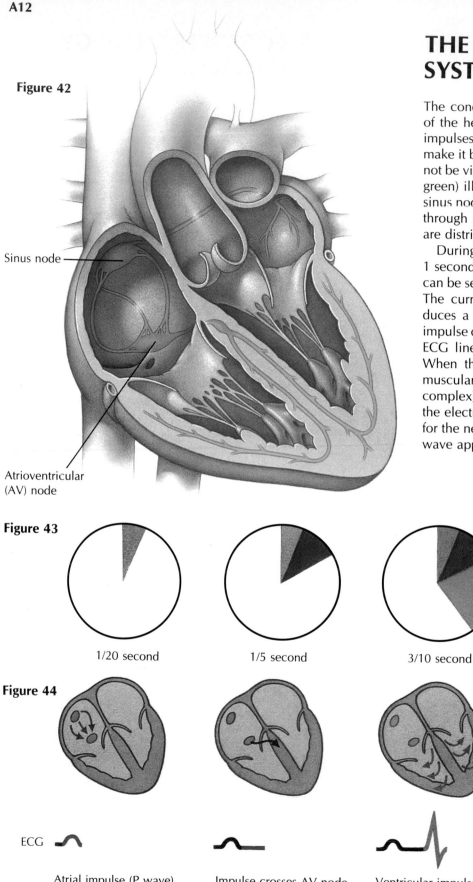

Sinus node

Atrioventricular (AV) node

Figure 43

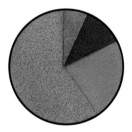

1/20 second   1/5 second   3/10 second   1 second

Figure 44

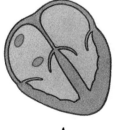

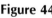
ECG

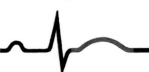

Atrial impulse (P wave)   Impulse crosses AV node (PR segment)   Ventricular impulse (QRS complex)   Recovery (T wave)

ELECTROPHYSIOLOGY CATHETERS

An electrophysiology test may be required for the evaluation of some heart rhythm problems. This test consists of inserting electrode wire catheters through veins into the right-sided chambers of the heart. Several wires are often required so that different parts of the conduction system can be evaluated at the same time. In this way, doctors can carefully assess the way in which electrical impulses travel through the heart and determine whether there are abnormalities that explain a person's rhythm problem or symptoms. The wires can be used to detect and record impulses in the heart (like an "internal ECG"), or they can be used to pace the heart or stimulate it into abnormal rhythms that can be examined.

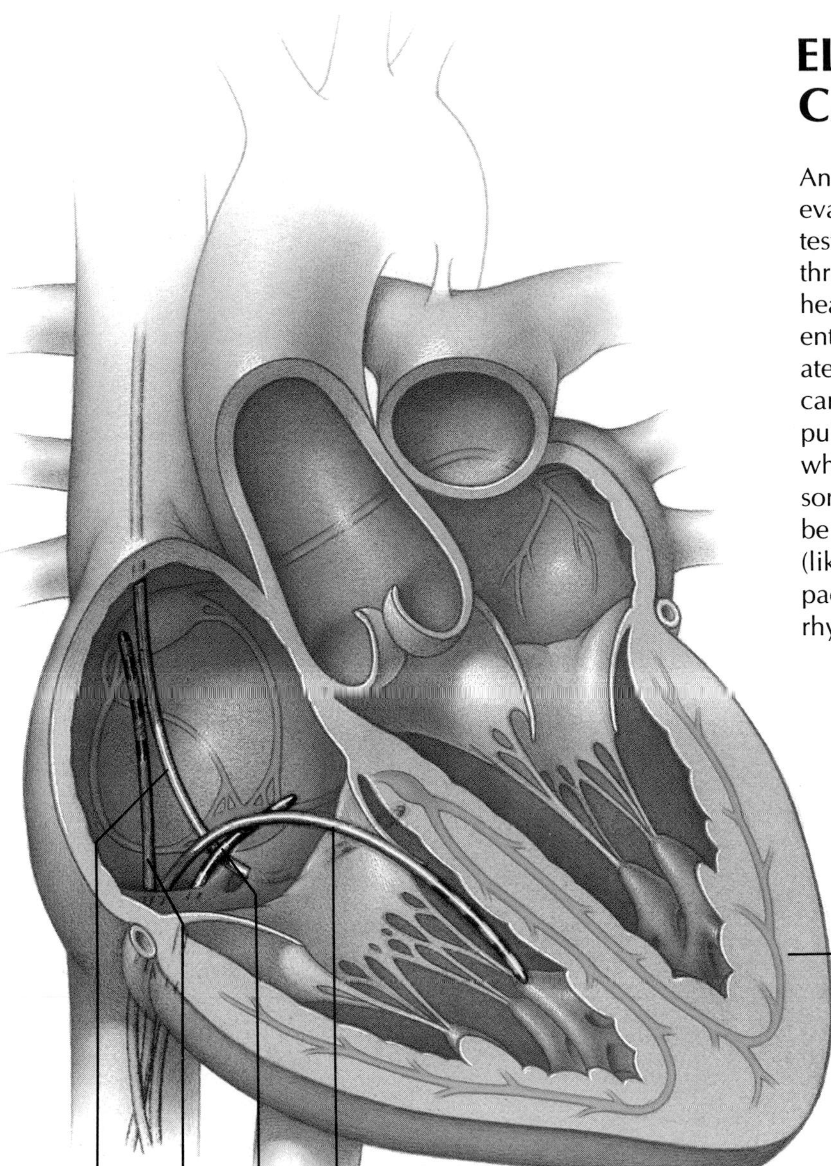

Figure 45: Cutaway view of heart showing typical location of electrode catheters in an electrophysiology test. Not every procedure requires all of the catheters.

Electrode threaded from the femoral vein to the right ventricle.

Electrode threaded from the femoral vein to the region of the atrioventricular node.

Electrode threaded from the femoral vein in the groin to the region of the sinus node.

Electrode threaded from the neck vein into the coronary sinus (the main coronary vein). This catheter detects impulses on the left side of the heart.

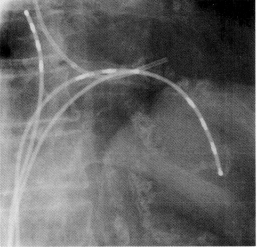

Figure 45A: An X-ray image of the electrophysiology catheters shown in the illustration.

PACEMAKERS AND DEFIBRILLATORS

Pacemakers produce small electrical impulses that stimulate the heart to beat. They are used when the natural heartbeat is too slow. Depending on the type of pacemaker, the impulses are carried by wires (leads) threaded through a vein into the right ventricle, the right atrium, or, as illustrated here, both chambers. Occasionally, wires can be placed surgically on the outer surface of the heart instead. Inserting a pacemaker with wires through the vein is a minor procedure that can be done with local anesthesia. The X-ray shows the appearance of a pacemaker system.

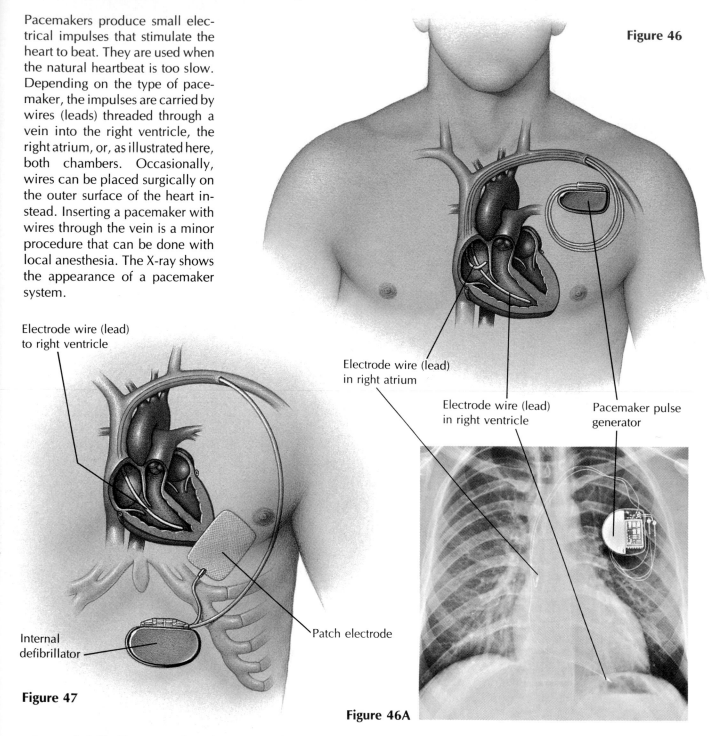

Figure 46

Electrode wire (lead) to right ventricle

Electrode wire (lead) in right atrium

Electrode wire (lead) in right ventricle

Pacemaker pulse generator

Internal defibrillator

Patch electrode

Figure 47

Figure 46A

Internal defibrillators produce larger stimuli that are capable of shocking a heart with ventricular fibrillation or ventricular tachycardia back to a more normal rhythm. These devices are larger and must be implanted under the muscle of the abdomen. Different types of defibrillators use different systems of leads. The one shown here has a wire in the right ventricle and a "patch" or "mesh" electrode under the skin of the chest, near the heart. The wire inside the heart monitors the rhythm. A computer in the device determines whether the rhythm is satisfactory or requires a shock. The shock is produced by an electrical current passed between the patch electrode and the wire in the heart.

DISEASES OF THE BLOOD VESSELS

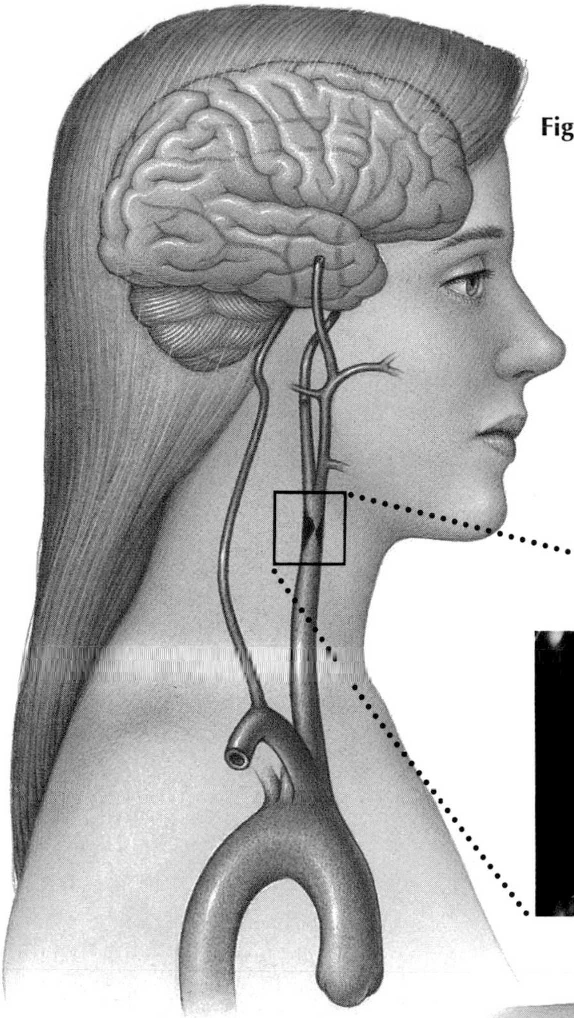

Figure 48

Several disorders of blood vessels are common. *Atherosclerosis* (deposits of cholesterol-containing plaques) in the arteries can cause partial or complete blockage of blood flow. Tissues downstream from the blockage receive insufficient oxygen-carrying blood. Atherosclerotic plaque in a carotid artery (at left) can impede blood flow to the brain. In addition, bits of blood clot or cholesterol can break off and plug smaller vessels in the brain, causing a stroke. One technique of detecting blockage in a vessel is Doppler ultrasonography (photograph inset): the *arrow* points to narrowing of the artery. Turbulence in the bloodstream, caused by the blockage, appears in blue in this Doppler image.

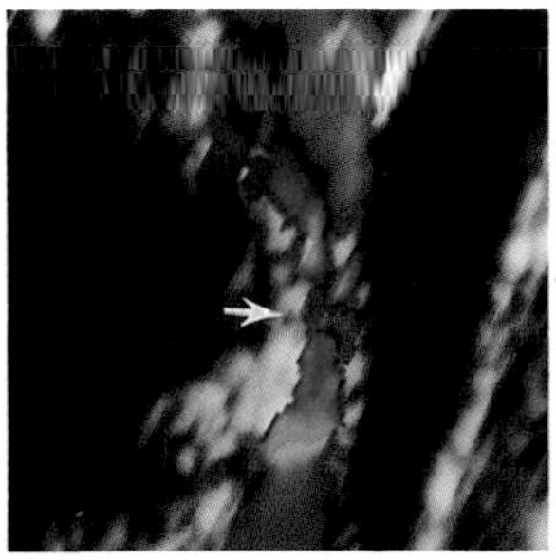

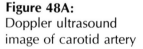

Figure 48A:
Doppler ultrasound image of carotid artery

Figure 49: *Abdominal aortic aneurysm* is an expanded region of the aorta which runs the risk of rupturing or forming a blood clot at the site of expansion. These aneurysms can be seen and accurately measured on ultrasound examination.

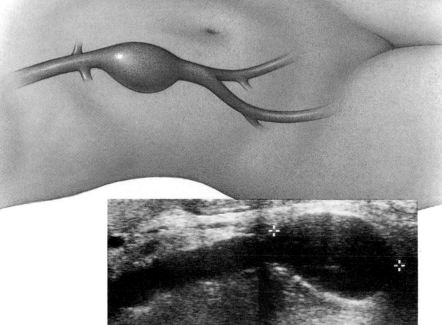

Figure 49A:
Ultrasound image of aneurysm.

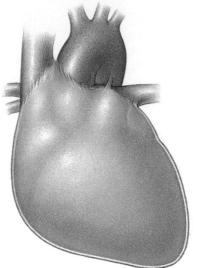

THE PERICARDIUM

Figure 50: The *pericardium* is a thin sac surrounding the heart. It consists of an inner and an outer layer. Normally, a small amount of fluid fills the space between the heart and pericardium.

Figure 51: Some conditions cause excess fluid to develop in the pericardial sac (*pericardial effusion*). If a large amount of fluid accumulates, it can push in on the walls of the heart, decreasing the ability of the heart to expand and take in blood during diastole. This condition, called *cardiac tamponade*, can diminish the effective pumping function of the heart. The fluid may need to be drained by a needle carefully inserted through the chest wall (*pericardiocentesis*).

Figure 52: Inflammation of the pericardium is called *pericarditis*, a condition that can cause chest pain. Some types of pericarditis can lead to thickening and stiffening of the pericardium over time, encasing the heart in a rigid container. This *constrictive pericarditis* also leads to inefficient functioning of the heart, and it may require surgical removal of the pericardium.

Figure 50: The normal pericardium forms a thin covering over the heart.

Figure 51: Fluid accumulation in the pericardium can lead to tamponade, a condition in which the pressure of the fluid prevents the heart from filling adequately.

Figure 52: Thickened, stiff pericardium of constrictive pericarditis.

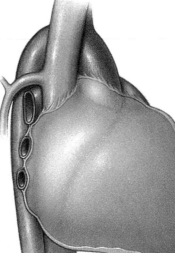

Figure 51A: On the chest X-ray, a pericardial effusion makes the heart look large.

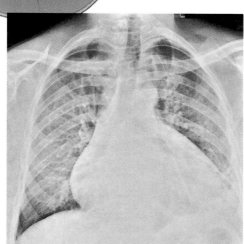

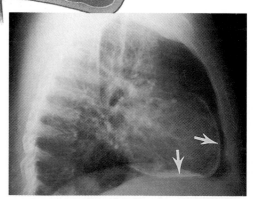

Figure 52A: In constrictive pericarditis, calcium sometimes deposits in the pericardium and can be seen on chest X-ray.

PART 1

Normal Heart and Blood Vessels

Every tissue in your body depends on your heart, but you may take for granted the perpetual beating that keeps you alive from the moment of birth until you die. How does this simple pump perform such an amazing task throughout your lifetime? As you gain a better understanding of how the normal heart works, you may also gain a sense of wonder at its elegant design.

The strength, rhythm, and speed of the heart's pumping action to a large extent determine your health. This chapter describes how the normal heart and circulation perform with precision and efficiency.

THE MYOCARDIUM (HEART MUSCLE)

Your heart, a muscular structure about the size of your fist, and a 60,000-mile network of blood vessels make up your cardiovascular system. The heart itself is the focal point because it performs the main function of the cardiovascular system: pumping blood to all the tissues of the body. The muscle responsible for pumping the blood is called the myocardium (*myo* means "muscle," *cardia* means "heart"). Although the myocardium is the driving force of the circulation, it could not function as a pump without all of the other components that combine with it to make up the cardiovascular system: the valves, the coronary vessels, the conduction (electrical) system, the arteries and veins throughout the body, and the pericardium (the sac around the heart).

Location of the Myocardium (Heart Muscle)

Your heart is located slightly to the left of the center of your chest, protected by the breastbone (sternum) in front, the spinal column in back, and the lungs on both sides (see Figure 1, page A1).

The right side of your heart projects toward the front of the chest, and the left side is toward the back. In an adult, the heart weighs about ¾ pound.

Both sides of the heart have an atrium (a small upper receiving chamber) and a ventricle (a large lower pumping chamber). The two sides of the heart are linked in a figure-eight loop connected by the arteries and veins of the lungs and the arteries and veins of the rest of the body (see Figure 4, page A2).

Structure of the Myocardium (Heart Muscle)

The heart is shaped like a cone, with the point (apex) at the bottom and the broader base at the top. The apex of the heart is the tip of the ventricles and points down to the left side of the chest. The wide upper part of the heart includes the right and left atria and the origins of the major blood vessels.

The heart has three layers of tissue: the myocardium, the epicardium, and the endocardium. The myocardium is the thick main layer of heart muscle. Its outside surface is covered by a thin, glossy membrane called the epicardium. Another smooth, glossy membrane, the endocardium, covers the inside surfaces of the four heart chambers, the valves, and the muscles that attach to the valves (see Figure 11, page A4).

Myocytes: The Cells of the Heart Muscle

The myocardium is composed of individual muscle cells called myocytes. These myocytes act together to contract and relax the heart chambers in the correct sequence to pump blood to the lungs and the body.

Although the cells are individual units, they are coordinated and work together. Remember, the purpose of the heart is to pump blood. It is able to accomplish this pumping in a coordinated manner because of the way the cells are arranged and because electrical messages can pass easily between the cells.

When filaments within the heart muscle cells contract, the cells shorten (see Figure 12, page A4). Shortening of the cells contracts the heart muscle and so makes the pumping chambers become smaller; as a result, blood is squeezed out. When the filaments within the cells relax, the cells lengthen and the heart muscle relaxes; the relaxation makes the pumping chambers expand. When the cham-

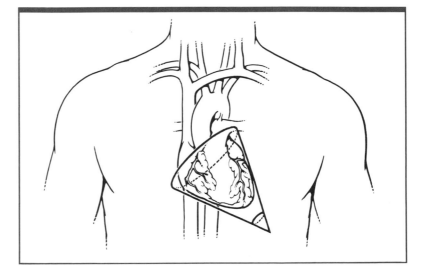

bers expand, blood flows back into them.

How the Heart Pumps

The cardiovascular pump operates by squeezing blood out of its chambers (contraction) and then expanding to allow blood in (relaxation). The action is as simple as squeezing water out of a soft plastic bottle while holding it under water and then releasing your grasp so that water is sucked back into the bottle as it reexpands.

This cycle of contraction and relaxation causes blood flow to be "pulsa-

The heart is somewhat cone-shaped, with the tips of the ventricles pointing down and to the left.

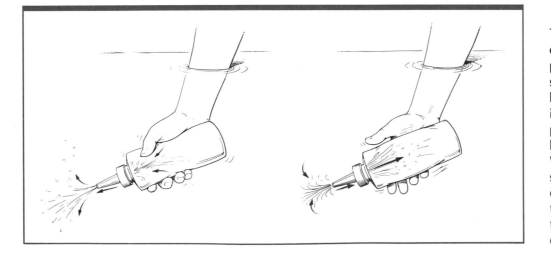

The basic principle of the heart's pumping action is similar to what happens when water is squirted out of a plastic bottle while held under water. When the bottle is squeezed, water is ejected, and when the bottle is allowed to reexpand, water is drawn back into it.

tile." You can feel your heart beat by touching your chest. The pulse of blood flow is also transmitted to your blood vessels, so you can feel your pulse at points where large arteries are close to the surface of your body, such as the wrist, neck, and groin.

Double Pump

Your heart is actually a double pump. The right side, made up of the right atrium and right ventricle (often called the "right heart" by doctors), pumps blood through your lungs, where it receives oxygen and rids itself of carbon dioxide. The left side, made up of the left atrium and left ventricle (the "left heart") receives the newly oxygenated blood and pumps it through the rest of your body, where it delivers oxygen and picks up the waste product carbon dioxide. The circulating blood also

performs many other "transportation" functions such as distributing nutrients and hormones and carrying other waste products to sites of elimination.

In a healthy heart, no blood passes directly between the right and left sides. The two atria are separated by a wall called the atrial septum, and the two ventricles are separated by the ventricular septum. Blood that returns from the tissues of the body to the right heart chambers must, therefore, circulate through the lungs before it can enter the left heart chambers.

The amount of blood that enters and leaves the left heart chambers is exactly the same amount as passes through the right heart. Thus, any increase or decrease in blood flow to the right heart will cause a similar change in the amount of blood pumped to the body by the left heart. Despite this similarity, the anatomy and functions of the right and left sides of the heart are different in many ways.

The Right Heart

The right side of your heart is responsible for pumping blood to your lungs (the pulmonary circulation).

"Used" blood from your body returns to the right side of your heart via two large veins: the superior vena cava (from the head and arms) and the inferior vena cava (from the legs and abdomen). The blood is a dark bluish red because it has delivered oxygen to the body and is "deoxygenated" (without much oxygen). The right side of your heart pumps this deoxygenated blood to the lungs, where it releases carbon dioxide and picks up oxygen. The carbon dioxide is expelled into the air as you breathe.

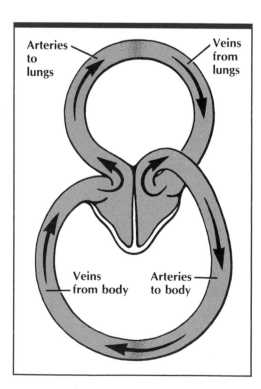

Arteries to lungs

Veins from lungs

Veins from body

Arteries to body

A figure-eight is a simple way to describe the route of blood flow through the body. One loop is the circulation to the lungs, where the blood receives oxygen (*top loop*). The other loop is the circulation to the body, where the blood delivers oxygen and nutrients to all the tissues and organs (*bottom loop*).

Relatively low pressure is required to push blood through the lungs. Therefore, the right side of your heart is less muscular and less powerful than the left side. Nevertheless, efficient performance of the right heart is important in ensuring optimal function of your whole cardiovascular system.

The Left Heart

When the hemoglobin in your red blood cells picks up oxygen in the lungs, your blood becomes bright red. The blood travels from the lungs to the left side of your heart, where it is pumped to the rest of your body through the aorta (the largest blood vessel in your body). The left side of the heart is responsible for pumping blood to the tissues and organs of the body to deliver oxygen from the lungs.

While the blood circulates throughout your body, substances other than oxygen and carbon dioxide are also transported from site to site. The blood carries hormones from glands to their sites of activity. Waste products other than carbon dioxide go to the kidneys and liver, where they can be removed or broken down. Blood picks up nutrients from your intestines and carries them to the liver and other points in your body where they are needed.

The pressure in the blood vessels throughout your body is relatively high compared with the pressure in the lung circulation. When you have your blood pressure checked, it is a measurement of the pressure in blood vessels throughout your body (see What Is Blood Pressure?, page 133). The left heart must have enough strength to push blood forward under higher pressure. Therefore, the left side of the heart is stronger and more muscular than the right side.

The Atria

The atria are the small receiving chambers for blood returning from the body (right atrium) or from the lungs (left atrium) (see Figure 3, page A1). Although the atria contract, their contraction is relatively weak and serves mainly to push blood into the ventricles.

Most people's hearts could pump sufficient blood throughout the body even if the atria did not contract at all. However, the beating of the atria contributes to the overall efficiency of the heart and allows it to pump more blood with less effort. This added efficiency is particularly important if disease damages other parts of the heart that are responsible for pumping.

Each atrium is about the size of a golf ball, or slightly larger. The walls of the right atrium are less than $1/8$ inch thick. The left atrial wall is thicker and more powerful than the right atrial wall, but its volume is about the same.

The Ventricles

The ventricles are the main pumping chambers that propel the blood to the lungs (from the right ventricle) and to the body (from the left ventricle) (see Figure 3, page A1). Each holds about $1/8$ cup of blood after the heart contracts and about $1/2$ cup after the heart is filled.

The walls of the right ventricle are $1/4$ inch thick. The walls of the left ventricle are three times thicker; the left ventricle is thus by far the most powerful chamber in the heart. The left ventricle must generate enough pressure to drive the blood to every part of the body.

The Cardiac Cycle

The period from the beginning of one heartbeat to the beginning of the next is called the cardiac cycle. The cardiac cycle consists of a period of contraction (called systole, SIS-toe-lee) followed by a period of relaxation (called diastole, die-ASS-toe-lee). The blood is pumped out of your heart during systole. During diastole, your heart relaxes and fills with blood. (During *systole*, the heart *squeezes* or pumps; during *diastole*, it *dilates* or relaxes.)

Your heart must relax fully before it can contract again. This allows the heart to fill with blood. At 70 beats per minute, the cardiac cycle lasts about 8/10 second.

In a healthy, resting adult the heart beats about 72 times per minute, about 104,000 times a day, or about 2½ billion times in a lifetime. It pumps about 3 ounces of blood with each beat, or about 5 or more quarts each minute. This amounts to approximately 2,000 gallons a day. An 18-foot-diameter swimming pool holds about 6,500 gallons—your heart could fill the pool in a little more than 3 days! The tens of millions of gallons of blood that your heart pumps in a lifetime is almost beyond comprehension. During strenuous exercise, the heart may have to pump four to seven times the amount of blood it pumps at rest.

The Heart's Work

No matter how forceful the contraction, your heart does not pump all the blood out of the ventricles with each beat. The portion of blood that is pumped out of a filled ventricle is referred to as the ejection fraction. A nor-

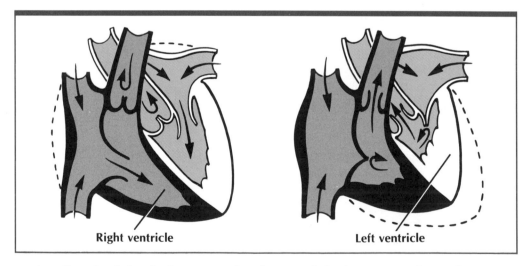

Right ventricle   Left ventricle

During diastole (left), the heart muscle relaxes and the heart expands to allow blood to flow into the pumping chambers (ventricles) from the upper holding chambers (atria). During systole (right), the muscle of the ventricles contracts, squeezing blood out of the chambers. The blood from the right (darker-outlined) ventricle is propelled into the circulation of the lungs. The blood leaving the left (lighter-outlined) ventricle goes to the rest of the body. Notice that blood begins to enter the atria while the ventricles are squeezing.

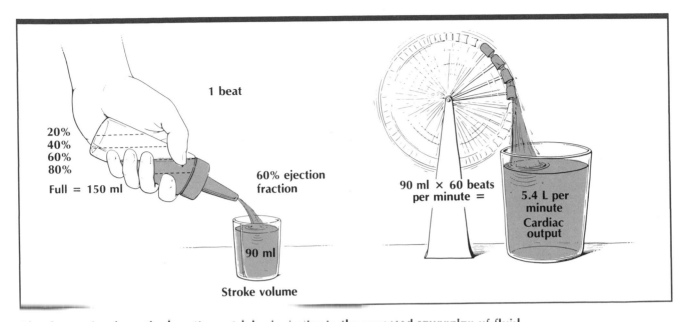

1 beat

20%
40%
60%
80%
Full = 150 ml

60% ejection fraction

90 ml

Stroke volume

90 ml × 60 beats per minute =

5.4 L per minute Cardiac output

Blood pumping from the heart's ventricles is similar to the repeated squeezing of fluid from a bottle (*left*). The amount of fluid (or blood) that squirts out into the cup (or artery) is the stroke volume. The stroke volume is a portion of the total volume of the bottle (or ventricle). This portion is called the ejection fraction. In this example, a stroke volume of 90 milliliters (ml) is squirted out of a 150-ml bottle. Thus, the ejection fraction is 60 percent (*right*). If the bottle is squirted (or the heart beats) 60 times each minute, the total volume of fluid ejected into cups over 1 minute is 5,400 ml (5.4 liters [L]). This amount is called the cardiac output.

mal ejection fraction is 50 percent or more; this value indicates that at least half the blood in the ventricle is pumped out on each beat. The ejection fraction is a good indicator of the overall function of the heart pump. In a healthy person, the ejection fraction increases about 5 percent with exercise. When ventricles are diseased, the ejection fraction can diminish to 20 to 30 percent or lower.

The actual amount of blood pumped by the left ventricle with one contraction is called the stroke volume. The stroke volume and the number of times the heart beats per minute (the heart rate) determine the cardiac output, which is the amount of blood the heart pumps through the circulatory system in 1 minute.

The heart has an automatic mechanism to ensure that it pumps out the same amount of blood that it receives. When more blood enters the heart, the cardiac muscle is stretched more. The more the muscle is stretched, the more

Amount of blood the heart pumps per minute*

- Normal output = 5 to 6 liters (a liter is roughly equivalent to a quart)
- Output without atria contracting = 4 to 6 liters
- Output of weakened heart with atria contracting = 3½ liters
- Output of weakened heart without atria contracting = 2½ liters

*Measurements taken at rest, not during exercise.

forceful will be the contraction, and the more blood will be pumped with each beat. Imagine what would happen without this simple but vital adjustment mechanism. If the heart took in just a tiny bit more blood than it pumped out on each beat, it would gradually swell to the point of being unable to function.

The heart can also increase the amount of blood it pumps by beating more times per minute, within limits. When the heart beats very fast, the strength of the heart muscle decreases and the period of diastole (when the heart relaxes between contractions and fills with blood) becomes too short for the heart chambers to fill adequately.

Although the pumping action of the heart seems simple, the mechanisms that make the pump perform are complex and elegant. Subsequent sections of this chapter describe how the valves, coronary vessels, conduction system, arteries and veins, and the pericardium are involved in the heart's work of pumping blood.

THE HEART VALVES

Although the pumping action of your heart is certainly effective at ejecting blood from the chambers, it alone would not ensure effective blood flow through the figure-eight circulatory loop. Any pumping system requires a

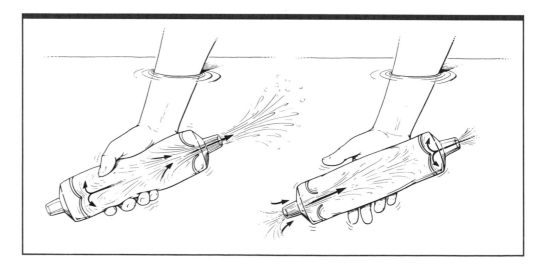

The heart muscle squeezes blood out of the ventricles, and the heart valves are situated to ensure that the blood moves in only one direction. The squeeze bottle again illustrates this principle.

During contraction (*left*), fluid is ejected through a one-way valve at one end of the bottle. Fluid cannot escape backward through the other end of the bottle because of a one-way valve preventing flow in that direction.

During expansion of the bottle (*right*), fluid now enters through the previously closed valve because the direction of flow is different. By the same token, the previously open valve closes to prevent the back leakage of fluid that was just squeezed out.

method to guarantee that the pumped fluid goes in the desired direction. This is the purpose of the valves.

Each valve in your heart opens and closes once with each heartbeat (or about once every second throughout your lifetime).

Location and Structure of the Valves

There are four valves in your heart: the tricuspid, mitral, pulmonary, and aortic (see Figure 3, page A1). The valves are strong, thin leaflets of tissue anchored to the myocardium. The leaflets consist of single sheets of fibrous tissue covered by endocardial cells. At the base of each valve leaflet, the fibrous layer merges with the myocardium to form a flexible hinge, called the annulus.

The Atrioventricular Valves

The atrioventricular valves are the tricuspid (on the right side of the heart) and mitral (on the left side of the heart). These valves regulate the flow of blood from the atria to the ventricles. Their leaflets are delicate flaps that open during ventricular diastole and close during systole. The leaflets are larger than needed to close the opening. Thus, some overlap and puckering of the leaflet tissue occur, ensuring a good seal when the valve is closed.

The leaflets are anchored and supported by chordae tendineae, strong cords that stretch from the valve edges to the myocardium and restrict how far the valve swings when it closes. They prevent the leaflets from flapping back into the atria during ventricular con-

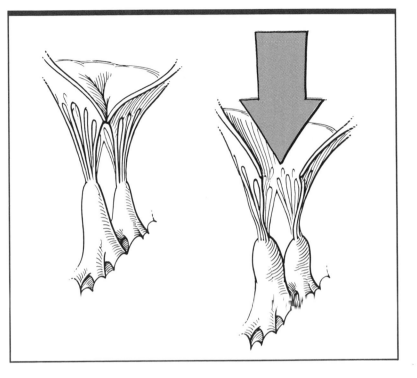

traction. These chordae are similar to the strings of a parachute in function and appearance.

The chordae insert into mounds of myocardium, known as papillary muscles, inside the ventricle.

The *tricuspid* valve, separating the right atrium and right ventricle, is named for its three tooth-shaped leaflets. Tricuspid leaflets tend to be thinner and more translucent than mitral leaflets, and tricuspid chordae tend to be thinner than mitral chordae.

The *mitral* valve (resembling the pointed shape of a bishop's miter) separates the left atrium and left ventricle. In contrast to the three other cardiac valves, which each have three leaflets, the mitral valve has only two.

During diastole when the ventricles relax and expand, the tricuspid and mitral valves open, allowing blood to flow into and refill the ventricles. When the ventricles contract again, blood pushes on the undersides of the

The atrioventricular (mitral and tricuspid) valves as they appear when closed (*left*) and open (*right*). When open, they allow blood to flow from the atria to the ventricles.

leaflets and forces them to close. At the same time, the tiny tendons pull on the edges of the leaflets to keep them from bulging back into the atria and letting blood leak backward.

The Semilunar Valves

The aortic and pulmonary valves are similar to one another in structure but are different from the atrioventricular valves. Their leaflets of delicate tissue are shaped like crescents, thus the name "semilunar" (half-moon) valves. The *pulmonary* valve is at the opening from the right ventricle to the pulmonary artery, and the *aortic* valve is at the opening from the left ventricle to the aorta.

In contrast to the atrioventricular valves, the semilunar valves have no chordae tendineae and are structurally simpler. The aortic valve leaflets are

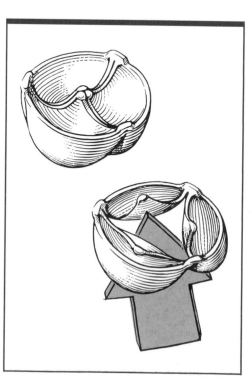

The semilunar (aortic and pulmonary) valves as they appear when closed (*top*) and open (*bottom*). When open, they allow blood to flow from the ventricles to the aorta and pulmonary arteries.

thicker and more opaque than the pulmonary valve leaflets.

Blood flowing from the ventricles pushes the leaflets of the semilunar valves toward the artery walls during contraction, allowing blood to pass through freely. When the blood flow from the ventricles decreases, the pressure in the ventricles falls. The pressure in the artery soon becomes higher than that in the ventricles. When this happens, the blood under higher pressure in the arteries presses the leaflets downward, and the valves snap closed.

One-Way Blood Flow

The valves are designed to allow blood to pass in only one direction. The valves do not actively open and close; that is, they do not automatically open when blood is approaching. Instead, they function like a gate that opens only when it is pushed and is built in such a way that it will open in only one direction. The valves open and close in response to the naturally occurring pressure differences that build up within the heart's chambers during the systolic and diastolic portions of each cardiac cycle.

For example, the aortic valve opens to allow blood to eject from the left ventricle into the aorta, because during systole (contraction) the pressure in the left ventricle is higher than that in the aorta. This pressure difference forces open the leaflets and allows blood to flow through the aortic valve.

During diastole, when the left ventricle relaxes, the pressure in the left ventricle becomes low again while the pressure in the aorta remains high. The valve is pushed closed by the pressure, and blood is prevented from leaking back.

THE CORONARY BLOOD VESSELS (THE FUEL LINES)

Like any other organ or tissue in the body, your heart requires its own blood supply to get the oxygen and nutrition it needs for energy to contract again and again. Although the chambers of the heart are filled with blood, the heart muscle does not extract oxygen and nutrients from the blood in its chambers. The heart receives its nourishing blood supply through the coronary arteries. Because of its heavy work load, the heart requires a particularly rich blood supply. At rest, the blood flow through the coronary arteries averages about 225 milliliters (more than 7 ounces) per minute. This amount is 4 to 5 percent of the blood pumped by the heart, even though the heart makes up less than 1 percent of the body's weight.

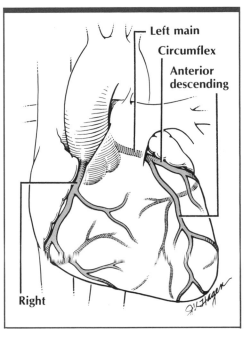

The coronary arteries emerge from the aorta and spread along the outer surface of the heart; from there they send smaller branches into the heart muscle.

Location of the Coronary Arteries

The coronary arteries branch off from the base of the aorta just above the aortic valve. They run along the surface of the heart, encircling the top and branching toward the bottom like a crown (*corona* means "crown," hence their name).

The coronary arteries each have many branches like a tree. The trunks and large branches of the arteries run along the outer surface of your heart. Each trunk is about the size of a soda straw. The smaller branches penetrate into the heart muscle, going from the outside toward the inner surface of the cardiac chambers to carry blood to the myocardial cells (see Figure 25, page A9).

The smaller arteries branch into even smaller vessels and ultimately into capillaries. The capillaries are the points at which oxygen and nutrients are exchanged for waste products.

Structure of the Coronary Arteries

Like other arteries in the body, the coronary arteries have three layers: the inner layer (intima), the muscular layer (media), and the outer layer (adventitia). The inner surface of the blood vessel is lined by a layer of cells called the endothelium. The cavity (channel) within the vessel in which blood flows is called the lumen.

The Major Coronary Arteries

The left coronary artery supplies the front, top, and part of the back side of the left ventricle. The right coronary artery supplies most of the right ventri-

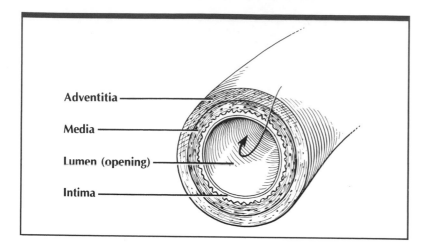

Adventitia

Media

Lumen (opening)

Intima

The coronary arteries, like all of the larger arteries of the body, are tubes with walls that have three layers: the inner (intima), the middle (media), and the outer (adventitia). Blood flows through the opening called the lumen.

cle and also a portion of the undersurface and back of the left ventricle in 80 to 90 percent of people.

The left main coronary artery divides into the anterior descending artery, which carries blood down the front of the heart to both ventricles, and the circumflex artery, which winds around the back of the heart to nourish that portion of the left ventricle and left atrium.

The right coronary artery curves around the front of the heart between the right atrium and right ventricle, sending one branch, the marginal artery, along the front to bring blood to

the right ventricle. The second branch, the posterior descending artery, travels along the undersurface of the heart, sending smaller arteries to both ventricles.

Each person has a unique coronary artery tree. The coronary arteries can have various numbers of branches, and the placement of those branches varies greatly from person to person.

The left coronary artery, in all but rare circumstances, is the major source of blood supply to the left ventricle (the main pumping chamber of the heart). The right coronary artery may vary in size from small to large, and its contribution to the overall blood supply to the heart, while always important, is somewhat variable. Usually, the left coronary artery supplies about 65 percent of the heart's blood flow (45 percent by the left anterior descending artery and 20 percent by the circumflex artery), and the right coronary artery supplies 35 percent.

How Do the Coronary Arteries Adjust Blood Flow?

Blood flow through the coronary arteries is closely related to the amount of oxygen that the myocardial cells need at the moment. Therefore, in normal coronary arteries, blood flow increases as the demand for oxygen increases, such as during exercise.

During exertion, when the heart beats faster and more vigorously, more oxygen is needed. To get more blood to the myocardium, the muscular layer of the arteries relaxes and allows the arteries to expand (get bigger), so more blood can flow through them. More blood can flow through a wide vessel than a small one in a given period, just

Common reasons why your heart may demand more oxygen

- Fast heart rate due to exercise, excitement, or heart rhythm abnormality
- Strong contractions of the heart due to exercise
- High pressure inside the heart chambers, especially the ventricles, due to high blood pressure or valve problems
- Enlarged heart chamber due to any condition that causes heart failure
- Increased muscle mass (thickening of the heart muscle) due to heart muscle abnormalities, high blood pressure, or valve problems

as more water can flow through a wide pipe than a small one in a given period.

The Coronary Veins

Although you rarely hear about the coronary veins because they are unlikely to cause any problems, the blood that supplies the heart must be returned for a fresh supply of oxygen. Capillaries lead to coronary veins, which converge into larger and larger vessels and ultimately become the coronary sinus, which drains into the right atrium. Most of the blood returning from the myocardium of the left ventricle flows through the coronary sinus.

THE CONDUCTION SYSTEM (ELECTRICAL SYSTEM)

An intricate timing system underlies the rhythmic contraction of the ventricles which results in the pulse. Obviously, the normal beating of the heart is vital to the heart fulfilling its function of pumping. If the pumping is interrupted or erratic, your heart may not deliver enough blood to your tissues.

To fulfill its pumping task, the heart must beat at an appropriate rate, and the chambers of the heart must contract in a coordinated fashion. The atria contract first to help blood flow into the ventricles. When this step is complete, the ventricles contract and propel the blood out to the arteries of the body.

The heart rate and sequence of contraction are mediated by the conduction system of the heart. The conduction system is like electrical wiring that conducts electrical impulses throughout the muscle of the heart. These electrical impulses stimulate the heart muscle to contract and squeeze blood out of the heart into the arteries.

Parts of the Conduction System

The sinus node, a group of cells in the upper part of the right atrium, is the normal origin of the electrical impulse.

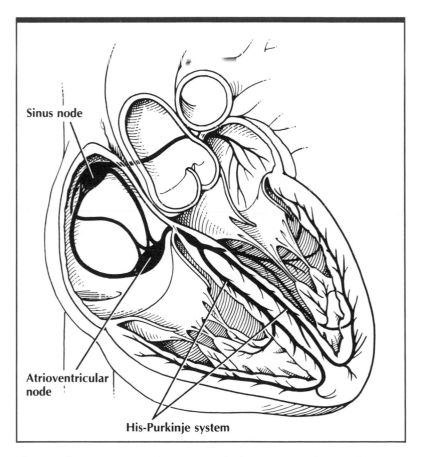

Sinus node

Atrioventricular node

His-Purkinje system

The conduction system is a network that carries electrical signals throughout the heart. The heartbeat originates in the sinus node, high in the right atrium. It travels through the atrial pathways to the atrioventricular node. There the signal briefly slows down as it is "funneled" into the electrical network of the ventricles, the His-Purkinje system. The conduction system permits the electrical signal to reach all parts of the heart in a timely fashion, so that the heartbeat is coordinated and occurs at a normal rate.

It is the heart's natural pacemaker. The impulse is channeled into the adjacent cells of the conduction system. This channeling, in effect, produces an electrical current that then passes from cell to cell down through the distant portions of the conduction system.

The second part of the conduction system is the electrical pathways in the atrium through which this electrical current preferentially travels on its journey throughout the atria and down to the ventricles.

The third portion of the conduction system is the atrioventricular (AV) node, which is a cluster of cells in the center of the heart between the atria and the ventricles. The AV node is like a gate that slows down the electrical current before it is allowed to pass through to the ventricles. This conduction delay at the AV node ensures that the atria contract a short time before the ventricles.

After it leaves the AV node, the current travels into specialized conduction tissue called the His-Purkinje system. This system of branching pathways of specialized electricity-conducting tissue rapidly distributes the current throughout the muscle cells of the left and right ventricles.

The interval from the initiation of the electrical impulse in the sinus node to completion of its delivery through the conduction system to the myocardial cells is brief, averaging about ¼ second when the heart is beating 72 beats per minute. More than half of this time is due to the built-in delay at the AV node (see Figure 43, page A12).

How the Conduction System Controls Heart Rate

In the conduction system, the flow of current in a cell is passed on to adjacent cells. In the heart muscle cells, the same thing happens, but in addition the electrical current activates the contractile apparatus of the muscle cell. When the contractile apparatus is activated, it initiates the pumping action of the heart muscle. Thus, the conduction system, from the sinus node on down, is responsible for controlling the speed and rhythm of your heart's contraction.

Unlike most other muscle cells of the body, cardiac cells can initiate their own electrical impulse and contraction. Although the nervous system can adjust the rate at which the heart beats, it is not the driving force that makes it beat. Even a heart that has been removed from the body, or cardiac cells that have been separated from one another, can continue to contract for a while. In fact, even if the sinus node fails, other sites can take over the pacemaking function.

The reason that the sinus node sets the pace is that its natural rate for formation of the electrical impulse is faster than the rates in other cells farther down in the conduction system, and the faster rate overrides the slower rates. As you go down the conduction system, the rate of spontaneous contraction gets slower and slower. For example, in an adult the usual sinus node rate at rest is 60 to 100 beats per minute. The spontaneous rate at the AV node is 40 to 60 beats per minute, and the rate in the ventricles is only 20 to 40 beats per minute.

Although the slower rate of impulse formation from an AV node site will keep you alive, your heart performs better under the direction of the sinus node. Likewise, if neither the sinus node nor the AV node is working, another backup system (in the ventricles) takes over. However, it is even slower and is not designed to do the job alone.

Regulation of Heart Rate

The normal heart rate in a resting adult is 60 to 100 beats per minute. Remember, "normal" means that *most* people have heart rates in this range *most* of the time. Small fluctuations outside the "normal" range do not necessarily indicate a problem. Some doctors might say the normal resting heart rate is 50 to 90 beats per minute.

As you run, climb stairs, or exercise, the sinus node responds and your heart rate speeds up. Your heart beats faster with increased activity to send more blood to nourish your muscles.

Along with exercise, several other things can increase the heart rate, including mental stress, tobacco, caffeine, alcohol, and certain prescription and nonprescription drugs. Alternatively, your heart rate normally slows during sleep and with some medications. Pulse rates in the range of 30 to 50 beats per minute are not unusual in healthy adults during sleep.

The Autonomic Nervous System

The message that prompts the sinus node to increase or decrease its rate is delivered by the autonomic nervous system. The autonomic nervous system automatically controls many functions in your body such as blood pressure, breathing, excretion, and heart rate. You do not have to decide consciously to breathe or to change your heart rate because the autonomic nervous system takes care of these decisions for you. It can make snap judgments. For instance, it can cause the sinus node to increase the heart rate to

Heart rates for different ages

Normal Heart Rates at Rest	
Age Group	**Beats per Minute**
Newborn	140
Young child	100 to 120
Adult	60 to 100
Maximal Attainable Heart Rates	
Age, Years	**Beats per Minute**
25	200
35	188
45	176
55	165
65	155

These are averages. The value for an individual person may be different.

twice its normal rate within only 3 to 5 seconds.

How Fast Can a Heart Beat?

As you age, it may seem as if your body is slowing down. In fact, your heart rate actually does slow with age. The decrease is not noticeable during everyday activities, but your maximal heart rate during exercise decreases as you grow older. For example, your maximal heart rate at age 25 is about 200 beats per minute. By age 65, your maximal heart rate is only about 155 beats per minute.

The heart rate may also slow as a desirable result of being in good physical condition. An athlete's heart often beats slower than normal because training has allowed the heart to contract more strongly and pump more blood with each beat. As a result, the heart does not need to beat as fast to produce normal blood flow.

THE ARTERIES AND VEINS

Your arteries and veins are essential for carrying the blood pumped by the heart to and from all parts of the body. The arteries carry blood away from the heart, and the veins bring blood back to the heart from the tissues in the body.

The arteries can be thought of as a "tree" in which a trunk branches into smaller and smaller branches and twigs (arterioles) until they finally become capillaries. Capillaries are only slightly wider than a single blood cell. Thus, they allow only a single-file column of blood cells to travel through at a time. It is through the thin wall of the capillaries that oxygen, carbon dioxide, nutrients, and waste products are exchanged (see Figures 7 and 9, page A3).

After the blood flows through the capillaries, it enters small veins (venules) that merge into larger and larger branches (veins) that go back to the atria.

The Main Arteries and Veins

The main artery in your body is the aorta. It carries bright red (oxygenated) blood to the tissues of the body. The ascending aorta emerges upward from your left ventricle. It makes a U-turn in the upper part of the chest and descends to become the abdominal aorta. Large branches lead from your aorta to your head, trunk, arms, and legs. The main arteries supplying your head are the carotid arteries. Your arms receive their blood supply through the axillary arteries, and your legs receive their blood supply through the femoral arteries. These main branches divide into smaller ones as they get farther away from the heart (see Figure 5, page A2).

Your pulmonary artery carries blood from your heart to your lungs. It arises from your right ventricle and transports dark bluish red (deoxygenated) blood to the lungs.

The main veins in your body are the superior and inferior venae cavae. They empty into the right atrium. The superior vena cava receives blood from your head through the jugular veins, and from your arms through the axillary veins. The inferior vena cava receives blood from several veins in the abdomen and from your legs through the femoral veins. As with the arteries, the veins branch into smaller ones as they get farther away from the heart. In this case, though, blood flows *from* the small vessels into the bigger ones and finally into the heart.

Your pulmonary vein carries newly oxygenated blood from your lungs to the left atrium of your heart.

At any given time, 9 percent of your blood is traveling to and from the lungs in your pulmonary vessels and about 7 percent is in your heart. By far the greatest volume of blood (84 percent) is in the vessels that travel to and from the rest of your body. These vessels are called the systemic arteries and veins (the systemic circulation). Within the systemic circulation, 64 percent of the blood in the body is in the veins, 13 percent is in the arteries, and 7 percent is in the tiny branching arterioles and capillaries.

Structure of the Arteries and Veins

The structure of the systemic blood vessels is the same as that of the coronary arteries. The outside of the vessel is the adventitia. The middle muscular layer is called the media, and the inner layer is called the intima. The opening (lumen) of the vessels is lined with endothelium (see the figure on page 12).

The blood vessels are more than just passive channels in which blood flows. They are a dynamic element of the circulatory system in their own right, and the individual layers interact in many ways. The adventitia carries the vasa vasorum (small blood vessels supplying necessary nourishment to the other layers). It also contains nerves that can signal the muscles in the media to contract. The endothelial lining of the inner layer senses and produces messages that tell the muscle layer to contract or expand. Contraction and relaxation of muscles in the media help to control blood pressure and the amount of blood distributed to the various organs. In these and other ways, the arteries and veins can have a major impact on the overall function of the body's circulation.

The Arteries

Because your arteries transport blood under high pressure, they have strong elastic walls, and the blood flows rapidly through them. The flow of blood in the arteries is said to be pulsatile. This means that the amount of blood flowing constantly increases and decreases as a result of the heart pumping a new volume of blood into the arteries 70 times per minute. This effect is what causes the pulse that you feel over the arteries in your wrists and neck.

The Arterioles

The arterioles also have strong muscular walls that can close off the arteriole

completely or dilate it greatly. This feature enables the arteriole to change the blood flow to the capillaries in response to the needs of your tissues. Muscles, for example, when active, may need as much as 20 to 30 times the blood flow that they need at rest. Because the heart can increase its output by only four to seven times, these tiny vessels continually monitor the needs in each tissue and control the blood flow in that portion of the body to the level required. When a large

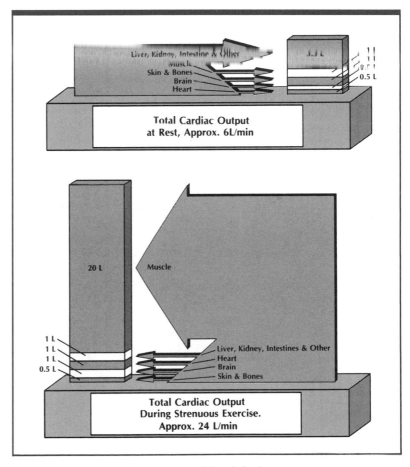

Cardiac output, or the amount of blood the heart pumps in 1 minute, varies depending on how much oxygen and nutrients are required by the body and on which organs have the greatest need. During strenuous exercise the total cardiac output can increase by as much as four times, and the proportion allotted to the working muscles increases as well. Although the *proportion* of blood going to the heart and brain decreases during maximal exercise, the actual *amount* of blood remains fairly stable.

increase is needed in one area (for example, exercising muscles), the proportion of flow to other organs is temporarily decreased.

The Capillaries

The capillary walls are very thin, allowing small molecules to pass through them. The role of the capillaries depends on the tissues in which they are located. Pulmonary capillaries release carbon dioxide from the blood into air sacs (alveoli) and at the same time absorb oxygen from the air sacs into the blood. The capillaries in the kidneys send waste products into tubules where urine is formed. In the walls of the intestines, nutrients are absorbed from broken-down food. Capillaries in the muscles exchange oxygen and nutrients for waste products and carbon dioxide.

The Veins

The pressure in your veins is very low, and their walls are thinner than the walls of the arteries. Your veins have valves that keep the blood flowing only toward the heart. Veins are capable of contracting and expanding in response to the needs of the body. They can act as a reservoir because their walls are 6 to 10 times as expandable as those of the arteries. When you need blood drawn for most diagnostic tests, it is taken from a vein.

The "Venous Pump"

When your move your legs or even tense your leg muscles, blood in your legs is propelled toward the heart. This mechanism is called the "venous pump." If you stand perfectly still for a long time, this pumping action is lost, and as much as 15 to 20 percent of your blood volume "pools" in your legs. Because that amount of "pooled" blood is diverted from the overall circulation, other organs may not get their "fair share." The first organ to feel the consequences is the topmost—the brain. This effect is frequently the reason some people may feel dizzy or even pass out after standing for a long time, such as soldiers standing at attention or people standing at church.

THE PERICARDIUM

The pericardium is a sac surrounding the heart (see Figure 50, page A16). It actually is two sacs, an inner one and an outer one, with a small amount of fluid between them to act as a lubricant. This allows the heart to beat with minimal friction.

The inner lining of the pericardium is a thin, moist membrane. The tough outer layer of the pericardial sac adheres to several areas in the chest cavity to anchor the heart in place.

Although the pericardium provides some support and lubrication for the heart, it is somewhat expendable (like the appendix or gallbladder). You can get along without it if it should ever have to be removed surgically.

PART 2

What Is Heart Disease?

Heart disease takes many forms and varies widely in severity. Some cause a few nuisance problems. Many cause major changes in your life. Still others cause death.

Some people are born with heart disease, and in many it develops later. Most people detect warning symptoms, but for others, heart disease strikes without the slightest clue.

SYMPTOMS: SIGNALS OF DISEASE

Sometimes, a specific symptom provides a warning. Or, you may be unable to pinpoint the specific problem but you just do not feel right. Your doctor may be the first to discover a suspicious test result or physical sign. In other cases, a heart attack is the earliest warning.

Malfunctions in your cardiovascular system may display themselves by causing various symptoms. The detective work of determining what problem is causing symptoms is the cornerstone of diagnosis, and an accurate diagnosis is the best chance of finding an effective treatment.

What Is a Symptom?

A symptom is a change in the way your body feels that may indicate illness or disease. A symptom is totally subjective. No one but you can experience it or detect it. A symptom is not the disease itself.

Doctors cannot detect a symptom; only you can do that. Doctors are trained to listen to your description of symptoms and to ask questions to determine the significance of each. Doctors also look for "signs"—outward manifestations of the disease or problem.

Although neither the symptoms nor the signs are the disease, they are clues to a potential underlying problem.

They are your body's way of telling you that something may be wrong.

An Early Warning System

Because many symptoms are an early warning of underlying disease, it is important to respond to them in the right way. It would be silly to dwell on every minor ache, pain, and twinge in your body. These symptoms do not signal a serious illness. Over the years, you have learned to ignore certain symptoms because experience has shown that they have little impact on your overall health.

However, you may have symptoms of an actual problem, but because you have become familiar with the symptoms, you know what to do about them. For example, a runny nose, stuffy head, sore throat, and cough suggest that you are coming down with a cold. People with colds usually take it easy and use a mild pain reliever and cough medicine as needed. A visit to the emergency room is unnecessary.

Questions may arise, though, when you experience a symptom for the first time or if it is worse than usual or accompanies other symptoms. When these situations occur, you might wonder whether an illness is present and whether you need medical attention. You ask yourself, "Do I need to see a doctor? How soon? Should I wait and see whether anything else happens? Is there anything I should do to deal with the situation myself?"

The first step in answering these questions is to understand what the symptoms may mean. One purpose of this book is to help provide that working knowledge.

The second step is to decide whether the symptom is related to an underlying medical problem. Even if you are uncertain, it is advisable to consult a doctor.

The third step is to decide how urgently you need medical attention. On the one hand, it probably would be inappropriate, time-consuming, and expensive to call an ambulance or go to the emergency room for a momentary jab of pain on the right side of the chest. However, it might be appropriate to set up an appointment with a doctor for an examination.

On the other hand, it would be folly to ignore sustained chest pressure or breathing difficulty. You might hope it will go away, and you might not want to bother the doctor in the middle of the night, but you could be having a heart attack.

Neither this book nor any other book can cover all the possible symptoms you may experience, nor can it presume to make diagnoses. Unfortunately, no system or formula tells you in advance whether a symptom is significant. The same symptom or symptoms may indicate widely differing and unrelated types of conditions in different people; conversely, many different symptoms may be caused by one illness. No one can be expected to determine a diagnosis or its significance before seeing a doctor.

In general, however, you should consider seeing a doctor soon if a symptom meets any of the following general criteria:

- The symptom is new.
- The symptom is severe.
- The symptom is worsening.
- The symptom provokes anxiety.
- The symptom is unrelieved by a previously recommended medication.
- The symptom is a repetition of a symptom that was associated with a previous serious problem. This may be an indication that the problem has recurred.

Beyond these general recommendations, specific symptoms have their own implications. Certain important symptoms or signs may indicate a possible problem in your heart or circulation. These include chest pain, shortness of breath, fatigue, swelling, loss of consciousness, light-headedness, palpitations, limb pain, skin discoloration or sores, shock, and sudden changes in vision, strength, coordination, speech, or sensation. This section will help you recognize these signs and symptoms and how they relate to different types of heart and blood vessel disease.

This book does not take the place of a doctor's evaluation. If you have any questions, you should ask your doctor directly for further advice.

How Should I Discuss Symptoms With My Doctor?

Because symptoms are such an important clue to underlying problems, and because no one except you can describe your symptoms, the better you can communicate your symptoms to your doctor, the more likely it is that the doctor can help you. Some doctors claim that 90 percent of the final diagnosis is revealed by what you tell them during your examination. Thus, you can save time, money, and effort, and increase the chances that your doctor will find an effective solution, by carefully describing your symptoms.

In view of this advice, the more clearly you can describe your symptoms, the more effective your evaluation will be. Admittedly, many symptoms are vague, but if you use precise terms and cover all the details of a symptom (see Symptoms: All the facts, below), you help the doctor find the problem.

Think about what you want to tell the doctor ahead of time. If you are vague, if you are quiet, or if you are unfocused, important information may be lost. Your doctor will ask questions

to fill in the gaps, but usually the information you volunteer contains the key clues to a correct diagnosis.

The descriptions of the main cardiovascular symptoms and signs that follow may help you communicate more clearly with your doctor. At this point, the focus is on the symptoms, rather than what causes them. Some of the problems the symptoms *suggest* will be mentioned.

As an aid to further reading about the possible diagnoses, a list is provided at the end of the descriptions of most symptoms. These "Diagnoses to Consider," as they are called, are not all-inclusive, but they are intended to facilitate your information-gathering about specific problems. Moreover, the list does not mean that you *necessarily* have one of those problems if you have that symptom.

Later in this chapter, you will find guides after each description of a disease that will direct you to information about possibly relevant testing procedures or treatments. Again, these lists do not mean that every or any test or treatment listed is *necessary* for that condition. Nor do they contain the only tests or treatments available. Ultimately, only your doctor can advise you about your diagnosis and the best course of evaluation and management for your specific circumstances.

Symptoms: All the facts

Just as a beginning reporter learns to cover the "who, what, when, where, and how" of a story, doctors are taught in medical school to seek certain information about symptoms. These bits of information help doctors get the full story about your symptoms. You may be able to describe your symptoms more clearly if you specify these details:

- Quality (How does it feel?)
- Location (Where does it bother you?)
- Severity (How bad is it?)
- Provocation (What brings on the symptom?)
- Relieving factors (What reduces or eliminates the symptom?)
- Duration (How long have you had it? How long does it last?)
- Frequency (How often does it occur?)
- Associated symptoms (Do you have other problems along with it?)

Symptoms Guide

CHEST PAIN. Chest pain is probably the symptom most commonly associated with heart disease. Cardiologists spend a large part of their time analyzing "chest pain." Ironically, the sensation associated with most types of heart disease is rarely described as pain. In fact, some people go out of their way to say that they are *not* experiencing pain, but rather a difficult-to-describe discomfort.

Chest pain usually falls into three categories: the chest pain due to angina (pain caused by an insufficient oxygen supply to the heart muscle), chest pain from other cardiac causes such as an inflammation of the pericardium (see page 112) or the tearing pain from dissection of an artery (see page 102), and chest pain from noncardiac problems such as gallbladder disease. This section focuses on angina and on chest pain from other cardiac causes.

Angina Pectoris. Angina pectoris is one of the most common symptoms of heart disease. Angina, like all symptoms, is not a diagnosis. In most cases it is associated with any condition in which the heart muscle does not get an adequate supply of blood and oxygen.

Qualities of Angina Pectoris. Angina pectoris is most often described as a constricting pressure or tightness of the chest. However, it can take many different forms, including aching or sharp pains. People experience angina pectoris in different ways, but in an individual the pattern is consistent.

Many people who experience angina have a difficult time explaining the nature of the discomfort to the doctor. Some people use images such as "like an elephant sitting on my chest" or "like my chest is in a vise." They often describe the pain as dull rather than sharp.

When asked to show where the discomfort is located, many people put their whole hand or a clenched fist on their chest, because it is not possible to localize the sensation by pointing a finger. (This is a classic sign called "Levine's sign.")

Symptoms and signs commonly associated with heart disease

The symptoms and signs most commonly associated with heart and blood vessel disease are the following:

- Chest pain (angina pectoris)
- Shortness of breath (dyspnea)
- General fatigue
- Swelling (edema)
- Loss of consciousness (syncope)
- Light-headedness (presyncope)
- Palpitations
- Limb pain or tiredness (claudication)
- Abnormal skin color
- Sores on skin (ulceration)
- Shock (collapse)
- Sudden change in vision, strength, coordination, speech, or sensation

Location. The discomfort of angina pectoris is often described as spreading throughout the chest and occasionally radiating into the back, neck, shoulders, and arms, especially on the left side. Sometimes the discomfort is located only in the arm or the jaw, and not in the chest. Believe it or not, some people with angina have consulted with their dentist initially in the mis-

Terms people use to describe angina

- Crushing
- Constricting
- Vise-like
- Strangling
- Pressure
- Heaviness
- Fullness
- Feeling like a weight

- Squeezing
- Burning
- Ache
- Like gas
- Tight
- Like indigestion
- Choking
- Coldness with perspiration or weakness

taken (but understandable) belief that the cause of their jaw pain was dental.

Provocation.   Angina pectoris is typically provoked by either mental or physical stress. Mental stress can be brought about by anxiety, fright, or other strong emotions. Physical stress can be brought about by walking (especially up a hill), stair climbing, running, housework, sexual intercourse, or other activities. The added stress requires more work from the heart, which produces a greater need for oxygen in the coronary arteries. If this need is not met, angina results.

Angina is provoked more easily by performing physical activities in cold weather or after a meal. Cold temperatures and digestion require more work from the heart. In the cold, your body sends more blood to your arms and legs to keep warm. Digestion is a kind of "internal exercise" that requires more blood be supplied to the digestive tract. As a result, your heart must work harder—perhaps hard enough to outstrip its supply of oxygen.

Duration.   Angina that is caused by a temporary insufficiency of the coronary blood supply typically lasts a matter of minutes, as opposed to momentary twinges. If you have angina that lasts more than 5 to 10 minutes, you could be having a heart attack. You should seek medical attention immediately.

Relief.   If angina occurs during exercise, it will usually disappear within minutes of stopping the exercise or other stressful activity. People who have experienced the discomfort before or who have been diagnosed as having angina may take nitroglycerin when they experience the symptoms. Relief usually comes within 2 or 3 minutes.

Associated   Symptoms.   Occasionally, chest discomfort that turns out to be angina pectoris due to coronary artery disease is associated with other symptoms. Other symptoms include shortness of breath (air hunger), anxiety, palpitations, nausea, sweating, and light-headedness.

Angina pectoris is usually experienced as discomfort, tightness, or pressure in the chest or in some regions of the back, neck, jaw, shoulders, and arms (especially the left arm). In some persons the discomfort is limited to a specific area, whereas in others it can radiate to various sites throughout the upper body.

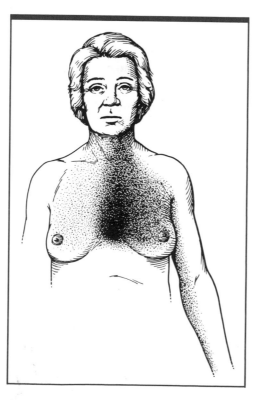

Angina: Diagnoses to Consider

Coronary artery disease
  (see page 70)
Hypertrophic cardiomyopathy
  (see page 43)
Valve disease, especially aortic
  stenosis
  (see page 65)
Pulmonary hypertension
  (see page 110)

Other Possible Causes. Although some people have a classic constellation of symptoms suggesting angina pectoris, more often only some of the features point to angina, and others may be absent or atypical. Accordingly, you and your doctor must keep in mind possible diagnoses other than those associated with angina.

Not all chest pain is angina by any means. The less the symptoms sound like angina, the less likely the symptoms are caused by insufficient blood supply to the heart muscle. Other types of chest pain may signal the presence of other heart problems.

Sharp pain over the breastbone or front chest wall that becomes worse with breathing in or with lying down may point to inflammation of the pericardium (the sac that surrounds the heart).

Chest Pain Due to Problems Other Than Angina. Chest pain can have many causes. Some causes are related to the heart and blood vessels. Others have nothing to do with the cardiovascular system but may be important nevertheless. The doctor considers a list of different possible causes, a process referred to as a differential diagnosis. Your careful description of the pain can often eliminate other possibilities.

Sometimes a person has alarming chest pain and yet has no identifiable problem with the heart. Conditions that often turn out to be present, although heart disease was suspected, include stomach disorders such as heartburn (esophageal reflux), stomach or duodenal ulcer, or gallstones with gallbladder irritation or inflammation. Other conditions that can mimic angina include chest wall pain (caused by soreness of the muscles between the ribs or the immovable joints

between the ribs and breastbone), a pinched nerve in the neck, inflammation of the membranes around the lung (pleuritis), blood clots in the pulmonary arteries, and shingles (herpes zoster).

SHORTNESS OF BREATH (DYSPNEA). Shortness of breath is another common symptom associated with some types of heart disease. Actually, it is a difficult symptom to describe. Usually it implies a sense of hunger for air that cannot be satisfied. Dyspnea (*dys* means "abnormal," *pnea* means "breathing" or "ventilation") is the medical term used to describe an abnormally uncomfortable awareness of breathing (which could mean labored, shallow, or rapid breathing).

Some people cannot distinguish dyspnea from chest discomfort, and dyspnea and angina sometimes occur together.

Shortness of Breath With Various Levels of Activity. Of course, everyone becomes short of breath after strenuous exertion. If you are not used to exercise, you may become short of breath with only moderate exertion. Therefore, this symptom is abnormal only when it occurs at rest or at a level of activity that is not expected to cause shortness of breath. It is important to distinguish when shortness of breath is due to actual health problems and when it is caused by being out of shape. You are the best judge of when your degree of breathlessness is abnormal for you.

For example, if you usually engage in an average amount of activity but find that you feel short of breath after climbing one flight of stairs, you may have an underlying disease process.

Doctors refer to this as "dyspnea on exertion" ("DOE"). Many doctors evaluate the degree of dyspnea by asking how many blocks you can walk at a normal pace, or how many flights of stairs you can climb. Shortness of breath at rest usually indicates a more advanced level of underlying disease.

Other factors may make you feel short of breath without an active underlying disease necessarily being present. For example, if you are overweight, you must carry that additional weight for any activity, which in itself may cause shortness of breath at an early stage of exercise.

Shortness of breath may occur in different patterns, which can help determine the underlying cause.

Shortness of Breath at Night (Paroxysmal Nocturnal Dyspnea).

"Paroxysmal" means a sudden onset, and "nocturnal" means occurring in the night. One classic pattern of shortness of breath occurs at night when you are asleep and lying down. You awake abruptly gasping for air and may sit up and fling open a window to try to catch your breath. Sometimes the episode is accompanied by coughing, wheezing, or a smothering sensation. To get any relief, you ultimately must sit straight up. Finally the symptoms subside, and you are able to return to bed and sleep for the rest of the night. If not, you may have to sleep sitting up in a chair.

This pattern of shortness of breath is a classic clue to the presence of heart failure (see page 36). Often, people who experience this find they can minimize the symptom by sleeping with their trunk and head in an upright position, either bolstered by pillows or sleeping in a chair or recliner. Difficulty breathing except in an upright position is called orthopnea (*ortho* means "straight" or "upright").

Rapid Breathing (Tachypnea).

Any condition that makes a person short of breath tends to lead to more rapid breathing. Rapid breathing is called tachypnea (*tachy* means "fast"). Tachypnea occurs partly in an effort to get more oxygen and also because of anxiety.

Hyperventilation.

Labored, shallow, or rapid breathing as signs of underlying heart or lung disease must be distinguished from the sense of breathlessness and rapid breathing associated with hyperventilation. In hyperventilation, the problem (rather than the consequence) is anxiety. Hyperventilation due to anxiety is sometimes a repetitive sighing type of breathing and sometimes continued rapid breathing. You feel as though you cannot breathe deeply enough. Your arms and hands may tingle during hyperventilation.

The effect of hyperventilation is to reduce the carbon dioxide in the bloodstream to abnormally low levels. This can make you feel light-headed or tingly (especially around the mouth), and muscle cramps may develop. An effective way of counteracting the low carbon dioxide level is to rebreathe the same air you breathed out, because it contains a lot of carbon dioxide. Do this by placing a small paper bag over your mouth and nose and breathing into it. Ultimately, the psychological causes for your hyperventilation should be addressed in order to prevent its recurrence.

Associated Symptoms.

Other signs and symptoms may occur with shortness of breath and provide clues as to the origin of the problem. Swelling of the feet and legs (edema), abdominal bloating, or shortness of breath while lying down suggests severe congestive heart failure. If you have these symptoms, you should promptly see your doctor.

If your shortness of breath is associated with angina, the dyspnea may be related to coronary artery disease. Sudden onset of shortness of breath may be a clue to various possible problems, including a blood clot in the lungs, fluid in the pericardium (the sac that surrounds the heart), heart attack, or anxiety-induced hyperventilation.

Other Possible Causes. Of course, shortness of breath can be related to problems with the lungs or lung circulation, including emphysema, chronic bronchitis, and pulmonary hypertension. In contrast to cardiac dyspnea, the dyspnea of chronic obstructive lung disease or emphysema often occurs when you are in a position that prevents your lungs from expanding, such as when you bend over to tie your shoes.

Shortness of Breath: Diagnoses to Consider

Heart failure (see page 36)
Valve problems (see page 57)
Coronary artery disease
  (see page 70)
Congenital heart disease
  (see page 48)
Pulmonary embolism
  (see page 107)
Pulmonary hypertension
  (see page 110)
Lung disease
Anxiety

FATIGUE.   Many people complain of a generalized sense of fatigue, or of being tired, that is not necessarily associated with shortness of breath or actual muscle weakness. Although fatigue certainly affects your life and may make you worry about heart disease, it is rarely associated with heart disease unless you also have other, more specific symptoms. If you are tired when you awaken and stay tired all day, the cause is most likely not your heart.

Nevertheless, if you complain of fatigue, especially if it has developed over a short time, your doctor will search for an underlying cause, among which heart disease is one possibility. Other possibilities include a low red blood cell count (anemia), low thyroid activity (hypothyroidism), various infections, and a disordered sleep pattern. In most people with isolated fatigue, though, a specific cause cannot be identified.

SWELLING (EDEMA). Swelling (edema) is the leakage of fluid from the bloodstream into the surrounding tissue, like coffee through a coffee filter. Edema can occur for several reasons, including congestive heart failure, obstruction of the veins, and kidney failure. In all these cases, the fluid tends to collect at the lowest points because gravity forces fluid out of the lowest blood vessels.

You may first notice swelling in the feet and ankles, especially after a long day of standing or sitting, such as during a long plane trip. Crossing your legs, which partially obstructs the flow of blood from your feet, may make the condition even worse. A mild amount of this type of edema may not mean that anything is wrong.

As the condition causing swelling worsens, the edema may ascend to the thighs and even the trunk. If you are confined to bed most of the time, the most significant edema may be in the lower back, again because gravity forces the fluid out at the lowest point.

In the early stages you may notice that your shoes and socks are leaving a more prominent impression than usual over your ankles and calves. As the edema becomes more severe, it is actually possible to indent the skin and leave an impression with your finger. (Doctors refer to this as "pitting edema.")

Edema may cause bloating of the stomach and poor digestion because of fluid in the walls of the intestinal tract. It can occur in the lungs (pulmonary edema), which is the basis for shortness of breath in congestive heart failure.

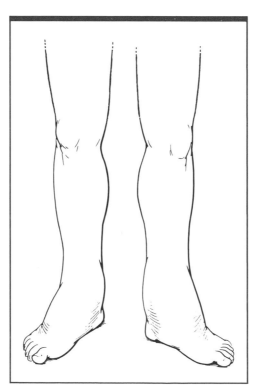

Swollen feet and ankles indicate edema, or leakage of fluid from the bloodstream into the surrounding tissues.

Edema Caused by Heart Disease. When edema is caused by a heart problem, it is because the heart cannot pump effectively. As the heart performs less and less efficiently as a pump, it becomes more and more of a dam. The fluid that was previously being pumped effectively through the bloodstream now collects behind the dam as though in a reservoir.

Tissues that are "sponge-like," such as the layers of tissue under the skin, the liver, and the lungs, are prone to "soak up" the excess fluid. Thus, people with decreased pumping function experience swelling of the legs, swelling and pain in the region of the liver under the right side of the rib cage, and shortness of breath from fluid in the lung air sacs.

Eventually, inadequate heart pumping decreases the amount of blood flow to your kidneys. Your kidneys respond in the same way they would respond if you were losing blood through an injury—they "hold onto" fluid rather than excreting it as urine. Thus, you will gradually accumulate extra fluid in your body, which will show up as a weight gain. You can retain a lot of fluid—as much as 10 pounds in some people—before you can detect edema in the arms and legs from heart failure.

Other Possible Causes. Another cause of edema is blockage of veins with a blood clot (thrombus). The most common site of vein blockage is in the legs (deep venous thrombosis). Even after the blockage is resolved, damage to the veins caused by the blood clot and damage to the valves within the veins may cause an ongoing problem with edema in the legs and ankles.

Less common sites of vein blockage are the arms or under a collarbone. Blockage in these sites can cause swelling of the hand or arm. If the main vein that returns blood from the arms and head to the heart is blocked, both arms and the face may have swelling.

When your kidneys fail, your body cannot remove fluids, and the proteins that hold fluid in the bloodstream are reduced. Proteins can also be reduced in other diseases. When the proteins are low, fluid is more likely to leak from the bloodstream, as though through a sieve, into the surrounding tissues.

Swelling (Edema): Diagnoses to Consider

Heart failure (see page 36)
Venous obstruction or
   incompetence
   (see pages 105, 109)
Kidney failure
Liver disease
Low blood proteins
Excess sodium (salt) ingestion
   (see page 150)
Shock (see page 34)

LOSS OF CONSCIOUSNESS (SYN-COPE).   One of the most alarming symptoms is sudden loss of consciousness (syncope). You lose consciousness when your brain does not get enough blood and oxygen. Heart disease can cause syncope if it reduces your heart's ability to pump enough blood to your brain. Heart problems that can cause syncope are related to rhythm disturbances, obstructed blood flow, a sudden fall in blood pressure,

or severe heart muscle disease causing congestive heart failure.

Pattern of Syncope.   Loss of consciousness can occur with or without warning. For example, it may be preceded by a sense of light-headedness (presyncope), sweating, nausea, palpitations, or a pale appearance, or it may occur suddenly with no warning whatsoever. It may occur during any activity, such as household chores or even while driving.

Provocation and Relief.   In some cases, syncope is entirely unprovoked. In other situations, a factor or factors can be identified (such as fear, the sight of blood, stress, pain) that are related to the episode. Some unusual types of syncope occur during urination, defecation, or coughing.

What we typically think of as a simple faint (called vasovagal or vasodepressor syncope) can be resolved by lying down. After you lie flat, the blood flow to your brain is restored, and you regain consciousness. All people who faint should be placed in a lying-down position, preferably with their legs raised so their feet are 6 to 8 inches above the ground. This helps blood flow to the brain.

You may have occasionally felt light-headed from standing up quickly after lying down. In this case, the blood pressure control mechanism does not keep up with the need to pump blood "uphill" to the brain. Some people have particularly poor control mechanisms and may pass out or become very light-headed when they stand up—a condition called orthostatic hypotension.

Duration. The duration of the loss of consciousness can be so short that you hardly know whether you lost consciousness. You just find yourself on the floor for no apparent reason. Little or no damage occurs to your brain from lack of oxygen if you quickly regain consciousness. Actually, the most serious risk is bodily injury from the fall itself.

Other episodes can be more sustained. The more prolonged the unconsciousness, the more likely that it will become permanent and that death (sudden cardiac death) will occur unless cardiopulmonary resuscitation (CPR) is initiated. Anyone who remains unconscious for more than several seconds requires on-the-spot evaluation to determine whether CPR is required. This involves answering the following questions: Is a pulse present? Is the person breathing? (See page 241.)

Frequency. Syncope can happen once in a lifetime, or it can occur repeatedly. The major thrust of evaluating a person who has experienced syncope is determining the likelihood of it happening again. Obviously, if the chances are high, then a more aggressive approach to prevention is required.

Associated Symptoms. Sweating, nausea, and pallor often precede fainting.

Palpitations leading up to a syncopal attack suggest an irregular or rapid heartbeat as the cause of this spell. Sudden, unexpected loss of consciousness is usually related to a heartbeat abnormality that is so severe that the brain suddenly is deprived of its circulation and oxygen.

Other Possible Causes. Convulsions associated with loss of consciousness suggest a primary problem with the brain such as epilepsy, stroke, bleeding into the brain (cerebral hemorrhage), or tumor. However, convulsions can sometimes occur as a result of oxygen deprivation due to a heartbeat irregularity. Therefore, the presence of a seizure or convulsions does not rule out a heart-related basis for the episode.

Other noncardiac causes of syncope include a low blood sugar level (hypoglycemia), hyperventilation, and migraine headache.

Loss of Consciousness (Syncope): Diagnoses to Consider

Arrhythmia (see page 82)
Hypotension (very low blood
    pressure)
Shock (see page 34)
Hypertrophic cardiomyopathy
    (see page 43)
Aortic stenosis (see page 65)
Stroke (see page 100)
Seizure
Pulmonary hypertension
    (see page 110)

LIGHT-HEADEDNESS (PRESYNCOPE). Some people experience a sense that they will pass out but actually do not. The symptom is usually described as light-headedness and is referred to by doctors as presyncope or near-syncope.

Light-Headedness Versus Dizziness. Many people use the word "dizziness" to refer to light-headedness. However, a careful distinction must be drawn between light-headedness, which is the sensation that you are about to pass out, and true dizziness (vertigo), which is a sense that you are spinning or whirling around as if you just got off a merry-go-round.

Light-headedness may have many different causes, including heart rhythm abnormalities. The heart rhythm abnormalities responsible for the symptom of light-headedness usually are less severe and of shorter duration than those that lead to syncope.

Other Possible Causes. The symptom of vertigo suggests either an abnormality of the inner ear's balance mechanism or a brain-related problem. Occasionally, no specific cause for vertigo can be found.

Light-Headedness (Presyncope): Diagnoses to Consider

Arrhythmia (see page 82)
Hypotension
Hypertrophic cardiomyopathy
   (see page 43)
Aortic stenosis (see page 65)
Pulmonary hypertension
   (see page 110)

PALPITATIONS. Palpitations are an uncomfortable sensation of your heartbeat or a thumping sensation in your chest. The symptom may or may not be associated with heart disease, and it is the most common symptom in people who have an abnormal heartbeat (arrhythmia). However, as people age, extra beats (extrasystoles) tend to increase. These may be felt in people with otherwise apparently normal hearts.

Pertinent features of the thumping are the rate at which it is occurring, whether it is regular or irregular, whether there are individual thumps and how frequent they are, or whether there are strings of rapid thumps. If the palpitations occur in series or strings, they may develop gradually and accelerate, or they may suddenly take off rapidly.

These characteristics are important in distinguishing the different types of heart rhythms that may be causing the palpitations, so you should describe them to the doctor with some care. A good descriptive technique is simply to tap out with your hand the pattern of palpitations as you recall it. All too often, palpitations do not occur when you are in the doctor's office or being monitored, so an accurate description becomes all the more important.

Provocation and Relief. You should note whether anything provokes or stops the episodes. Some people find that certain types of rapid, regular palpitations can be interrupted by holding their breath or bearing down as though they were straining at a bowel movement (Valsalva's maneuver). Sometimes a change in position will bring on or stop the palpitations.

Your doctor will want to know whether things such as exercise,

---

Ways that people describe palpitations

■ Fluttering in the chest	■ Missing a heartbeat
■ Thumping in the chest	■ Skipping a heartbeat
■ Flip-flops	■ An extra heartbeat
■ Pounding in the chest	■ Racing in the chest
■ Feeling the heartbeat in the neck	■ Fast heartbeat

eating, emotion, alcohol use, or medication have any effect on your palpitations.

Associated Symptoms. Key features helpful in diagnosing the cause of the palpitations and any underlying heart problems include the association of chest pain or pressure, light-headedness or syncope, or shortness of breath.

Other Possible Causes. Although the apparent cause for thumping in the chest would seem to be the heartbeat, this is not always the case. Some people have a normal heart rate during their palpitations. Presumably, they are either anxious or experiencing chest wall twitching that is mistaken for the heartbeat.

Some people describe "skipped heartbeats" or a sense of "vacancy" in the chest that quickly passes. The usual cause is early extra heartbeats (premature contractions or extrasystoles). After a beat comes a little too soon (premature), your heart waits a little longer before it beats again (this is called a compensatory pause). You may be sensing the beat after the pause because it tends to be a bit stronger than the average heartbeat.

Palpitations: Diagnoses to Consider

Arrhythmia (see page 82)
Anxiety

LIMB PAIN OR TIREDNESS (CLAUDICATION). Leg pain can develop in the calves and feet with certain kinds of circulatory problems.

Depending on the underlying cause, the pain may be crampy, sudden, and severe, or you may experience numbness. The location of the pain also depends on the location of the circulatory problem.

People with partially or totally blocked circulation to the legs have an insufficient oxygen supply to their muscles for the work that is required for walking. They typically complain of a sense of muscle fatigue, aching, or cramping when they use these muscles for walking, climbing stairs, or other activities.

Provocation and Relief. Depending on the degree of obstruction, the symptoms occur at various levels of exercise. The discomfort can usually be relieved by resting.

When the arteries become sufficiently blocked, the discomfort may persist and continue even if you rest. Simply elevating the legs may provoke pain if the circulation is blocked to a sufficient degree.

Location. The site of the tiredness or cramping depends on where the artery is blocked. If the blockage is at the knee level or below, the discomfort may be confined to the foot, especially the instep. If the blockage is at the thigh level, the calf muscles are mainly affected. Blockage at the level of the groin or above results in cramping and fatigue in the muscles of the thigh and below, and the discomfort may also be felt in the buttock.

Other Possible Causes. Conditions other than arterial blockage can cause similar symptoms, and it is important for your doctor to make this distinction. For example, aching or pain in the legs that does not go away when you stop walking but actually requires you to sit or lie down may be caused by abnormalities of the spine that pinch the spinal cord.

---

*Limb Pain or Tiredness
(Claudication):
Diagnosis to Consider*

Arterial obstruction
(see page 99)

ABNORMAL SKIN COLOR. Skin color abnormalities can provide clues to underlying cardiovascular problems. Technically, skin color is a sign rather than a symptom. But if you notice a change in skin color, you may want to see your doctor.

Skin color can vary from normal in several ways. It may be unusually white or pale (pallor), bluish (cyanosis), reddish (erythema), or black (necrosis, or tissue death).

Location. Diffuse pallor may be caused by general depression of the circulation such as in shock (see page 34) or a fainting episode. Localized pallor is commonly caused by obstructed blood flow to a region that prevents adequate red (oxygenated) blood from reaching the skin. However, your skin may look red in areas where blood flow is abnormally abundant, as occurs in areas of an inflamed arthritic joint.

The location of skin color changes will lead your doctor to a conclusion about where the blood flow abnormality is and what blood vessels are involved. One classic constellation of symptoms is the occurrence of sequen-

tial white, blue, and red discoloration of one or more fingers, especially when exposed to cold. This is caused by spasm of the small vessels in the fingers. It is referred to as "Raynaud's phenomenon." It may occur as an isolated "disease" in itself, or it may be associated with other illnesses.

Duration. If the obstruction to blood flow is temporary, the pallor will disappear and the pinkish hue of the skin will return. However, if the blockage is prolonged, the skin may turn bluish (cyanotic) from lack of oxygen. If blood flow resumes after this stage, the skin may turn abnormally pinkish (erythematous). If the blockage is permanent and uncorrected, the tissue of the muscle and skin will eventually die and turn black (necrotic).

SORES ON THE SKIN. Nonhealing sores on the skin (ulceration) can also be a consequence of inadequate blood flow to the skin because an artery or vein is blocked or damaged. If tissue does not receive enough blood, it is vulnerable to even minor injury and infection. If the tissue does not receive enough oxygen and nutrients from the blood, it cannot heal.

Gangrene is the actual death of tissue. It usually appears as an area of black, shrunken skin in the region affected by the blockage.

Associated Symptoms. Pain, paleness or other skin discolorations, and coldness may also accompany nonhealing sores on the skin. Insufficient blood supply may cause inflammation and damage to the nerves (neuritis), which may cause burning, pain, and numbness. (These problems may occur in people with diabetes.)

SHOCK.   Shock is a constellation of dramatic symptoms and signs that imply a very serious circulatory abnormality. A person in shock has many problems:

- Very low blood pressure
- Confusion and altered consciousness (including possible unconsciousness)
- Generalized pallor and cold, clammy skin
- Evidence of malfunction of other organs because they are not getting enough blood
- Poor breathing function
- Low urine formation and inability to remove waste products

Shock can be due to various causes, including heart attack, trauma, hemorrhage, and overwhelming infection. If your heart's ability to meet your body's needs is limited, blood flow is directed to certain vital organs (the heart and the brain) at the expense of other organs such as skin, muscle, kidneys, and liver.

The constellation of symptoms from shock requires an emergency response by a medical team, including intravenous medication and fluids, help with breathing, blood transfusions if necessary, and urgent searching for the underlying cause so that it can be corrected if possible.

Shock: Diagnoses to Consider

Heart attack (see page 75)
Trauma
Hemorrhage (bleeding)
Infection

SUDDEN CHANGE IN VISION, STRENGTH, COORDINATION, SPEECH, OR SENSATION. A particular combination of symptoms indicates inadequate supply of blood to the brain. Depending on the duration of the symptoms, they may indicate a transient ischemic attack (TIA) or stroke (see page 100). Specifically, the symptoms can include the following:

- Weakness, tingling, numbness, or paralysis typically involving one side of the body (or one limb or side of the face). Both sides of the body may be affected
- Vision loss or double vision
- Speech difficulty, slurred speech
- Incoordination, dizziness, severe headache

Two key factors that distinguish these symptoms from others are their rapid onset and their duration. Vision, speech, or sensation deteriorates over minutes to hours. If the episode lasts only a few minutes, it is classified as a TIA. The symptoms come on rapidly and last briefly, and then you return to normal. TIAs indicate a temporary deficiency of blood supply to the brain. TIAs are regarded as a warning that a stroke may occur in the not-too-distant future. They warrant immediate evaluation by a doctor so that appropriate treatment can be started as soon as possible.

Another warning sign of stroke is amaurosis fugax. This is a temporary visual defect caused by inadequate blood flow to the eye. It may seem like a curtain is descending or rising over your field of vision, usually in one eye. Again, such a symptom requires immediate medical evaluation.

The symptoms of a stroke can be extremely varied because they correspond to the area of the brain that has been injured because of inadequate blood supply. In some cases, blood can be supplied to the injured area by way of another artery. This may explain, in part, the partial recovery after some strokes.

> *Sudden Change in Vision, Strength, Coordination, Speech, or Sensation: Diagnoses to Consider*
>
> Stroke (see page 100)
> Transient ischemic attack
> (see page 100)

TYPES OF HEART DISEASE

Heart disease can affect any and all parts of the cardiovascular system (see Part 1, "Normal Heart and Blood Vessels")—the myocardium, the valves, the coronary arteries, the conduction system, the arteries and veins, and the pericardium. Disease in any of these areas may be called "heart (or cardiovascular) disease."

You Can Have More Than One Type of Heart Disease

The process of diagnosing heart disease is complicated. To begin with, more than one type of cardiovascular disease or problem can occur at the same time in the same person. In fact, this is often the case. However, one problem may overshadow the others. This problem may be the most direct cause of symptoms, or it may have the greatest effect on your overall health and life span.

When more than one problem occurs, the conditions can sometimes be related to a single underlying cause. For example, "hardening of the arteries" due to cholesterol plaque deposits (atherosclerosis) can occur in your coronary arteries (arteries to the heart muscle itself), carotid arteries (arteries carrying blood to the brain), aorta (the main artery leading from the heart), and leg arteries. Thus, you could have symptoms of angina (chest pain), stroke (brain injury), and claudication (limb pain or tiredness), all of which are caused by insufficient blood flow due to atherosclerosis.

Knowing that certain problems occur together, doctors must sometimes piece together evidence of associated disease even if you have only one symptom or evidence of only one problem. Suppose, for example, that your doctor has detected an abdominal aortic aneurysm (see page 102) and recommends an operation to repair it. Experience has shown that coronary artery disease is present in more than 50 percent of people with aortic aneurysms, *even* if it is not causing symptoms of angina. Because coronary artery disease might make the aneurysm operation risky, your doctor may recommend tests to see whether serious coronary artery disease is present. Looking for and treating the coronary artery disease first make the operation for the aneurysm less risky.

One Type of Heart Disease Can Cause Another

Another complexity in diagnosis is that one type of heart disease can actually cause another, which in turn may become the main problem. For example, coronary artery disease can cause a heart attack (see page 75), which may damage enough heart muscle that the heart becomes too weak to pump efficiently. After that, you may have no further symptoms directly from the coronary arteries (such as angina), but you may experience symptoms from the weak pumping of the ventricles (such as congestive heart failure, see page 37).

As another example of one kind of heart disease causing another, a baby can be born with a hole in the heart wall separating the right and left ventricles (a ventricular septal defect). High blood pressure in the arteries to the lungs (pulmonary hypertension) may develop if the defect is large enough and is not closed soon enough by an operation. Pulmonary hypertension may cause shortness of breath (dyspnea) and blue discoloration of the skin (cyanosis). Thus, dyspnea and cyanosis caused by a lack of oxygen in the bloodstream become the prominent symptoms. In some cases, they may be the first signs of the original defect.

This section describes the gamut of things that can go wrong in each part of the cardiovascular system. Keep in mind that the problems can be—and often are—interrelated.

Heart Failure

The term "heart failure" is frightening, and heart failure is a serious problem, but it does not mean that the heart is not working at all. Heart failure means that the heart is unable to circulate enough blood to meet the needs of the body. Heart failure has various degrees of severity, depending on what the problem is and how long the problem has existed.

Unfortunately, heart failure is common, affecting 1 of every 100 people in the United States, or more than 2 million people. The impact of such widespread illness is enormous. Aside from suffering due to the symptoms, 35 percent of all people with heart failure require hospitalization each year. Obviously, the expense to the nation is considerable. Despite advanced medical care, 15 percent of all people with heart failure die in 1 year, and 50 percent of those with advanced symptoms die in 1 year.

Heart failure is not a specific disease. It is a shorthand way of describing a group of symptoms caused by diseases in which the heart is unable to circulate enough blood to meet the body's requirements.

CAUSES OF HEART FAILURE.

Heart failure can be caused by anything that impairs the heart's ability to pump effectively, including congenital heart disease, valvular disease, and heart muscle disease (such as from a heart attack). But these diseases are not the same as heart failure. You can have congenital heart disease, problems with the valves, or a heart attack and not have heart failure. But if one of these problems prevents your heart from pumping enough blood to your body, you are said to have heart failure.

Heart failure refers to the symptoms that occur when the heart muscle is weakened or when the work load is too great for the heart muscle to perform its task of pumping enough blood to meet the demands of the body. In either case, two things happen:

1. The heart cannot pump enough blood to provide the tissues with all of the nutrition, oxygen, and waste removal functions that they need.
2. Back pressure builds up in the veins because the heart does not efficiently pump blood through the arteries. In other words, as the heart becomes less and less a pump, it becomes more and more a dam.

SYMPTOMS OF HEART FAILURE. These two consequences of inadequate pumping function lead to all of the symptoms associated with heart failure: shortness of breath (dyspnea) and fatigue with exertion; shortness of breath at rest and especially when lying down (orthopnea) because of fluid accumulation in the lungs; swelling or accumulation of fluid in the feet, legs, and trunk; and general fatigue. Because many of the symptoms of heart failure are caused by congestion of the tissues and lungs with fluid, it is often called congestive heart failure.

With mild heart failure, you may not have any symptoms while sitting and resting. You may not be short of breath until you engage in physical activity. With severe heart failure, you may experience distress even at rest, including shortness of breath, pale skin color, coolness in the arms and legs, and blue color of the lips, fingers, and toes (cyanosis). These symptoms may become worse when you lie down.

With severe heart failure, you are also prone to various irregular heart rhythms and may experience palpitations or syncope (see pages 20–35 for a review of symptoms). Another symptom with advanced heart failure may be what is termed ''Cheyne-Stokes'' respiration, which is characterized by alternating periods of slow breathing with pauses and periods of rapid, deep breathing.

RIGHT AND LEFT HEART FAILURE. You may also hear doctors refer to right heart failure or left heart failure, depending on which side of the heart is most severely affected. In left heart failure, blood flow to the body is decreased and fluid accumulates in the lungs. These conditions develop because the left side of the heart becomes more like a dam, and the reservoir behind it is mainly the lungs. The congestion in the lungs is responsible for the sensation of breathlessness that is common in congestive heart failure.

When the left side of the heart functions inadequately as a pump, back pressure leads to congestion (*shown in the shaded areas*) of the lungs. Fluid accumulates in the lung tissue and air sacs, making breathing more difficult.

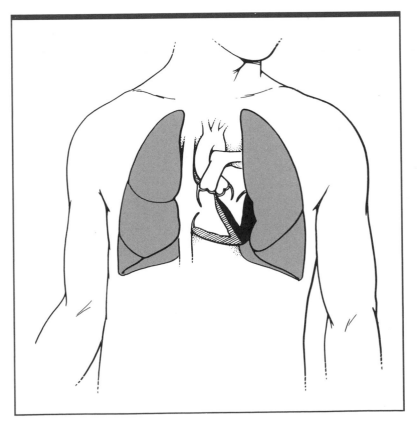

Right heart failure also causes decreased blood flow, but the reservoir for the right side of the heart is mainly the rest of the body, so swelling occurs in the legs and abdominal organs, including the liver. Right heart failure can cause pain on the upper right side of the abdomen from liver engorge-

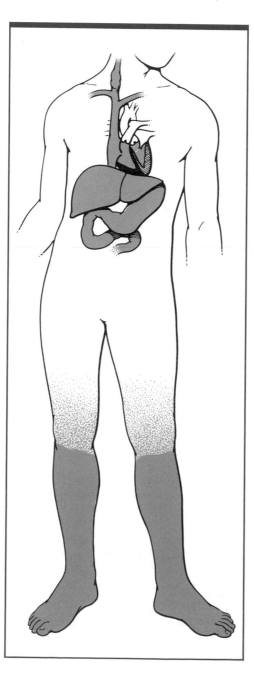

When the right side of the heart functions inadequately as a pump, back pressure leads to congestion (*shown in the shaded areas*) of the body's tissues. The veins in the neck may become engorged, the liver enlarges and may be tender, the walls of the intestines thicken and nausea or loss of appetite occurs, and the feet and legs swell.

ment, as well as loss of appetite, nausea, and bloating.

LOW OUTPUT FAILURE. In some people the consequences of heart failure are related to inadequate blood flow rather than to accumulation of fluid (congestion). Doctors often refer to this as low output failure.

- If your kidneys do not receive enough blood flow, they do not produce enough urine; excess fluid and water accumulate in your body. This condition increases the swelling (edema).
- If your muscles do not receive enough blood flow, your endurance is reduced. The decreased endurance leads to early fatigue when you exert yourself.
- If your brain does not receive enough blood flow, you may become light-headed or confused.

HEART FAILURE DUE TO CARDIO-MYOPATHY. Loss of the pumping efficiency of the heart has many causes. These include a mechanical problem (congenital or valvular), prolonged high blood pressure (which increases the work load on the heart), damaged sections of muscle tissue in the heart from coronary artery disease (heart attack), and diseases directly affecting the entire heart muscle (cardiomyopathy).

This section discusses heart failure that is caused by cardiomyopathy, or diseases of the pumping muscle of the heart (myocardium). Heart failure from other causes is covered in other sections.

Cardiomyopathy (*cardio* means "heart," *myo* means "muscle," *pathy* means "disease") is a disease of heart muscle. Cardiomyopathy can be further described by its cause (if known) or by the type of pumping defect that is present. For example, cardiomyopathy caused by alcohol use is called alcoholic cardiomyopathy. In many cases, the cause of cardiomyopathy cannot be determined, and the condition is then referred to as idiopathic cardiomyopathy (idiopathic means self-diseased, that is, no other identifiable cause).

Deaths from cardiomyopathy constitute about 1 percent of heart disease deaths in the United States. Men and blacks have the highest rates of death from cardiomyopathy.

Types of Cardiomyopathy.
There are three basic types of cardiomyopathy, which are distinguished by the kind of muscle problem involved:

1. Dilated cardiomyopathy, in which the heart muscle becomes weak and the heart chambers subsequently enlarge (dilate)
2. Hypertrophic (*hyper* means "over," *trophic* means "nourishment") cardiomyopathy, in which the heart muscle itself is much thicker than normal
3. Restrictive cardiomyopathy, in which the heart becomes stiff and cannot fill efficiently during diastole, the period of the heartbeat when the chambers fill with blood (see page 6)

Dilated Cardiomyopathy (Weakened Squeezing Capacity)

Charles is a 42-year-old commercial artist who recalls missing 2 days of work 4 months ago because of a "bad cold" with a runny nose, sore throat,

The most common causes of heart failure in the United States

- Coronary artery disease
- Disease of the heart muscle (cardiomyopathy)
- High blood pressure (hypertension)
- Valvular heart disease

and cough. Although these symptoms subsided, he never felt back to normal because he tended to be tired all the time. Six weeks ago he felt distinctly short-winded during a softball game at a company picnic; he stopped playing early so he could sit and catch his breath. Since then he has noted shortness of breath when climbing one flight of stairs. One week ago he began waking up in the middle of the night feeling breathless, which he found he could minimize by propping himself up on three pillows. For the past 2 days his ankles have been conspicuously swollen. Now he has been brought to the emergency room because he awoke gasping from an after-dinner nap and has been unable to catch his breath. The doctor told him and his wife that his lungs are filled with fluid and his heart is enlarged. He was given an intravenous injection of a diuretic to increase elimination of fluid by the kidneys and was admitted to the hospital for evaluation.

Dilated cardiomyopathy refers to overall enlargement (dilatation) of the heart chambers, especially the ventricles (see Figure 13, page A4). Although this enlargement is a key part of dilated cardiomyopathy, it is not the initial problem but rather the heart's own response to a weakness of heart muscle and poor pumping ability. The weakness of the heart muscle in this condition is generalized ("global"); all parts of the myocardium are affected about equally. Enlargement of the heart is the heart's way of trying to compensate for the weakness of its muscle. This is called a compensatory mechanism.

If the heart muscle is weak, it is unable to pump out the same portion of blood that it could at normal strength. But our bodies have an impressive capability of adjusting to changes. Rather than simply "accepting" the limitations of decreased pumping ability, the heart and other organs of the body undergo compensatory changes to try to maximize their efforts.

Think of the heart chambers expanding and contracting like a soft plastic bottle being squeezed while being held under water (see illustration on page 3). If your grip has become weakened, you cannot squeeze very much of the water out. Let's say that at normal strength you could squeeze out

60 percent of the water that flowed into the bottle when you let it expand under water. Similarly, a heart may pump out 60 percent of the blood it contained at the end of diastole.

With your weakened grip, however, you may be able to squeeze out only 20 percent of the water in the bottle. Likewise, weakened heart muscle may be able to pump only 20 percent of the blood it contains. Obviously, the volume of blood being pumped out of the heart with each beat would be much less.

However, if you got a bigger bottle, it would hold more water. Consequently, even with your weakened grip, if you squeezed out 20 percent of the water, that would be a greater total volume than 20 percent of the smaller bottle.

The same concept applies when the heart enlarges. There is a much larger volume of blood in the chambers dur-

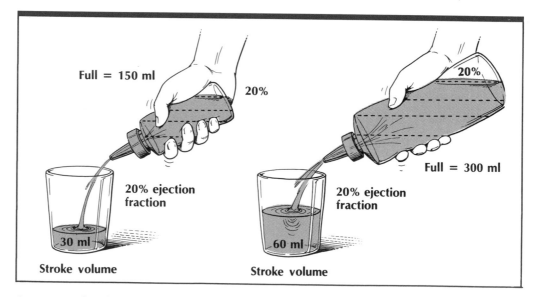

A squeeze bottle illustrates how the heart adapts to weakened pumping action by enlarging. The 150-ml bottle on the left can squeeze only 20 percent of its fluid out, much less than the normal amount of about 60 percent (see figure on page 7). Thus its stroke volume is only 30 ml. The larger bottle holds 300 ml, so even with a reduced ejection fraction of 20 percent, it produces a stroke volume of 60 ml, which is an improvement.

ing diastole. Even if the heart pumps out only 20 percent of the blood it contains, the total volume pumped is larger.

Our bodies have other compensatory mechanisms, too. It is one of the basic ''laws of the heart'' that the more you stretch heart muscle (up to a limit), the more forcefully it will squeeze on the next beat (this is also known as Starling's law, after one of its discoverers). When the heart enlarges, it stretches more to increase the pumping force.

Other organs also attempt to compensate for a weak heart muscle. The kidneys and various hormonal mechanisms changes that increase the volume of blood and fluid. Maintaining a high volume of blood in the heart is important for stretching the heart muscle to maintain the amount of blood that is pumped with each stroke.

The heart rate may also increase in response to signals from your nervous system. The heart tries to maintain its output by pumping faster.

However, all of these compensatory mechanisms can work only up to a point. They eventually are unable to keep up as the heart increasingly weakens. Ironically, in severe cardiomyopathy, the effects of the compensatory mechanisms lead to many of the problems of heart failure.

For example, the hormonal and kidney adjustments that occur, which try to maintain or increase blood and fluid volume, account in large part for the swelling in the legs and abdomen and for the fluid in the lungs in heart failure. Elevated levels of certain hormones, such as epinephrine (adrenaline), can cause constriction of blood vessels. This increases the resistance and pressure against which the weakened heart must pump.

Conditions that can lead to dilated cardiomyopathy

- High blood pressure
- Infections
- Toxic agents, especially alcohol and certain cancer-treating drugs
- Heart valve defects
- Chronic (sustained) fast heart rate
- Nutritional deficiency
- Abnormalities of metabolism
- Blood diseases
- Neurologic disorders
- Pregnancy
- Hereditary (genetic) tendency
- Unknown (idiopathic) conditions

Ultimately, much of the treatment for heart failure may be to reverse some of the effects of these compensatory mechanisms.

Causes of Dilated Cardiomyopathy.
Idiopathic.   A major group of dilated cardiomyopathies are those that are caused by unknown factors. These are called idiopathic dilated cardiomyopathies. Many experts believe these idiopathic types are due to a viral infection of the heart (perhaps one that occurred in the past and is no longer detectable) that has left the heart weakened. Idiopathic dilated cardiomyopathy may occur at any age. It occurs more often in blacks than in whites, and in men more often than in women. Rarely, this type of cardiomyopathy develops in a woman during pregnancy and persists even afterward.

Toxins and Drugs.   Many toxic substances can cause weakening of the heart muscle. The most common one is excessive alcohol intake, which can result in a severe dilated cardiomyopathy. In some instances, this can be reversed if alcohol intake is stopped.

Myocarditis. Occasionally, a heart biopsy (see page 220) may show inflammation of the heart muscle, or myocarditis (*itis* means "inflammation"). Myocarditis is probably due to an active viral infection.

Signs and symptoms of myocarditis include fever, vague chest pain, joint pain, and an abnormally rapid heart rate. A person with myocarditis may improve as the inflammation goes away, but it is also possible that the myocarditis will leave the heart in a severely weakened condition.

One of the main goals of your doctor, of course, is to try to promote the healing of myocarditis successfully, and the means of doing this most effectively are still under careful study.

Coronary Artery Disease. Although coronary artery disease is the most common cause of weakened heart pumping, enlargement of the ventricles, and symptoms of heart failure, it does not cause a true dilated cardiomyopathy. Rather than causing generalized global damage of all heart muscle cells, coronary artery disease reduces the blood and oxygen supply to areas of heart muscle (myocardial ischemia) and damages zones of the heart. This regional damage then leads to inefficient pumping. The result is similar to what occurs in dilated cardiomyopathy, so some doctors refer to it as "ischemic cardiomyopathy" (related to an insufficient blood supply).

The most common problem occurs when the heart muscle is scarred and the heart is dilated because of a previous heart attack or heart attacks, in which case the damage is irreversible.

However, less commonly, the weakened heart muscle is due to constant poor circulation to the heart without heart attacks; then there is some chance that pumping function can be improved if circulation is restored. This condition of reduced pumping function has been given the name "hibernating myocardium." Obviously, because one condition is reversible and the other is not, it is important to distinguish between the two. This may require sophisticated tests.

Symptoms of Dilated Cardiomyopathy.   In some people, symptoms of dilated cardiomyopathy may develop gradually over months or years. In others, symptoms appear suddenly after a respiratory or flu-like illness.

You may get short of breath with activity, when you lie down, or during the night when you are sleeping. Your legs may swell, and you may have abdominal pain from congestion in your liver. About 10 percent of people with dilated cardiomyopathy have chest pain. In short, dilated cardiomyopathy causes the constellation of symptoms referred to as heart failure (see page 36).

How Serious Is Dilated Cardiomyopathy?   Unfortunately, once the overt signs of heart failure become evident in people with dilated cardiomyopathy, up to 50 percent die within 1 year, and more than 75 percent die within 5 years. However, research in heart failure has shown that treatment can affect the outcome. Indeed, treatment methods are becoming increasingly effective at controlling symptoms and extending life, including careful tailoring of medications and appropriate use of heart transplantation.

Dilated Cardiomyopathy

Possible Tests

Electrocardiography
(see page 192)

Chest X-ray (see page 200)

Radionuclide ventriculography
(see page 204)

Echocardiography
(see page 209)

Cardiac catheterization and
cardiac angiography
(see page 216)

Hemodynamic measurements
(see page 268)

Left ventriculography
(see page 218)

Myocardial biopsy
(see page 219)

Possible Treatment

Sodium restriction
(see page 150)

Medications
(see pages 251 and 305)

Transplantation
(see page 254)

Hypertrophic Cardiomyopathy (Overgrowth of Heart Muscle).

Rick is a 35-year-old teacher who has noticed the general development of breathlessness and chest heaviness during exertion. At first these symptoms were very vague, so he is not sure when they started, although he thinks they may have developed perhaps 2 years ago. Yesterday, he ran upstairs from his basement to answer the doorbell; when he reached the top of the stairs and opened the door, he almost passed out and had to lie down.

Hypertrophic cardiomyopathy is an overgrowth of heart muscle that can impair blood flow both into and out of the heart. This type of cardiomyopathy is less common than dilated cardiomyopathy, but it is not rare and has been the focus of much medical interest.

Hypertrophic cardiomyopathy results from abnormal thickening of the heart wall. The thickening can occur in several places throughout the ventricles. Most commonly it occurs in the

Below left, **Normal structure of the heart.**
Below right, **A heart with idiopathic hypertrophic subaortic stenosis (IHSS). Notice the thickened septal wall between the left and right ventricles. The thickening makes the heart stiffer so it relaxes less efficiently to let blood enter the ventricle. When the ventricle squeezes, the bulge may partially block blood flow through the aortic valve.**

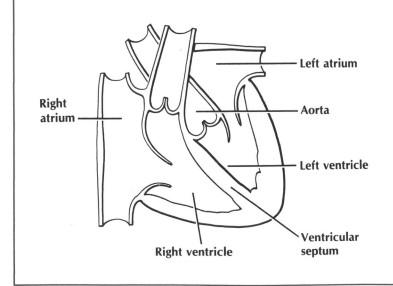

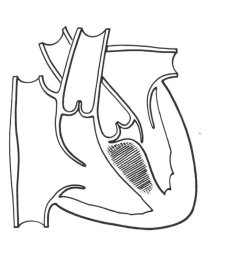

This heart has hypertrophy (excessive wall thickening) limited to the tips of the ventricles.

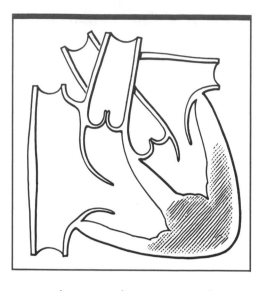

septum between the two ventricles just beneath the aortic valve. The septum may be 1½ or more times as thick as the outer wall of the heart. With a thicker muscle wall, the cavity of the ventricle may be smaller. Thus, the volume of blood in the ventricle may be normal or decreased.

This thicker wall is unable to stretch as well during the diastolic (filling) phase of the heartbeat, although contraction during systole is normal or even exaggerated.

Hypertrophic cardiomyopathy is sometimes called idiopathic hyper-

Hypertrophy can also be widespread throughout the muscle of the ventricle. This type of condition may develop as a result of uncontrolled high blood pressure. High blood pressure is like weight lifting for the heart—it results in a bigger muscle. Unfortunately, hypertrophied heart muscle is less, rather than more, efficient.

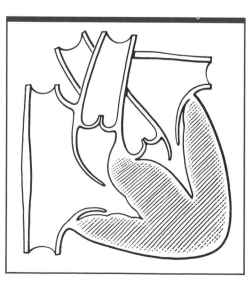

trophic subaortic (beneath the aorta) stenosis, abbreviated IHSS. This overgrowth creates a bulge that protrudes into the ventricular chamber and impedes the flow of blood from your heart to the aorta and the rest of your body.

When this obstruction is present, the cardiomyopathy is also called hypertrophic obstructive cardiomyopathy (HOCM, often pronounced "HOkum"). In this condition, the problem is not that the heart muscle is weak but that the overgrown heart muscle impedes the flow of blood through and out of the heart.

If the example of the plastic bottle is used, the sides of the bottle have thickened, especially near the opening. The thickening decreases the space inside the bottle and gets in the way of the opening.

With HOCM, one of the leaflets of the mitral valve between the left atrium and the left ventricle moves forward during contraction, and this, along with the thicker septum between the ventricles, obstructs blood flow. Ironically, the obstruction to blood flow may worsen the harder the heart squeezes, because the thickened septum protrudes even farther into the pathway of the blood trying to flow out of the heart.

Hypertrophic cardiomyopathy does not always affect the area beneath the aortic valve. Sometimes the condition occurs down near the apex (tip) of the heart, and in other individuals the overgrowth is distributed more or less evenly throughout the heart muscle. These cases can be likened to the plastic walls of the bottle becoming thickened all over and making squeezing less effective. In those situations, the problem is not due to obstruction. The thickened muscle is simply inefficient at pumping and especially at relaxing. The blood flow can decrease because of this, and heart rhythms are a problem as well.

Causes of Hypertrophic Cardiomyopathy. True hypertrophic cardiomyopathy is of unknown cause (idiopathic). Similar conditions can arise from a long history of high blood pressure leading to overgrowth of the heart muscle. The heart muscle builds up the same way a weight lifter builds up the biceps with repeated weight lifting, because high blood pressure imposes a high work load on the heart muscle. In a sense, the heart muscle is lifting a heavy load for a long time. Unfortunately, overgrowth of the heart muscle is not conducive to increased efficiency. Valve problems, especially aortic stenosis (see page 65), can also lead to overgrowth (hypertrophy) of heart muscle.

Symptoms of Hypertrophic Cardiomyopathy. The three major symptoms of hypertrophic cardiomyopathy are shortness of breath, chest pain, and loss of consciousness with exertion, along with other symptoms of heart failure, including shortness of breath while lying down and palpitations. Some people may die suddenly.

Now that echocardiography is commonly performed, many people are being diagnosed with hypertrophic cardiomyopathy even when the condition is not causing symptoms.

Chest pain (angina) is a common symptom of hypertrophic cardiomyopathy; about three-quarters of people with hypertrophic cardiomyopathy experience it. The angina is caused when the normal coronary arteries cannot provide the enlarged heart muscle with enough oxygen. Some people have chest pain that lasts longer than typical angina, and it often happens right after, not during, exercise.

Shortness of breath is present at some point in about 9 of 10 people with symptomatic hypertrophic cardiomyopathy.

About half of all people with hypertrophic cardiomyopathy experience light-headedness or loss of consciousness, because blood flow is so severely impaired that it is not sufficient for the rest of the body, including the brain. When you exert yourself, this is especially likely to happen. During exercise, the heart contracts harder and the overgrown bulge protrudes even farther into the already narrowed pathway. The condition can be made even worse if the mitral valve contributes to the blocking action itself or allows blood to leak backward because of the high pressure in the ventricle. Some people with hypertrophic cardiomyopathy have syncope or sudden cardiac death because they are prone to heart rhythm abnormalities.

Who Is Affected by Hypertrophic Cardiomyopathy? Hypertrophic cardiomyopathy can occasionally run in families. Symptoms of hypertrophic cardiomyopathy may occur at any age, but most start in the teens and 20s. In most people with hypertrophic cardiomyopathy who develop symptoms, the symptoms develop by age 35 years.

Hypertrophic cardiomyopathy is present in 2 percent to 6 percent of people with cardiomyopathy and is more common in men than women and in blacks than whites.

How Serious Is Hypertrophic Cardiomyopathy? Three to 5 percent of people with hypertrophic cardiomyopathy will die in 1 year, and 50 to 90 percent of deaths will be sudden, presumably from rhythm disturbances. People with hypertrophic cardiomyopathy should avoid strenuous exercise because of the risk of sudden death.

Luckily, in half to three-fourths of people with newly diagnosed hypertrophic cardiomyopathy, the condition does not get any worse over the next several years. Deterioration to heart failure is uncommon, happening in only 7 percent of people with hypertrophic cardiomyopathy. When it does progress to heart failure, features of dilated cardiomyopathy may be present as well.

Medications can relieve some of the symptoms of hypertrophic cardiomyopathy and can reduce the irregular rhythms, but it is not clear that they help you live longer. Surgical removal of the obstructing portion of myocardial overgrowth can be very effective in severe forms of this disorder.

Hypertrophic Cardiomyopathy

Possible Tests
Electrocardiography
   (see page 192)
Chest X-ray (see page 200)
Echocardiography
   (see page 209)
Cardiac catheterization—
   hemodynamics
   (see page 216)

Possible Treatment
Medications (see page 251)
Myotomy/myectomy
   (see page 259)
Pacemaker (see page 280)

Restrictive Cardiomyopathy (Stiffness of the Heart). The least common type of cardiomyopathy, and probably the least understood, is restrictive cardiomyopathy. In this condition, the heart muscle is too stiff to allow enough blood in from the pulmonary veins. Obviously, blood has to get into the heart before it can be pumped out to the body. The heart cannot pump out blood that it does not receive.

In restrictive cardiomyopathy, filling of the ventricle is rapid but ends abruptly when the stiff heart stops expanding. As mentioned, restricted inflow is also part of the problem of hypertrophic cardiomyopathy in some people, because thick muscle does not relax as well as normal muscle.

Because the "inflow" of blood into the heart is compromised in restrictive cardiomyopathy, symptoms of heart failure can ensue.

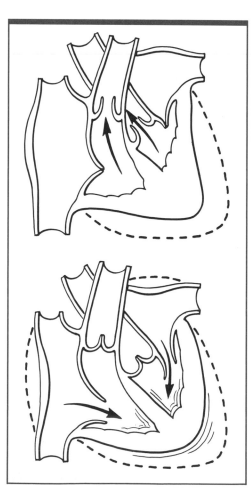

Restrictive heart muscle disease results in problems during the relaxing phase of the heartbeat. The broken lines show how the heart should look when it is fully relaxed in diastole. During contraction (*top*), the heart squeezes normally. But during diastole (*bottom*), it does not relax efficiently. The result is that the ventricles do not fill with as much blood as they should for the next contraction.

Causes of Restrictive Cardiomyopathy. In most cases, pure restrictive cardiomyopathy does not have a well-recognized cause, so it is idiopathic. But any condition that can cause extensive scarring in the myocardium or thickening of the endocardium can restrict filling of the ventricles. For example, your heart may have reactions to radiation or drugs for cancer, or to the cancer itself, which result in stiffening of the muscle. Diseases that affect connective tissue throughout the body, such as progressive systemic sclerosis (scleroderma) and pseudoxanthoma elasticum, may also cause fibrosis or stiffening.

Amyloidosis. A recognized cause of restrictive cardiomyopathy is deposits of abnormal material into the heart muscle. One example of this is the condition known as amyloidosis, in which certain blood cells produce excessive protein material that deposits in the tissues. Sometimes the heart is the main tissue affected, and in this case the condition is called cardiac amyloidosis. In other conditions the heart is only one of several organs involved, including the kidneys, liver, skin, blood vessels, and intestinal tract. Amyloidosis can also lead to the dilated form of cardiomyopathy. Medical treatment for amyloidosis is not very effective.

Hemochromatosis

Jerry is a 54-year-old county administrator. He has had diabetes for 2 years. One year ago he reported to his family physician that he had become unable to function sexually. He reports that over the past several months he has felt generally ill, tired, and short-winded. Now his ankles are beginning to swell and he has lost his appetite. His wife wonders why he has begun to look so "tan" even though he never goes outside. Jerry's physician obtains a test, which discloses a very excessive amount of iron in the blood.

A defect in iron metabolism permits iron to build up in the body. This disorder is called hemochromatosis. Iron can build up in the heart muscle (as well as other organs) and cause stiffening.

Like amyloidosis, hemochromatosis can also lead to dilated cardiomyopathy. Hemochromatosis can occasionally be substantially helped by medications that "leech" the iron out of tissues and by repeated removal of pints of blood (the procedure for removing the blood is the same as that used when you donate blood). The removal of blood decreases the amount of iron, because the blood cells contain a large quantity of iron.

Symptoms of Restrictive Cardiomyopathy. With restrictive cardiomyopathy, you may experience weakness, shortness of breath, and occasionally chest pain. These symptoms reflect the inability of the ventricle to fill during diastole and to provide an increase in blood flow when needed. Edema, right upper abdominal discomfort, and loss of appetite are symptoms of reduced filling of the right ventricle.

Who Is Affected by Restrictive Cardiomyopathy? Men and women are equally affected by restrictive cardiomyopathy. The disease may occur at any adult age, but the average age at onset is in the 50s.

How Serious Is Restrictive Cardiomyopathy? With effective treatment of the cause of restrictive cardiomyopathy, the myocardium can regain function, and long-term survival is possible. Unfortunately, most causes of restrictive cardiomyopathy do not have good, specific treatment. Once heart failure or rhythm disturbances occur, long-term survival rates are not encouraging. For example, most people with hemochromatosis will die within a year once heart failure and rhythm disturbances occur, unless they have treatment to remove the excess iron.

Restrictive Cardiomyopathy

Possible Tests
Electrocardiography
   (see page 192)
Chest X-ray (see page 200)
Echocardiography
   (see page 209)
Cardiac catheterization—
   hemodynamics
   (see page 216)
Myocardial biopsy
   (see page 219)

Possible Treatment
Medications (see page 251)
Transplantation (see page 254)

Congenital Heart Disease

Congenital heart disease refers to defects of the heart that are present at birth. About 6 to 8 babies out of every 1,000 who are born alive have a congenital heart defect.

When you consider that 3 weeks after conception the heart consists of a tiny tube that folds, fuses, excavates, and molds itself so that all of its basic structures are present by the eighth week of development, it is more amazing that things turn out right as often as they do.

If your child has a congenital heart defect, you probably have many questions. What exactly is wrong? How did it happen? How will it affect your child's life? What can be done about it? Your doctor will answer these questions specifically as they relate to your family, but this section provides a general background to help you understand the information.

CONTINUING PROGRESS. The ability to stop the heart temporarily by using a machine to take over the function of the heart and lungs (cardiopulmonary bypass) led to spectacular advances in the treatment of congenital heart disease. At the Mayo Clinic, open heart surgery for congenital heart disease was first performed in 1955. More than 10,000 open heart operations, mostly for congenital heart disease, were performed during the next one-and-a-half decades. Remarkable strides continue to be made in the detection, evaluation, and treatment of congenital heart disease. As a result, large numbers of people are alive and well who formerly would have died early in life. Evidence of this progress is provided by the many girls who have surgery to repair congenital heart problems and then grow up to have children of their own.

Progress is still being made. For example, ultrasound examination can now detect some problems before your baby is born. This may allow increasing use of operations inside the uterus before birth. Because of these great strides, we can be much more optimistic about the future for people with congenital heart disease.

CLASSIFICATION OF CONGENITAL DEFECTS. Any part of the cardiovascular system can be affected by congenital problems, and more than one defect can occur in the same heart. Some defects are mild enough to go unnoticed at birth. Others cause major problems shortly after the baby is born. Common defects include the following:

- Abnormally formed blood vessels that impede the flow of blood
- Valves that obstruct blood flow, allow backward leakage, or are missing
- Incorrect or reversed connections between the main arteries and the heart or between the main veins and the heart
- Defects in the partition between the atria or the ventricles that allow blood to flow from the right side to the left side of the heart without going through the lungs, or from the left side to the right side without going through the rest of the body

Doctors often think of congenital defects in terms of whether they cause blueness of the skin (cyanosis). You have probably heard of "blue babies." Some of their blood circulates through their body without passing through the lungs to pick up more oxygen, and as a result their skin has a bluish tint.

WHAT CAUSES CONGENITAL HEART DISEASE? The exact cause of most congenital heart defects is rarely identified. Most experts believe that abnormal genes interact with environmental factors during the development of the embryo to produce congenital disease. Often an environmental cause, if any, cannot be detected. Most often, there are no easy answers.

Abnormalities in the chromosomes, including the one that causes Down's syndrome, are associated with some heart defects. Infections such as German measles in the mother during early pregnancy increase the risk as well.

If you have a child or another person in your family with a congenital heart defect, you probably wonder what the chances are of problems in future children. Unless a specific chromosomal problem is identified, or a clear pattern of hereditary heart disease is seen in a family tree, most experts believe the risk of occurrence in your next baby is about 2 percent to 5 percent—less than 1 in 20. Or, put in a more positive framework, chances are 19 in 20 that your next baby will be fine.

MANAGEMENT OF CONGENITAL HEART DISEASE Many types of congenital heart disease can cause major problems starting immediately or soon after birth. Some of them may even lead to irreversible changes that might prevent surgical correction. Therefore, there has been a trend over the years to operate on children with congenital heart disease at earlier ages.

For example, an opening in the partition separating the ventricles (ventricular septal defect) can lead to an increase in blood flow to the lungs and hence to elevation of the blood pressure in the lungs. The high blood pressure can become an irreversible problem on its own. This complication, called Eisenmenger's complex, may occur in early childhood, or it can develop progressively over many years, depending on the severity of the defect. When Eisenmenger's complex develops, it is no longer helpful to close the ventricular septal defect.

Operations can be curative (or as close to a cure as possible) or palliative. With palliative operations, the problem is not fixed, but adjustments are made to let the circulation work as well as possible under adverse circumstances. In some cases palliation is done at a young age to allow the heart and circulation to develop enough so a curative operation can be done later. Sometimes a palliative operation is all that can be done.

One of the earliest palliative operations to be developed is the Blalock-Taussig procedure, which improves (palliates) the condition of patients with cyanotic heart disease. (The operation was named after the surgeon and pediatric cardiologist at the Johns Hopkins Hospital who developed it.) In cyanotic heart disease, not enough blood can flow through the lungs to pick up the needed oxygen to supply the body. The Blalock-Taussig operation increases the flow of blood through the lungs by making a connection (shunt) outside the heart between a large artery to one of the arms and a large artery to the lungs. Thus, the shunt operation does not correct the defects inside the heart that cause the severe reduction in blood flow through the lungs. Rather, it only relieves (palliates) the blueness and tiredness by increasing the flow of blood through the lungs.

The Blalock-Taussig operation may still be performed when complete correction is not feasible, or when the overall risks might be lessened by first doing a preparatory palliative shunt operation in anticipation of complete correction later on.

WHAT IS THE OUTLOOK?   As you might expect, congenital heart defects can result in the widest range of disabilities. They can be so severe that life cannot be maintained, or they can be so mild that trouble is not even suspected. A list of such minor defects would include an aortic valve that has only two cusps (bicuspid) instead of the normal three, mitral valve prolapse, or a small atrial septal defect.

Sometimes these abnormalities never do cause problems. Other times they become more abnormal with aging and then cause problems. For example, a child with a bicuspid aortic valve may have satisfactory function of the valve. As the child ages, the valve may thicken and calcify and lead to narrowing (stenosis), or it may retract and result in backward leakage (regur-

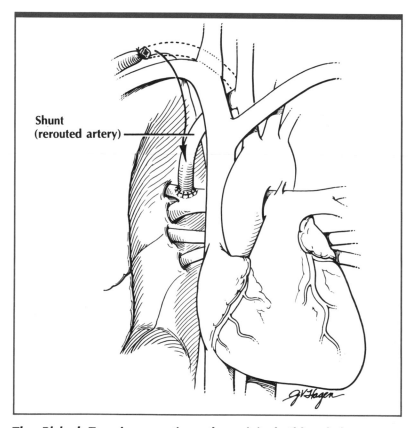

Shunt (rerouted artery)

The Blalock-Taussig operation—the original "blue baby operation"—is a way to reroute blood that has bypassed the lungs and therefore missed picking up vital oxygen. The surgeon redirects (shunts) blood from an arm artery to a pulmonary (lung) artery. This improves conditions such as severe tetralogy of Fallot (see figure on page 56), in which some blood that returns from the body misses going through the lungs because of a hole in the septum between the two ventricles. With this operation, some of this "blue" blood is returned to the lungs to pick up oxygen. Although this operation does not correct the original problem, it can improve the situation.

gitation). These changes may not produce symptoms until middle age or even later.

Many congenital heart defects can be surgically corrected at a young age, and your child can thus have a normal life. However, even after corrective surgery for congenital heart disease, residual problems can remain or crop up later, so your child will need continued medical observation. Heart rhythm disorders (see Arrhythmias, page 82) and endocarditis (see page 58) remain potential threats, even many years later.

Sometimes your doctor may recommend waiting for a time before repairing a defect. Reasons for this delay include the following:

■ The problem will not get any worse if you wait for a limited time.
■ The baby is too small. The operation will be easier at an older age.

In such cases, delaying an operation would be expected to have no adverse effect on the outcome for your child. In other cases, surgery may be delayed not by choice but because the problem was not found or the diagnosis was incorrect. Some congenital problems are very hard to diagnose without difficult, risky, and expensive tests, which are done only if there is a high suspicion of an abnormality. If the defect is not causing obvious problems, the likelihood increases that it might be overlooked at routine examinations.

With some congenital defects such as ventricular septal defect, if an operation to close the defect is postponed too long, the excess blood that shunts through the defect and through the lungs may damage the small end branches of the pulmonary artery. The damage might become so severe that

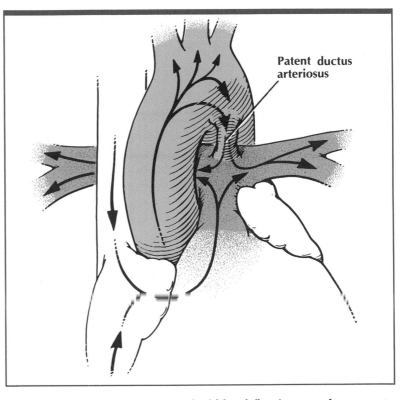

Patent ductus arteriosus. **Instead of blood flowing out the aorta to the body, some blood is directed back to the lungs through an opening that normally closes at birth. The heart is overworked because it must pump enough blood out of the left ventricle to supply the body with oxygen, plus allow for the amount that returns directly to the lungs.**

an operation to close the septal defect would no longer be helpful. Lung transplantation would then be the last possibility to help.

SPECIFIC EXAMPLES OF CONGENITAL HEART DISEASE.   Some defects may occur by themselves, and others may occur in combination. Following are descriptions of just a few of the many types of congenital heart defects.

Abnormal Artery Near the Heart. Patent Ductus Arteriosus.   The ductus arteriosus is an artery that allows blood in the fetus to bypass the lungs until the lungs expand at the time of birth. It normally closes soon after birth. When it remains open (patent), blood can flow from the aorta to the pulmonary artery. This defect overworks the heart, causes excess blood flow in the lungs, and can lead to heart failure. It is more common in infants whose mothers had German measles in early pregnancy and in infants who were born prematurely or at high altitude.

In premature babies, the patent ductus arteriosus often closes spontaneously within weeks or months after birth. If the ductus remains open and heart failure does not respond to medical treatment, surgical closure may be required, even during infancy. Once the ductus has closed, no further problems are typically encountered. New methods of closing the patent ductus with a plug or "double umbrella" through a catheter (a tube passed through a major blood vessel to the heart) are currently being explored.

Coarctation of the Aorta. Coarctation (constriction) of the aorta is a narrowing that impedes blood flow from the heart to the lower part of the body and increases blood pressure. If heart failure develops, even during infancy, removal of the narrowed segment may be necessary. Experience is now accumulating with the technique of dilating the narrowed segment with an inflatable balloon catheter guided inside the narrowed zone of the aorta. Even for children in whom heart failure has not yet developed, removal of the narrowed segment should not be delayed indefinitely, because the high blood pressure can become irreversible. Survival beyond age 50 years is unusual in people who do not have their coarctation repaired; most die by the mid-30s.

Coarctation of the aorta accounts for 15 percent of congenital heart problems in adults. (More people with coarctation of the aorta are being identified in blood pressure screening programs.) Twice as many men have it as women.

Incorrect Connections of the Main Arteries and the Heart.
Transposition of the Great Arteries. In this defect, the origins of the two arteries from the heart are reversed: the aorta comes from the right ventricle and the pulmonary artery emerges from the left ventricle. Thus, a portion of the person's blood recirculates through the right heart and lungs without ever passing through the body. Likewise, the remaining portion of the person's blood recirculates through the left heart and the body without passing through the lungs. Obviously, if oxygen-carrying blood does not reach your body, you cannot live. For survival, there must be a connection between the two systems. The two systems may connect if there is an associated defect such as patent ductus arteriosus, atrial septal defect, or ven-

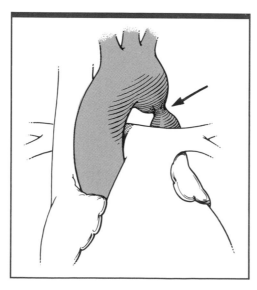

Coarctation of the aorta. The aorta is narrowed (*arrow*), usually below the branches to the head and arms. The heart must work harder to pump blood, and blood pressure is often higher in the arms (*above the narrowing*) than in the legs (*below the narrowing*).

tricular septal defect. If such a connection is not present, a palliative septal defect can be created between the two atria with a special catheter.

Although the correction of this complicated condition proved challenging for a long while, several surgical procedures are now available to relieve this problem and help affected infants. Without treatment, 30 percent of these babies die in the first week of life. By the first year, 90 percent of the infants die if they do not have surgery.

Truncus Arteriosus.   In truncus arteriosus, the pulmonary arteries (that go to the lungs), the aorta, and the coronary arteries all originate from a single large artery, or trunk. Thus, all the blood, both oxygenated and poorly oxygenated, must mix together as it flows through the single exit valve and through the single truncus arteriosus (arterial trunk).

Truncus arteriosus is not common. It accounts for about 1 percent of all cases of congenital heart disease.

Surgery should be performed within the first 6 months of life. It involves sewing a flexible tube on the heart that carries blood from the right ventricle to the pulmonary arteries. This tube also contains a valve, made of animal tissue or artificial material, which substitutes for the deficient exit valve. Continued careful medical evaluation is required even after successful correction. Without correction, few children with this defect reach adulthood.

Defects in Valves.
Aortic or Pulmonary Valve Stenosis.   Narrowing of the aortic or pulmonary valves is among the most common congenital heart defects. These valve problems are described on pages 57–70.

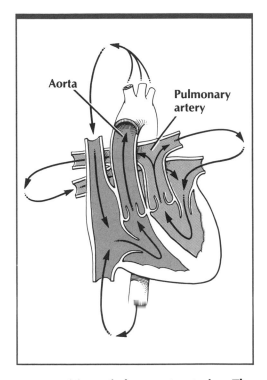

Aorta

Pulmonary artery

Transposition of the great arteries. **The great arteries (the aorta and the pulmonary artery) are in reversed positions (transposed). The aorta emerges from the right ventricle and the pulmonary artery comes from the left ventricle. Instead of a figure-eight circulation (see figure on page 4), the circulation is now two separate circles: blood returning to the heart from the lungs (*shaded red*) is pumped right back to the lungs, and blood returning from the body (*shaded gray*) is pumped right back to the body. Unless the two circles are connected, for example by a ventricular septal defect (see figure on page 55), no oxygen can get into the blood going to the person's body—a fatal condition.**

Ebstein's Anomaly.   This rare congenital heart defect accounts for less than 1 percent of all forms of congenital heart disease. It affects males and females equally.

Ebstein's anomaly involves abnormally developed tricuspid valve

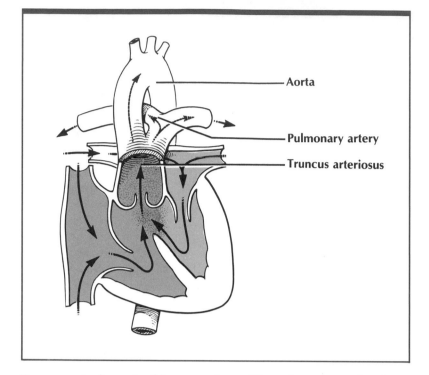

- Aorta
- Pulmonary artery
- Truncus arteriosus

Truncus arteriosus. **In this unusual condition, the aorta and pulmonary artery emerge from the heart in a single tube (trunk) that gets blood flow from both the right and the left ventricles. The result is that some oxygenated blood returns directly to the lungs, and some deoxygenated blood returns to the body without going through the lungs first.**

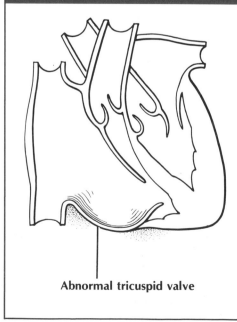

Ebstein's anomaly. **The tricuspid valve is misshapen so that it does not properly prevent back leakage of blood from the right ventricle to the right atrium.**

Abnormal tricuspid valve

leaflets. (The tricuspid valve prevents backward blood flow from the right ventricle to the right atrium.) The leaflets are attached abnormally and have other related problems that produce back leakage of blood through the valve and make additional work for the heart. Episodes of excessively fast heartbeats complicate Ebstein's anomaly in about one of four patients.

In some people with Ebstein's anomaly, symptoms develop gradually. Some live into their 60s and 70s, even in the presence of significant disease. Others die in infancy or early childhood.

Surgery is usually postponed until the onset of disability, because the long-term results are uncertain. But in people who have indications of increased risk, there are good results with surgical reconstruction or replacement of the tricuspid valve.

Septal Defects.

Atrial Septal Defect. This is a hole in the wall between the two atria (the upper chambers of the heart) that allows abnormal blood flow. Girls with atrial septal defect outnumber boys 3 to 1.

The location and size of the hole are variable, but in all uncomplicated atrial septal defects, blood is shunted from the left to the right atrium during diastole (when the heart fills with blood), and blood flow to the lungs is increased. Often, the presence of an atrial septal defect is not recognized because symptoms may be nonexistent early in life and it is not easy to detect by physical examination alone. The defect may be found when your doctor hears an abnormal pattern of blood flow during a routine checkup. It accounts for about 25 percent of congenital heart conditions detected in adults.

If the defect is recognized early, it is usually closed surgically between the ages of 1 and 6 years. The risks of surgery are low, and the long-term results are excellent. After surgery, a normal life-style with no restrictions is usually possible.

The outlook for people who do not have the problem repaired is not encouraging. Almost half die before age 40 years, most often from heart failure.

Ventricular Septal Defect.   This is an opening between the ventricles (the pumping chambers of the heart) that increases blood flow, under high pressure, to the lungs. Increased blood flow to the lungs overworks the heart; this may lead to high blood pressure in the lung arteries or congestive heart failure. If the defect is not repaired, eventually the blood shunts from the right to the left side of the heart, causing blueness from inadequate oxygen in the tissues.

Ventricular septal defect is the most common heart malformation, accounting for 25 percent of the cases of congenital heart disease. Almost 50 percent of all ventricular septal defects close by themselves without an operation, mostly during the first few months after birth, because they are small.

Small ventricular septal defects that do not cause symptoms usually do not require surgery, but people with ventricular septal defects should receive preventive antibiotics before dental and certain surgical procedures (see Endocarditis, page 58).

In children with large defects, major problems, including heart failure, may develop in early infancy. Treatment for these babies is aimed at controlling the heart failure with drugs. If this is unsuccessful, surgery to close the defect is usually done before age 1 year. After

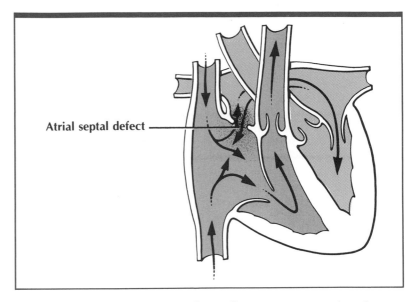

Atrial septal defect. A hole in the wall (septum) separating the two atria permits mixing of oxygenated blood and deoxygenated blood. Usually, the direction of blood flow through the hole is mainly from the left atrium to the right, and the result is excessive flow of blood through the lungs.

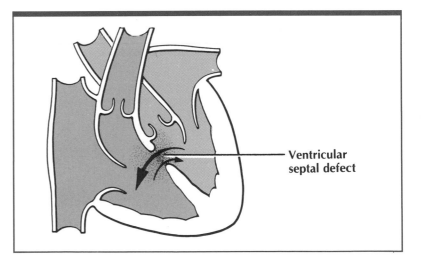

Ventricular septal defect. A hole in the wall (septum) separating the two ventricles permits mixing of oxygenated blood and deoxygenated blood. Initially, the direction of blood flow through the hole is mainly from the left ventricle to the right, and the result is excessive flow of blood through the lungs. With time, the blood pressure in the lungs becomes excessively high, forcing the direction of flow through the hole to reverse (this is called Eisenmenger's complex). Some deoxygenated blood now goes through the hole into the left ventricle and out to the body, causing a bluish tinge to the skin (cyanosis).

successful closure, a normal life-style is usual.

Combination of Defects.
Tetralogy of Fallot. A French physician, Etienne Fallot, described this defect in 1888. Tetralogy of Fallot is really four defects in combination. First, the septum that divides the two ventricles is incomplete (so there is a ventricular septal defect), and oxygen-poor blood is thus allowed to mix with oxygen-rich blood. Second, the passageway from the right ventricle to the lungs is markedly narrowed. Third, the origin of the aorta is shifted toward the right side of the heart from the left. Fourth, the muscle in the wall of the right ventricle is thickened and stiffened. Only the first two of these defects cause significant trouble or require an operation. These defects result in decreased blood flow to the lungs and circulation of blue (unoxygenated) blood to the body tissues;

both of these effects cause bluish skin (cyanosis), clubbing (bulging of the nailbeds) of the fingers and toes, and extreme tiredness.

Tetralogy of Fallot constitutes 10 percent of all congenital heart disease. It is the most common cyanotic heart defect; nearly 3,000 new cases a year occur in the United States. Infants may require palliative surgery (for example, the Blalock-Taussig shunt procedure; see page 50) to improve blood flow to the lungs and decrease cyanosis. Once the child is past infancy, corrective open heart surgery is performed. The results of successful complete repair of tetralogy of Fallot are good: cyanosis disappears, exercise tolerance improves, and people lead normal lives. Without an operation, only 30 percent of people with tetralogy of Fallot would survive to the age of 40 years. Surgery results in almost 90 percent of patients surviving for *at least* 25 years from the time of surgery; generally, the

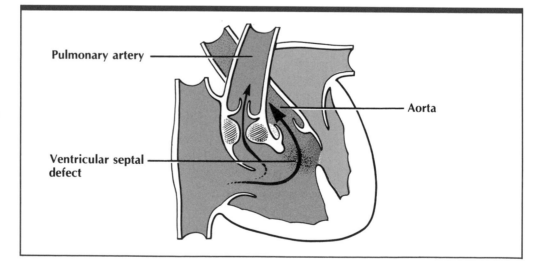

Tetralogy of Fallot. **This heart defect is complex, but relatively common. Its features are ventricular septal defect, obstruction to blood flow beneath the pulmonary valve, an aorta that is shifted rightward, and a thickened right ventricular wall. The overall result is usually that some deoxygenated blood is shunted into the aorta. If the septal defect is small or the obstruction is mild, babies with this condition may be "pink" rather than "blue."**

results are best if the defect is corrected before the patient is 12 years old.

Congenital Heart Disease

Possible Tests
Electrocardiography
(see page 192)
Chest X-ray (see page 200)
Echocardiography
(see page 209)
Cardiac catheterization
(see page 216)

Possible Treatment
Palliative or corrective surgery
(see page 259)

Defects of Valves

The valves keep the blood flowing in one direction, like one-way gates. They open when the pressure of the blood pushes them in the forward direction, and they close when the pressure on the other side of the valve pushes them back. Diseased valves may be too stiff to open easily or they may fail to close completely. Each of the four valves (mitral and aortic on the left side of the heart, and tricuspid and pulmonary on the right side) may be subject to obstruction (stenosis) if they are too stiff and to back leakage (regurgitation) if they fail to close.

A valve opening can become narrowed and "tight" (stenotic), a condition that limits the blood flow through it and causes the blood and fluid behind it to back up as if behind a dam. The backup leads to symptoms of congestive heart failure, heart chamber enlargement, and overgrowth of heart muscle, which can lead to angina. Various heart rhythm disorders can also develop.

Innocent heart murmurs

If your doctor tells you that your child has an "innocent" heart murmur, there is no need to worry. Innocent murmurs, by definition, do not cause problems.

Innocent murmurs are common in children. They may disappear and reappear, but they are harmless. Most innocent murmurs will disappear permanently when your child reaches adulthood.

Your child's doctor can hear innocent murmurs by listening to your child's heart through a stethoscope. Murmurs are sounds made by turbulent blood moving through the chambers and valves of the heart or through the blood vessels near the heart. Your doctor may also call them "functional murmurs" or "vibratory murmurs."

Your doctor may want to have your child undergo other tests to be sure that the murmur is innocent. Once they are done and if you are told that the murmur is innocent, you can relax. Your child does not have a heart problem. No restrictions or limitations in activity are necessary, because your child is normal and healthy.

Valves may not close properly and therefore allow blood to leak back in the wrong direction (regurgitation). This causes the heart chambers to enlarge and pump blood inefficiently, because excess blood must be pumped forward to compensate for the amount that leaks back with each heartbeat. Again, this can lead to congestive heart failure, tiredness, and some rhythm disorders. A "leaky" valve does not mean that blood leaks out of the heart, but that blood leaks backward through the valve.

Causes of valve disease range from congenital defects, to calcium deposits that accumulate on the valves as you age, to infections.

It may take decades before damage to valves shows up. Oddly, you can have advanced valve disease before any symptoms develop, because your

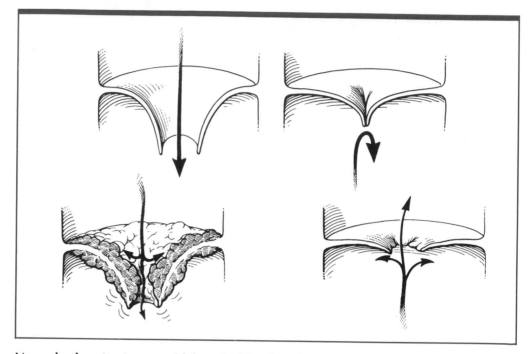

Normal valves (*top*) open widely to let blood easily flow forward, and they close tightly to prevent blood from leaking backward.

A valve with stenosis (*bottom left*) is unable to open widely and blood flow is partially obstructed. In this example, thick deposits of calcium prevent the valve from opening very widely.

In valve regurgitation (*bottom right*), a valve is not closing well enough to prevent back leakage. In this example, a portion of the valve has been destroyed by infection (endocarditis).

body compensates or adapts. However, as explained earlier, these adaptations eventually may be overwhelmed, leading to heart failure.

Therefore, if you develop valve disease, it is important that the problem be treated before it becomes so advanced that repair or replacement of the valve is no longer possible. The timing of procedures to repair or replace the damaged valve is important, because your doctor has to weigh the potential risks of surgery against the possibility that the problem will become too advanced to fix.

ENDOCARDITIS. Damaged or weakened valves are vulnerable to an infec-

tion called endocarditis. Infective endocarditis is inflammation of the endocardium, the membrane that lines the inside of the four chambers and valves of your heart. Usually, the inflammation is caused by actual infection of a valve with bacteria or other germs. Endocarditis can occur whenever bacteria circulate in the bloodstream. Bacteria (and other microorganisms) tend to settle on and then multiply on the misshapen valves where blood flow is turbulent.

Endocarditis is a major illness and can be fatal. It almost always results in a worse valve condition because of further destruction of the valve (see Figure 18A, page A7). Because of its severity, endocarditis may require 6 weeks or more of intravenous administration of antibiotics in the hospital, often followed by surgical treatment.

What Causes Endocarditis? Endocarditis may be caused by certain bacteria that are often present in the mouth and upper respiratory tract. The organisms may enter your bloodstream during dental or surgical procedures such as getting a tooth pulled or having your tonsils removed.

Bacteria in your intestinal tract, called enterococci, may also enter your bloodstream during an examination of, or surgical procedure in, the prostate, bladder, rectum, or female pelvic organs.

Endocarditis may also develop in drug abusers who use unsterilized needles to inject drugs into a vein.

In people with inadequate immunity to infection, endocarditis can develop from other organisms, such as fungus.

Who Is at Risk for Endocarditis? If your heart is healthy and normal, you are unlikely to develop endocarditis. The organisms tend to congregate and multiply in valves that are malformed or that have been damaged from rheumatic fever (see page 60).

You are at risk for infective endocarditis if:

- You were born with a defect in your heart or heart valves
- Your heart valves have become scarred from rheumatic fever
- You have an artificial heart valve

Even if your heart condition has not caused you any problems, or even if the defect has been repaired and you

---

Precautions for people at risk for endocarditis

Dental Procedures, Oral or Respiratory Tract Surgery
Before you undergo any procedure on your mouth (including routine cleaning at the dentist's office) or throat that may cause bleeding, your doctor or dentist will probably prescribe amoxicillin taken orally. You should take it 1 hour before the procedure and again 6 hours afterward.

People who are allergic to penicillin (amoxicillin is a type of penicillin) may take another antibiotic such as erythromycin. An injectable antibiotic may be necessary if you have already had valve surgery.

Urologic Procedures, Gastrointestinal Surgery, or Examination With Instruments
Urologic procedures include bladder operations, transurethral resection of the prostate, and dilation and curettage (D and C). Gastrointestinal procedures are, for example, hemorrhoid removal, polyp removal, or colon resection.

The germs in your intestine often are resistant to penicillin-type antibiotics. Your doctor may prescribe a combination of injectable antibiotics just before and again 8 hours after the procedure. Occasionally, antibiotics taken by mouth may suffice.

Lung and Skin Infections
If you develop a lung or skin infection, your doctor may prescribe antibiotic treatment to prevent endocarditis.

Think Prevention
It is important to use good oral hygiene every day and to have regular professional dental care. This involves routinely brushing and flossing your teeth and gums and getting regular checkups.

Your dentist and each of your doctors should be aware that you are at risk for endocarditis.

---

are healthy, you may still be at risk for this serious infection that could threaten your life. Your doctor is the best person to advise you about this.

How Serious Is Endocarditis? Endocarditis is a very dangerous disease that was nearly always fatal before the development of antibiotics. Although powerful antibiotics are now available, treatment can be difficult, and the results are uncertain. Therefore, doctors believe that prevention is the best approach.

How Can You Prevent Endocarditis?   Antibiotics can protect you from infective endocarditis by destroying or controlling the harmful bacteria. Many experts advise using these drugs before and after procedures that may allow bacteria to enter your bloodstream, travel to your heart, and cause an infection.

RHEUMATIC FEVER. In addition to congenital abnormalities and infections, valves may be damaged by rheumatic fever. Although rheumatic fever is not nearly as common in the United States as it was 40 years ago before the widespread use of penicillin, several outbreaks were reported in U.S. cities during the late 1980s. Rheumatic fever is still very common in Third World countries.

Forty to 60 percent of people having a first attack of rheumatic fever have heart inflammation. The mitral valve is involved in about 85 percent of cases, the aortic valve is involved in about 44 percent of cases, the tricuspid valve is involved in 10 percent to 16 percent, and the pulmonary valve is rarely involved. More than one valve is frequently affected.

Causes of Rheumatic Fever. Rheumatic fever seems to be the result of a reaction of your body to specific strains of the streptococcal bacteria. Symptoms of rheumatic fever generally appear about 2 to 4 weeks after an untreated "strep throat" infection.

Thus, antibiotics to treat strep throat infections can prevent rheumatic fever. The damage to the heart valve seems to be related to antibodies the body produces to fight the throat infection, or to toxic substances produced by the bacteria. It is not caused by an actual infection of the valve.

Strep throat usually comes on suddenly, especially with painful swallowing, fever, and tender, swollen glands under the jaw. Laboratory tests (throat culture) are needed to confirm that the sore throat is due to a streptococcal infection.

Symptoms of Rheumatic Fever. Symptoms of this disease include fever, rapid heartbeat, chills, joint pain that tends to migrate from one joint to another, a characteristic rash, fatigue, weakness, irritability, and occasional uncontrollable movement of the limbs. You may have raised, red patches on the skin or lumps under the skin.

Who Is Affected by Rheumatic Fever?   Rheumatic fever usually occurs in young people age 5 to 15. It rarely affects adults. Once you have had it, you are more susceptible to another attack. Doctors usually prescribe penicillin or another antibiotic continuously until adulthood after the first bout of rheumatic fever.

How Serious Is Rheumatic Fever? The heart inflammation from rheumatic fever does not always cause permanent damage. However, one or more of your valves may be scarred. The damage to your heart valves may take 10 to 30 years to show up. Serious complications may develop, and you may need surgery to repair or replace the damaged valves. In rare instances, the heart muscle itself can be severely inflamed, and this condition can lead to heart failure.

Most cases of strep throat do not lead to rheumatic fever. However, if you have strep throat, take all of the medication your doctor prescribes, even if your sore throat is gone in a day or two. That approach is the best way to prevent rheumatic fever.

VALVE DISEASE CAN BE SERIOUS, BUT SUBTLE. Even in advanced stages of valve malfunction, you may not experience symptoms. One reason is that the heart, circulation, and other parts of the body adapt to the problem and overcome it to some extent. But these adaptive or compensatory mechanisms can perform only up to a certain point. Then the problem becomes too overwhelming, and symptoms develop.

Sometimes you may not recognize symptoms because they develop so slowly. For example, intolerance of exercise may develop gradually. You may simply get used to it, so you do not recognize that you are restricted in any way.

Symptoms do not always correlate with the severity of the valve problem. Anyone with a valve problem must see a doctor regularly to monitor changes in the valves.

The problems brought on by valve disease vary depending on which valve is affected, whether it is too tight or too loose, and how advanced the disease is. Often, different types of valve problems occur together in the same person. For example, mitral stenosis and regurgitation can coexist, and the treatment is frequently different than for mitral stenosis alone.

Some combinations make the heart particularly inefficient. For example, with both aortic stenosis and mitral regurgitation, the blood not only has a hard time going forward during systole through the tight aortic valve but also is inclined to go backward through the leaky mitral valve. With these conditions, much of the blood will take the "easy path" and leak backward rather than going forward through the narrowed valve.

DEFECTS IN VALVES ON THE LEFT SIDE OF THE HEART. The most common valve problems involve the mitral and aortic valves on the left side of the heart. The oxygen-rich blood from the lungs enters the left atrium, passes through the mitral valve into the left ventricle, and leaves the ventricle through the aortic valve on its way to the rest of the body. Both the mitral and aortic valves can have damage that leads to obstruction (stenosis) or back leakage (regurgitation).

Mitral Stenosis

Ann, a 39-year-old homemaker, missed several months of third grade when she was a child because of rheumatic fever. She returned to good health, but during pregnancy with her third child at age 32 years she experienced shortness of breath with congestion in her lungs. Her physician diagnosed a "valve problem," but no treatment was advised. One year ago, Ann suddenly became very short of breath and went to the emergency room; the diagnosis was atrial fibrillation. Fortunately, a normal heart rhythm was restored with an injection of medication. For the past 2 months or so, she has felt distinctly tired and notices breathlessness when she climbs the basement stairs. After a medical examination, she is told she has mitral stenosis.

When the mitral valve is tight (stenotic), blood has a difficult time flowing from the left atrium to the left ventricle (see Figure 18B, page A7). The result is that the pressure of blood in the left atrium increases. The left atrium may enlarge because of the back pressure. Eventually that back pressure can cause leakage of fluid into the lungs (pulmonary edema). The left atrium is prone to develop rhythm irregularities (atrial fibrillation) (see page 92), which can further decrease the efficiency of the heart. You may suddenly experience symptoms, or mild symptoms may become worse.

Also, blood clots tend to form in the enlarged and fibrillating atrium. If a small fragment of the blood clot breaks loose, it can travel to other parts of the body and lead to blockage in an artery. One of the most serious risks is a blood clot traveling to the brain and causing a stroke.

Causes of Mitral Stenosis. Rheumatic fever in childhood is by far the most common cause of mitral stenosis. It can damage the heart valve and cause scarring, which results in problems later in life, usually in young adulthood.

More rarely, mitral stenosis can occur from congenital heart disease or from calcium deposits that accumulate over years. Some experts speculate about a viral cause, but no proof has been found.

Symptoms of Mitral Stenosis. You may not have any symptoms for years, even with significant mitral stenosis. When symptoms develop (commonly in the 30s), they include the symptoms of congestive heart failure. Inefficient circulation causes fatigue and shortness of breath (especially after exercise, at night, or when lying down). You may experience chest discomfort or palpitations. You may have frequent bouts of bronchitis. There is also the possibility of stroke.

Who Is Affected by Mitral Stenosis? Mitral stenosis is less common today than it was several decades ago, because the most common cause, rheumatic fever, has largely been eradicated in the United States. However, it remains a frequent problem in Third World countries. It is more common in women than in men.

How Serious Is Mitral Stenosis? If you have mild mitral stenosis, you may remain well, or have only mild symptoms, for decades. Eventually, symptoms of fatigue and breathlessness may become problems if the deformity of the valve is severe. Mitral stenosis carries a risk of rhythm abnormalities (atrial fibrillation) in which the atrium beats in a rapid and uncoordinated manner. Atrial fibrillation can lead to the formation of dangerous blood clots.

In general, mitral stenosis does not need to be corrected until symptoms develop (see page 260). Proper preventive measures against infective endocarditis are essential (see page 58).

Mitral Regurgitation

Martha is a 63-year-old lawyer who was told she had a heart murmur during a physical examination about 12 years ago. She was advised to take antibiotics at the time of dental appointments and to get regular medical checkups. Three years ago she was told her heart was enlarged, but in retrospect it was large on the chest X-ray from 9 years previously and had not changed much. Echocardiography was done, but no new treatment was prescribed. Now, her echocardiogram shows further heart enlargement and some decrease in pumping strength. The diagnosis (as before) is chronic mitral regurgitation. Martha feels she is wearing out a bit "from getting old," but otherwise feels all right. However, operation on the valve was recommended.

Mitral regurgitation is a much more common problem than mitral stenosis. In mitral regurgitation, the mitral valve leaflets do not close properly so that the blood leaks back (regurgitates) into the atrium when the left ventricle contracts (see Figure 19B, page A7). The leakage decreases the blood flow to the rest of the body and increases the work load of the left side of the heart.

Closing the mitral valve and opening the aortic valve during systole (squeezing) should result in forward flow of the blood. With mitral regurgitation, a portion of the blood in the ventricle is squeezed backward in addition to the portion that is squeezed forward through the aortic valve. This condition leads to inefficient functioning of the heart.

Causes of Mitral Regurgitation. Mitral regurgitation can be caused by rheumatic fever, but this is a rare cause. The usual causes are mitral valve prolapse that has worsened (see page 64), infection of the valve (endocarditis, see page 58), heart attacks that involve the heart wall where the mitral valve leaflets are tethered for support, and deterioration of the valve with aging. Despite the fact that mitral valve prolapse is very common, only very few people with it ever develop a worrisome degree of mitral regurgitation.

Symptoms of Mitral Regurgitation. If mitral regurgitation develops and progresses slowly (chronically), you may not notice any symptoms. However, some people experience symptoms of congestive heart failure (fatigue, weakness, shortness of breath with exercise or at night, swelling in the ankles) and irregular heart rhythms that may cause palpitations.

If severe mitral regurgitation develops rapidly (acutely), these symptoms can develop immediately and be very marked.

Andrew is a 61-year-old accountant who has always been healthy. While doing yard work he suddenly became extremely short of breath and began gasping. He was able to walk slowly into the house, but if he lay on the couch he felt like he was smothering. His wife called the ambulance. In the emergency room a diagnosis of acute mitral regurgitation was established by listening with a stethoscope and viewing an echocardiogram. The problem was rupture of the chordae tendineae (cords that anchor and support the valve). Oxygen and injection of medication to remove fluid that had accumulated in the lungs helped while arrangements were made for urgent surgical repair of the valve.

How Serious Is Mitral Regurgitation? You may not have any symptoms for 20 years or more with mitral regurgitation. Often symptoms appear in middle age or beyond.

Strange as it may seem, you may have very bad chronic mitral regurgitation and deteriorated pumping function and yet feel entirely well. The cardiovascular system is generally very adept at counteracting the deficiencies caused by the leaky valve. The prob-

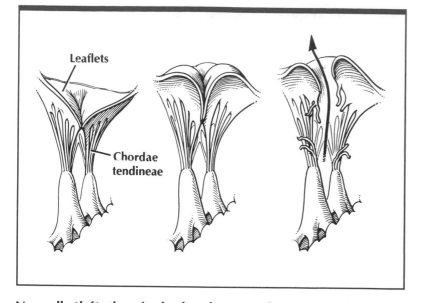

Normally (*left*), the mitral valve closes snugly to prevent back leakage of blood when the left ventricle contracts. The leaflets are tethered to the wall of the heart by stringlike chordae tendineae and papillary muscles.

In mitral valve prolapse (*center*), the valve leaflets bulge (prolapse) upward during closure. This is due to leaflets that are too large or chordae tendineae that are too long. The valve usually prevents back leakage of blood anyway.

In uncommon cases, when some chordae tendineae break (*right*), the valve leaflets may "flail" and allow back leakage to develop.

lem is that if the valve is not fixed or replaced, the strength of the heart muscle may decline so far that even when the valve is operated on, the problem with the weakened pump remains. Thus, it is important to operate early enough.

Consequently, one of the most difficult decisions in cardiology is deciding when to operate for mitral regurgitation. Despite extensive research, the ideal timing of surgery is still unknown. One of the biggest problems is that the ejection fraction (see page 6) is not a reliable way of determining the strength of the heart muscle in people with mitral regurgitation. It can seem "normal" (more than 50 percent) despite weakness of the

heart muscle. Doctors usually recommend operation for mitral regurgitation before the heart weakens to the point that the ejection fraction of the left ventricle is below 50 to 55 percent. Also, surgery is advisable as soon as symptoms develop.

Naturally, if you have mitral regurgitation, it is difficult for you to accept that a major operation may be advisable even though you feel well. However, this may be one of the most dramatic examples of "a stitch in time saves nine!"

Mitral Valve Prolapse. Mitral valve prolapse is usually harmless. The condition may be present in as many as 1 in 10 Americans, although some experts believe that mitral valve prolapse is overdiagnosed.

In mitral valve prolapse, the leaflets of the mitral valve between the left atrium and left ventricle bulge (prolapse) into the left atrium like a parachute during the heart's contraction. This condition may keep the leaflets from closing tightly and may allow some blood to leak back into the atrium from the ventricle.

Mitral valve prolapse is often called the "click-murmur syndrome" because your doctor may hear an extra clicking sound from the leaflets ballooning out and a murmur from the backward flow of blood (regurgitation).

Symptoms of Mitral Valve Prolapse. Most people with mitral valve prolapse do not have any symptoms. Some people may have brief episodes of rapid heartbeat (palpitation) or chest pain that is not typical of angina. A few may experience fatigue, shortness of breath, light-headedness, or loss of consciousness; an extremely rare occurrence is sudden death.

Many people with mitral valve prolapse suffer from undue anxiety. Perhaps this anxiety is in some ways explainable. Many people come to their doctors with otherwise inexplicable aches or pains or strange sensations. By default, in those who have mitral valve prolapse the condition becomes a scapegoat. Naturally, the patient becomes concerned. However, the mitral valve prolapse actually is not the source of all the problems.

Who Is Affected by Mitral Valve Prolapse? Mitral valve prolapse is somewhat more common in women than men. It also occurs more often in women who have scoliosis or other skeletal abnormalities. It appears to occur more often in some families than others.

How Serious Is Mitral Valve Prolapse? Most people with mitral valve prolapse have no problems. If you have mitral valve prolapse, you have a normal life expectancy and do not have to make any changes in your activities.

About 15 percent of people with mitral valve prolapse may experience symptoms of valve leakage that are significant enough to require careful evaluation of the mitral valve and consideration of valve surgery. In rare individuals with mitral valve prolapse (like Andrew, page 63), sudden mitral regurgitation can develop from breakage of chordae tendineae, which tether the valve leaflets (see page 64). In these cases, symptoms (shortness of breath) can develop rapidly.

If your doctor diagnoses mitral valve prolapse, you may have a risk of infective endocarditis. Although it is a small risk, endocarditis is such a serious complication that you should take preventive antibiotics before and after dental and some surgical procedures if your doctor recommends them (see Precautions for people at risk for endocarditis, page 59).

Aortic Stenosis

Jacob is a 70-year-old retired librarian. Five years ago an echocardiogram showed aortic stenosis that was "moderately severe." The aortic valve had heavy deposits of calcium on it. He was advised to use antibiotics at the time of dental examinations. He remained busy at work and home without difficulty. One year ago, an echocardiogram showed "severe" aortic stenosis, but he felt fine. During the past 6 weeks he has noticed chest tightness when working in his yard, and on one occasion he felt like he was about to black out. His doctor advised further evaluation and presented plans to replace his aortic valve with an artificial valve.

The aortic valve controls blood flow from the left ventricle to the aorta and the rest of the body. It opens when the ventricle contracts and closes when the ventricle relaxes.

Aortic stenosis means the aortic valve has become narrowed (see Figure 19A, page A7). The result is that the left ventricle must squeeze harder to get a sufficient amount of blood through the aortic valve with each beat. (Imagine trying to push the same amount of water through a small syringe needle as through a hose—it would take a lot more muscle power.) This increased work load makes the muscle of the left ventricle grow thicker (hypertrophy). Eventually the heart muscle cannot keep up with the work load and begins to fail.

Causes of Aortic Stenosis.   Aortic stenosis may be present at birth or develop as a result of rheumatic fever (see page 60). Some people are born with an aortic valve that has only two cusps instead of three. This abnormal valve seems to be more susceptible to calcium deposits that cause the valve to stiffen and narrow. Even a normal valve may become calcified as you age.

Symptoms of Aortic Stenosis.   Aortic stenosis does not always cause symptoms immediately, even though the valve can be tight. When the heart begins to fail, symptoms of congestive heart failure can develop (fatigue, weakness, shortness of breath with exercise or at night, swelling in the ankles).

Other symptoms associated with aortic stenosis are angina and spells of passing out. Some of these spells may be due to rhythm abnormalities, but a more likely explanation is that the tight aortic valve does not allow enough blood to pass into the arteries of the body. The regulatory mechanisms of the body normally can adjust the blood flow to the various organs. If you needed increased blood flow—for example, to the muscles during exertion—the tight aortic valve could not let enough blood out to fill the blood vessels in the muscles, which have dilated to promote increased blood flow. The result is a drop in blood pressure that could deprive the brain of enough blood flow (and oxygen), and you would pass out.

Who Is Affected by Aortic Stenosis?   Aortic stenosis can occur at any age (because the causes are different at different ages). People in their 20s and 30s may have murmurs, but symptoms might not occur until age 50 or 60 years. The condition is three times more common in men than women.

How Serious Is Aortic Stenosis? There is a long lag period in which you could have mild or moderate obstruction of blood flow and no symptoms (like Jacob). Your doctor may diagnose aortic stenosis by hearing a murmur at a checkup and confirming it with appropriate tests. People without symptoms should be carefully monitored, but experts believe that surgery usually is unnecessary until you begin to experience symptoms or show evidence of decreased pumping function of the heart. You may have to limit strenuous physical activity to avoid overworking the heart.

Once heart failure, angina, or passing out develops, survival is likely limited to 2 or 3 years or less unless you have surgery. This should be done without delay. After the operation, you will have no special limitations in activities.

If you have aortic stenosis, you are at risk for endocarditis and should take preventive antibiotics before and after dental and certain surgical procedures (see Precautions for people at risk for endocarditis, page 59).

Aortic Regurgitation
Betty is a 55-year-old television network executive who was told she had a murmur when she was 25 years old. Eight years ago, an echocardiogram showed back leakage of blood through an aortic valve that had only two cusps, instead of the usual three. Subsequent examinations and echocardiograms have shown gradual enlargement of

the left ventricle, although it still has almost normal pumping function. She feels well and uses antibiotics for dental procedures. Her physician is recommending continued regular examinations for now.

Aortic regurgitation is leakage of blood backward through the aortic valve, which controls the blood flow from the left ventricle into the aorta and the rest of the body (see Figure 18A, page A7). The aortic valve should close tightly to prevent blood from leaking back from the aorta into the left ventricle.

When the aortic valve does not close efficiently, some blood leaks back during diastole, when the ventricle is relaxing. Thus, blood enters the ventricle from the left atrium through the mitral valve (as it should) and also flows back from the aorta through the aortic valve. The heart has to work harder, which leads to enlargement of the left ventricle and inefficient functioning.

Causes of Aortic Regurgitation. The usual causes of aortic regurgitation are degeneration of a valve that has two cusps instead of the normal three cusps, degeneration with aging, infection (endocarditis or rheumatic fever), and abnormal expansion of the aorta above the valve.

Symptoms of Aortic Regurgitation. Symptoms of aortic regurgitation, when they develop, are usually those of congestive heart failure (fatigue, weakness, shortness of breath with exercise or at night, swelling in the ankles). You might also experience palpitations, night sweating, and angina.

How Serious Is Aortic Regurgitation? If you have aortic regurgitation, you can remain free of symptoms for a long time. If the aortic regurgitation is caused by rheumatic fever, symptoms may develop slowly over 10 to 30 years. If it is caused by endocarditis, symptoms may develop much more quickly and be more severe.

Paul is a 33-year-old manager of a fast-food franchise who has had a diagnosis of a bicuspid aortic valve since age 19 years, when an echocardiogram was done to evaluate a murmur. Four weeks ago he had three cavities filled. For the past 2 weeks he has felt tired and had a fever on most days, often with chills. During the past 2 days he has become short of breath and cannot lie flat without making the shortness of breath worse. Evaluation confirms the doctor's impression that he had an infection of the aortic valve and acute aortic regurgitation.

Much of the decision-making difficulty associated with mitral regurgitation also applies to aortic regurgitation. You can have minimal symptoms and yet your pumping function can deteriorate to a point that even if the valve is replaced, you may not improve as much as you might have if an operation had been undertaken earlier. However, an operation for even very advanced aortic regurgitation is still likely to yield a good result.

DEFECTS IN VALVES ON THE RIGHT SIDE OF THE HEART. The valves on the right side of the heart (tricuspid and pulmonary) are much less frequently affected by disease than those on the left side, and when they are, the disease is better tolerated in many cases.

Blood returning from the body flows into the right atrium, through the tricuspid valve, and into the right ventricle. From the right ventricle, the blood flows through the pulmonary valve to the pulmonary artery, which carries the blood to the lungs to receive oxygen. Both the tricuspid and the pulmonary valves can be affected by tightening (stenosis) or back leakage (regurgitation).

Tricuspid Stenosis. The tricuspid valve is the largest of the four valves in the heart. When it is affected by stenosis, it limits the blood flow from the right atrium to the right ventricle. Tricuspid stenosis is rare and usually occurs with other valve problems.

Causes of Tricuspid Stenosis. Tricuspid stenosis is usually caused by rheumatic fever or congenital heart disease. Rarely, it can be caused by deposits of a type of cancer cell called carcinoid.

Symptoms of Tricuspid Stenosis. Symptoms of tricuspid stenosis include generalized weakness and discomfort in the upper right abdomen due to back pressure in the liver. In most cases the symptoms are related to associated disease in the mitral or aortic valve. These symptoms include fatigue, shortness of breath, and fluid retention.

How Serious Is Tricuspid Stenosis? Because tricuspid stenosis tends to occur along with other valve problems, the other valve problems determine the outcome more than the tricuspid stenosis. If the function of the valve is badly deteriorated, surgery may be necessary.

If you have tricuspid stenosis, you are at risk for endocarditis and should take preventive antibiotics before and after dental and certain surgical procedures (see Precautions for people at risk for endocarditis, page 59).

Tricuspid Regurgitation. Tricuspid regurgitation allows blood to leak back into the right atrium from the right ventricle.

Causes of Tricuspid Regurgitation. Tricuspid regurgitation is usually caused by congenital heart disease and rarely occurs by itself. It may also result from rheumatic fever or endocarditis.

Tricuspid regurgitation can occasionally be a result of blunt trauma to the chest, such as hitting the steering wheel in a car accident.

Prolapse of the tricuspid valve can occur, just as it does with the mitral valve (see page 65). One rare but important cause of tricuspid regurgitation is deposits of a type of cancer cell called carcinoid.

Symptoms of Tricuspid Regurgitation. If there is right-sided heart failure, you may feel tired and short of breath and have swelling in the arms, legs, and liver, along with nausea and vomiting.

How Serious Is Tricuspid Regurgitation? Tricuspid disease is usually associated with other valve problems, and these will determine how serious the condition may be.

With the advent of sensitive tests that can look at blood flow in the heart (see Echocardiography, pages 209–216), a small amount of tricuspid regurgitation can be seen in almost all normal individuals. Thus, although the valves normally work extremely well, they do not completely seal off a small amount of back leakage.

If you have tricuspid regurgitation, you are at risk for endocarditis and should take preventive antibiotics before and after dental and certain surgical procedures (see Precautions for people at risk for endocarditis, page 59).

Pulmonary Stenosis. The pulmonary valve controls the flow of blood from the right ventricle to the pulmonary artery, which leads to the lungs. If the valve is tight, it limits the amount of blood that flows to the lungs.

Causes of Pulmonary Stenosis. When it occurs, pulmonary stenosis is almost always a part of a series of congenital heart problems. Rarely, it is caused by rheumatic fever or deposits of carcinoid tumor cells on the valve. Sometimes a tumor or aneurysm may compress the valve.

Symptoms of Pulmonary Stenosis. Symptoms occur only if the pulmonary stenosis is moderate to severe. They include fatigue, shortness of breath with exercise, light-headedness, and loss of consciousness. If the obstruction is severe, symptoms of right ventricular heart failure appear (swelling in arms, legs, and abdomen and a tender, enlarged liver). Bluish skin (cyanosis) may be present if the outflow of blood is substantially reduced or if there is associated shunting of blood from the right side of the heart to the left (see Tetralogy of Fallot, page 56).

How Serious Is Pulmonary Stenosis? Pulmonary stenosis, when severe, can lead to failure of the right ventricle and, ultimately, to death before 30 years of age. Thus, people with pulmonary stenosis may require surgery.

If you have pulmonary stenosis, you are at risk for endocarditis and should take preventive antibiotics before and after dental and certain surgical procedures (see Precautions for people at risk for endocarditis, page 59).

Pulmonary Regurgitation. Pulmonary regurgitation allows some of the blood to leak back into the right ventricle from the pulmonary artery.

Causes of Pulmonary Regurgitation. Pulmonary regurgitation can be caused by congenital disease or be a consequence of high blood pressure in the lungs. It is rarely caused by endocarditis.

Symptoms of Pulmonary Regurgitation. People with pulmonary regurgitation usually have no symptoms unless severe regurgitation develops with right ventricular enlargement and heart failure. If these occur, you may feel generally tired and have shortness of breath with exercise, loss of appetite, nausea, vomiting, and discomfort in the upper right part of your abdomen (from liver congestion). You may also have swelling in the arms and legs.

How Serious Is Pulmonary Regurgitation? Pulmonary regurgitation seems to be very well tolerated by the body. Indeed, there is evidence that some people can function perfectly well with their pulmonary valve entirely removed.

If symptoms of right ventricular failure appear, surgery to repair or replace the valve may be done.

If you have significant pulmonary regurgitation due to structural abnormalities, take preventive antibiotics before and after dental and certain surgical procedures to prevent endocarditis (see Precautions for people at risk for endocarditis, page 59).

Valve Disease

Possible Tests
Electrocardiography
   (see page 192)
Chest X-ray (see page 200)
Echocardiography
   (see page 209)
Radionuclide ventriculography
   (see page 208)
Cardiac catheterization—
   hemodynamics
   (see page 216)

Possible Treatment
Valve repair (see page 261)
Valve replacement
   (see page 262)
Balloon valvuloplasty
   (see page 261)

Coronary Blockages and Heart Attack

More than 6 million Americans experience symptoms due to coronary artery disease. As many as 1,500,000 Americans will have a heart attack this year, and about 500,000 will die. Blockage of the coronary arteries supplying the heart muscle (coronary artery disease, which can lead to heart attack) causes more deaths, disability, and economic loss than any other type of heart disease.

More than 200,000 to 300,000 people will undergo coronary artery bypass graft operations, and about 300,000 people will have percutaneous transluminal coronary angioplasties to try to reroute or reopen clogged coronary arteries (see page 270). Approximately 100,000 thrombolytic procedures are done each year to try to dissolve clots blocking coronary arteries in people having heart attacks (see page 266). The American Heart Association estimates that in 1993 all forms of cardiovascular disease cost the nation's economy $117.4 billion.

As dismal as these statistics sound, the past decade has seen dramatic declines in cardiovascular disease in this country and elsewhere. The death rate from coronary artery disease has decreased by more than 40 percent since 1978.

Although no one can say exactly why this decline has occurred, it is likely that better control of high blood pressure, a decline in cigarette smoking, more emphasis on physical activity, and better diets (less fat) have all played a role. Beyond these factors, progress in the diagnosis and treatment of coronary artery disease has also had an impact.

CORONARY ARTERY DISEASE. The coronary arteries are the heart's own circulatory system. They supply the heart itself with blood, oxygen, and nutrients. The heart uses this blood supply for energy to perform its continuous task of pumping.

Coronary artery disease can take many different forms, but they all have the same effect: The heart muscle does not get enough blood and oxygen through the coronary arteries. Consequently, the heart's own demands for oxygen and nutrients are not met. This condition can be either temporary or permanent.

Most coronary artery disease is caused by atherosclerosis (commonly called hardening of the arteries). The term "atherosclerosis" comes from the Greek *ather* (meaning "porridge") and *sklerosis* (meaning "hardening"). Fatty deposits collect in and on the lining of the artery walls, primarily the large coronary arteries, producing narrowing. If the narrowing is severe enough, blood flow within the coronary artery can be obstructed (see Figures 32 and 33, page A10).

Atherosclerosis (Hardening of the Arteries). Healthy arteries are flexible, strong, and elastic. The inner layer of arteries is smooth, enabling blood to flow freely.

As you age, your arteries normally become thicker and less elastic, and their calcium content increases. This "hardening" is believed to occur throughout the major artery system.

Atherosclerosis contrasts to this natural process, because it affects mainly the large arteries (including the coronary arteries). The inner layers of the artery walls become thick and irregular, and certain areas accumulate fats, cholesterol, and other materials. This gradual buildup of atherosclerotic plaque over a long time reduces the circulation of blood and increases the risk of heart attack, stroke, and other serious arterial diseases.

Initially the deposits are only streaks of fat-containing cells called fatty streaks. They are usually located at the points where arteries branch off. The fatty streaks can be found in the coronary arteries even as early as puberty.

As the fatty streaks enlarge, they invade some of the deeper layers of the artery walls, causing scarring and cal-

Definitions

Cardiovascular disease: any disease that affects the heart or the blood vessels

Coronary artery disease: blockage in the coronary arteries

Myocardial ischemia: blockage of the coronary arteries resulting in insufficient blood and oxygen reaching the heart muscle

Silent ischemia: myocardial ischemia that causes no symptoms

Angina: chest pain or pressure that results from myocardial ischemia

Myocardial infarction (heart attack): myocardial ischemia that lasts long enough to cause tissue death in the area of the heart supplied by a blocked coronary artery

cium deposits. Larger accumulations are called atheromas or plaques.

In atherosclerosis, blood cells called platelets often clump at microscopic sites of injury to the inner wall of the artery. Fat deposits also collect at these sites.

The plaque consists of a firm "shell" that may contain calcium with areas of fatty material, and the center consists of soft cholesterol. The shell portion may crack or fissure, exposing the inner portion. When this happens, a blood clot tends to develop at that site (see Figures 30 and 31, page A10). The clot may sufficiently reduce blood flow in the coronary arteries to cause angina (chest pain) or myocardial infarction (heart attack).

Causes of Atherosclerosis. The fatty streaks that are present very early in life do not necessarily grow into cholesterol-laden plaques. The mechanism that leads to the formation of blockages in the artery is still poorly understood. However, the risks of developing atherosclerosis are increased by certain identifiable factors, referred to as risk factors.

Some people are susceptible because of their genetic makeup or because they eat a high-fat diet. Other factors such as high blood pressure, high cholesterol levels in the blood, cigarette smoking, and diabetes can also lead to the development of fatty arterial plaques (see Modifiable Risk Factors, page 119).

Who Is Affected by Atherosclerosis? Atherosclerosis occurs mostly in middle-aged and elderly people. Up to about age 50 years, women lag behind men in the severity of atherosclerosis. After that, however, they catch up quickly.

High blood pressure, high blood cholesterol levels, and smoking encourage the development of atherosclerosis. Older age, a family history of coronary artery disease, diabetes, obesity, and a sedentary life-style also make you more susceptible to atherosclerosis (see Risk factors for coronary artery disease, page 116).

How Serious Is Atherosclerosis? When atherosclerosis occurs in the coronary arteries, it can lead to myocardial ischemia (insufficient blood supply to the heart). If the duration of ischemia is brief and your heart receives enough blood and oxygen and nutrients in time, the abnormalities caused by ischemia are reversible. However, if the duration of ischemia is longer than 40 to 60 minutes, significant irreversible injury may occur, and the parts of the heart muscle deprived of blood may become permanently damaged. This is a heart attack.

Symptoms Caused by Coronary Artery Disease. Coronary artery

disease can present as angina, myocardial infarction (heart attack), or sudden cardiac death. The most dramatic symptom of coronary artery disease is sudden death without prior warning. The most recognizable presentation of coronary artery disease is myocardial infarction, which can cause severe disability and death. At the other end of the spectrum is silent ischemia, which is significant coronary artery disease that causes no symptoms, at least for much of the time. Between those two ends of the spectrum is angina pectoris (chest pain).

Angina Pectoris
Bob was late for his meeting. He grabbed his briefcase and headed for the elevator. When it didn't come within a few seconds, he decided it would be faster to run up the three flights of stairs. After the second flight, he stopped, put his hand on his chest, and took some deep breaths. He had a tight feeling behind his breastbone and seemed unusually short of breath. After he rested a few minutes, the discomfort faded away.

Bob's description represents one of the most common patterns of symptoms in coronary artery disease—angina pectoris.

Causes of Angina Pectoris. Angina is the symptom that results from myocardial ischemia—insufficient blood and oxygen reaching the heart muscle because of blockage in the coronary arteries. The degree of coronary narrowing can vary, ranging from partial blockage in one vessel to extensive clogging of many vessels.

How Serious Is Angina Pectoris? If angina occurs only after unusual physical exertion, no dramatic change in life-style is required to prevent the pain. However, some people experience frequent bouts of angina during routine daily activities. They may change their daily routine so they do not have to do any strenuous exercise. Interestingly, the severity of symptoms does not relate directly to how many coronary arteries have blockages. A tight blockage in a small branch of a coronary artery can cause more discomfort in one person than severe narrowing of all three major coronary artery trunks in another person.

Some people with ischemia do not have typical anginal chest pain. Instead, they experience shortness of breath or, less commonly, fatigue or weakness as the only or main symptom of cardiac ischemia. Nevertheless, whatever the resulting symptoms, coronary artery disease represents ischemia in the heart muscle and should be monitored by your doctor.

Who Is Affected by Angina Pectoris? Angina is common, but only rarely occurs before age 30 years in men and later in women. About 3 million people in the United States have angina, and 300,000 new cases develop each year.

Types of Angina. Angina related to blockage in the coronary arteries can be subdivided according to whether it has had a predictable pattern for a prolonged time (stable angina) or is new or increasing (unstable angina). A third type of angina, variant angina, has nothing to do with plaque buildup in the arteries. Instead, it is caused by spasm of the muscle encircling the coronary arteries.

Stable Angina. When the pattern of chest pain has remained unchanged in terms of severity, frequency, and dura-

The pain of angina

> When the heart muscle does not get enough oxygen and nutrients, the heart cells use their own stores of energy for pumping. However, this process can work for only a short time before the heart cells are permanently damaged.
>
> Moreover, this process results in the buildup of by-products that cannot be removed efficiently because of the blocked blood flow—which caused the problem in the first place. This buildup of waste products (such as lactic acid) has been implicated as a cause of the pain in angina and heart attacks, just like the buildup of lactic acid in your other muscles causes pain when you overwork them.

tion for several weeks or months, it is referred to as stable angina. The symptoms are relatively predictable and occur with fairly consistent amounts of exertion or stress.

The main problem in stable angina is a fixed blockage to blood flow through one or more coronary arteries, caused by an atherosclerotic plaque (see Atherosclerosis, page 71). This narrows the diameter of the coronary artery so that only a limited amount of blood, carrying oxygen and nutrients, can reach the heart muscle.

Bob should have known that he would have trouble with the stairs. He has had that same chest pain every time he has overexerted himself for the past year.

The blood flow may be adequate for the heart when it is at rest, but when you exert yourself, the blockage does not allow the blood flow to increase as the demands of the heart increase. The heart's demand for oxygen outstrips the supply. Myocardial ischemia results, causing the symptoms of angina.

Unstable Angina. Unstable angina refers to a pattern of symptoms when angina is new, lasts longer, is more severe or frequent, is easier to provoke with less and less stress, occurs at rest, and responds less to medications that used to relieve the discomfort.

A month or so later, Bob started having his chest pain after only a few steps, and sometimes when he was just reading or watching television.

The presence of unstable angina implies that the underlying situation is fragile and worsening. Because this pattern often occurs before the development of a heart attack, it is sometimes called "preinfarction angina."

Researchers have not completely discovered what is happening during unstable angina. This is likely a phase of coronary artery disease in which the severity of the obstruction is intermittently getting worse and then better in a repeating cycle.

Some studies have shown that coronary arteries in people with stable angina have a smooth inner (endothelial) surface free of blood clots. People with worsening angina have ulceration and roughening of the endothelial lining, and people with unstable angina often have blood clots that form and dissolve sporadically.

When angina occurs at rest, the heart is not demanding extra oxygen, because there is no additional stress. Therefore, the problem must be a suddenly inadequate blood supply. This may be due to one of two things.

First, the coronary blood vessels, like all blood vessels, can dilate or constrict as a normal regulatory feature. When the nervous system tells an artery to constrict, and it is already severely blocked by atherosclerotic plaque, the blood flow—which is already inadequate—may be cut dramatically.

The second possible reason for inadequate blood supply is that the atherosclerotic plaque is at a point in the circulation where there is a great deal of turbulence (such as a bend in the artery) and the lining of the blood vessel (endothelium) is partly destroyed and malfunctioning. This damage leads to clumping of platelets on top of the atherosclerotic plaque. The additional clumping of debris impedes blood flow even further. After the platelets "pile up" to a certain point, the clump may dissolve or simply break up and move downstream, in which case blood flow can resume at its previous suboptimal level.

Either of these mechanisms may account for the waxing and waning pattern of unstable angina. Because unstable angina is a serious development, your doctor frequently will recommend hospitalization for stabilization, assessment, and further treatment.

Variant Angina. The muscle fibers encircling the coronary arteries may go into spasm in some individuals (see Figures 34 and 35, page A10). When that occurs, the lumen (the hollow part of the artery) at one point can severely narrow or even close off temporarily. Many problems can result, including silent ischemia, angina, and heart attack.

Variant angina (also called Prinzmetal's angina, after one of the first physicians to describe the pattern of symptoms) is different from the usual type of angina, in which demand for oxygen-rich blood outstrips supply. With variant angina, spasm can occur even in the absence of excess demand. In other words, the blood supply is cut off to a point less than the minimal requirements of the heart muscle even when it is at rest. Severe angina can occur with spasm, but some people experience no symptoms (silent ischemia).

The spasms may occur without apparent cause, but they also may result from strong emotional stress, exposure to cold, or inhaling cigarette smoke.

The symptoms of variant angina tend to be different from the pattern of stable or unstable angina. Variant angina is typically severe, lasts for a relatively brief time, and frequently occurs at night, waking you from sleep. Abnormal rhythm disorders are common during the periods of blood flow cutoff, which can cause you to pass out.

Angina

Possible Tests

Measurement of blood lipids
   (see page 190)
Electrocardiography
   (see page 192)
Exercise electrocardiography
   (see pages 196, 198)
Stress thallium scanning,
   exercise MUGA
   (see pages 198, 205)
Stress echocardiography
   (see pages 198, 215, 216)
Coronary angiography
   (see page 217)

Possible Treatment

Medications
   (see pages 263, 296, 298,
   299)
Percutaneous transluminal
   coronary angioplasty
   (see page 269)
Coronary artery bypass surgery
   (see page 272)

Myocardial Infarction (Heart Attack).
Sam was just finishing breakfast when it hit: severe, intolerable pressure in his chest. He wanted to think it was indigestion and that it would go away if he waited a few minutes, but it didn't stop. He had a vague feeling of uneasiness. Should he tell his wife about it? Something was definitely very wrong.

When he started sweating profusely and feeling nauseous, he decided to tell his wife. He had a feeling of impending doom. His wife called 911.

The doctors said it was lucky he came to the hospital: Sam was having a heart attack.

Myocardial infarction (heart attack) can be thought of as the end result of coronary artery blockage. An infarct is an area of tissue that has been permanently damaged because of starvation for oxygen and nutrients.

A heart attack occurs when a coronary artery is blocked permanently, or for longer than about 30 minutes to 2 hours. The region of the heart muscle (myocardium) supplied by that coronary artery is starved for oxygen and nutrition for so long that irreversible damage (necrosis) occurs (see Figure 29, page A10).

A heart attack generally causes severe anginal pain for longer than 15 minutes, but it is also possible to have a "silent" heart attack in which no symptoms occur. The evidence of a silent heart attack may show up on an electrocardiogram or other tests on the heart, or it may be discovered during an autopsy.

Causes of a Heart Attack.   Although physicians rarely have the chance to see coronary arteries at the exact moment of a heart attack (by doing coronary angiography, see page 217), evidence indicates that a heart attack is caused by the sudden blockage of the artery by a blood clot. The blood clot often forms at the site of a crack or rupture in an atherosclerotic plaque.

When angiography is done within several hours of a heart attack, a blood clot is frequently seen. If angiography is done later, however, there is less likelihood of seeing a blood clot. These angiographic findings suggest that blood clots tend to dissolve with time, although usually too late to prevent tissue necrosis.

Thus, one of the main treatments of heart attacks is the use of clot-dissolving medications (thrombolytic agents) (see page 301).

Most often, the clot that causes a heart attack forms in a coronary artery that has been narrowed by fatty deposits of atherosclerosis (see page 71). Rarely, blood clots can develop inside the heart in conditions such as mitral stenosis or in people who have previous heart damage. Clots can break off and enter the circulation of the coronary arteries, causing a heart attack if the blood clot lodges in a coronary artery and prevents blood flow from reaching the heart muscle. (This is the same way that a stroke is caused by a blood clot lodging in an artery in the brain.)

How Serious Is a Heart Attack? A heart attack may lead to immediate death either because so much of the heart dies that it can no longer function or because fatal rhythm disorders develop. However, many people survive a heart attack and are hospitalized.

If the area of damaged tissue (infarct) is small and the electrical system that controls your heart is not damaged, your chances of surviving a heart attack are good. The sooner you get to a hospital, the more can be done to limit the amount of tissue damage.

In general, damage to less than 10 percent of the ventricle muscle may lead to a decrease in the amount of blood that your heart can eject during each contraction. However, the reduction in heart function is mild, so a return to a reasonably normal life-style usually can be anticipated. If 25 percent or more of the heart muscle is damaged, your heart may enlarge and heart failure (see page 36) may develop. If 40 percent or more of the heart muscle is damaged, shock or death may occur (see Shock, page 34).

The location of the tissue damage can also affect the outcome. If the heart attack involves the front (anterior) por-

---

Factors that improve your chance for a favorable outcome after a heart attack

- Younger age
- No prior heart attack
- No recurrence of pain
- No congestive heart failure
- No heart rhythm disorders
- Normal blood pressure
- No diabetes
- No smoking
- Normal weight
- Male sex

Most people who are still alive 2 hours after their heart attack started will survive. However, there are possible complications. Approximately 7 percent to 12 percent of people who have a heart attack die during their hospitalization, although these rates are declining with new treatment techniques. Of those who survive to leave the hospital, about 5 percent to 15 percent die in the first year after a heart attack. About the same percentage have another heart attack within the next year.

tion of the heart, the consequences are likely to be more serious than if the tissue damage is along the lower (inferior) part of the heart muscle. Anterior heart attacks are usually more extensive.

Most people who die of heart attacks have severe blockages of more than one coronary artery so that a large portion of the heart muscle is damaged. Also, the pumping function of their left ventricle is impaired, which is associated with fatal rhythm disturbances.

Emergency Signs and Symptoms of a Heart Attack   Not all of the signs and symptoms mentioned below are present in all cases of heart attack, and some people do not have any symptoms. The more symptoms you have, the higher the likelihood that you are having a heart attack. Get help if you have any combination of these symptoms:

- Intense, prolonged chest pain (often a feeling of heavy pressure)
- Pain radiating from the chest to the left shoulder and arm, back, and even jaw
- Prolonged pain in the upper abdomen
- Shortness of breath
- Fainting
- Nausea, vomiting, intense sweating
- Frequent angina attacks that are not caused by exertion

People sometimes think back and realize that they did have a few signs that things were not quite right before they had their heart attack. A spouse or co-worker will often say the person looked older, paler, exhausted, or de-

Recognize a heart attack—you may save your life

Prompt, efficient treatment greatly improves your chances of surviving a heart attack. The first and most important step in treating a heart attack is your own recognition of what is occurring. The key to successful treatment is early treatment.

Unfortunately, too many people with heart attacks attribute the symptoms to something else or simply hope that the symptoms will disappear. They are putting themselves at an immediate disadvantage for effective treatment and survival. Of all people who die from their heart attacks, most of them (60 percent) die within the first hour after the onset of symptoms, before medical help is sought.

A heart attack is a medical emergency. It is important to reread the section on chest pain (see page 44) and recognize that if it lasts longer than 15 minutes and does not respond to nitroglycerin (if this medication has been prescribed for you), you must seek medical care at once.

pressed before the heart attack. Unfortunately, only about one-third of people with these symptoms consult their doctor.

If you think you or someone you are with is having a heart attack, find medical attention immediately. Fifteen percent of heart attack victims die suddenly within the first hour of symptoms. Sudden death can even be the first symptom of a heart attack. If you are with someone who stops breathing, begin cardiopulmonary resuscitation (CPR) immediately. After a person stops breathing, he or she can live only a few minutes without CPR. This limited time emphasizes the need for everyone to have training in CPR (see page 241).

Thousands of people die each year because they did not seek medical help in time. Don't worry about confusing a heart attack with indigestion or something else. Get immediate help. It may save your life.

Complications of a Heart Attack. The first problems associated with a heart attack—pain and discomfort, the risk of death, and permanent damage to the heart—may not be the last. Beyond these, a heart attack can lead to several other complications.

Congestive Heart Failure. After a heart attack, your heart may not pump as effectively, which may lead to symptoms of congestive heart failure. People with a severe decrease in blood flow and congestion in the lungs (pulmonary congestion) after a heart attack are at the highest risk of death.

Rhythm Abnormalities. Heart attacks can also lead to severe rhythm abnormalities. Rhythm disturbances account for more than one-half of all deaths from heart attack.

The most lethal rhythm abnormality is ventricular fibrillation, in which the contractions of the ventricles are very rapid and uncoordinated. Actually, the movement of the heart is more quivering than contracting. Without regular contractions, your heart cannot pump blood to the vital organs. You can see why this rhythm is lethal. It is often called "cardiac arrest," and it is the major mechanism for sudden cardiac death.

Other abnormalities in the sinus node (the heart's natural pacemaker, which initiates the heartbeat) and in the electrical system that conducts the heartbeat can result in a heartbeat that is too fast (tachycardia) (see page 93) or too slow (bradycardia) (see page 86).

Ventricular Septal Defect. Tissue death and rupture of the muscular wall (septum) between the two ventricles lead to ventricular septal defect (see page 55). Heart failure may develop suddenly in a previously stable person if the ventricular septum ruptures. If the problem is severe, immediate surgery to repair the septal defect is necessary.

Mitral Valve Regurgitation. A heart attack can destroy part of the mitral valve apparatus (such as a papillary muscle that supports the valve) and lead to severe, sudden regurgitation (back leakage) of blood from the left ventricle back into the left atrium. Severe congestive heart failure and death will follow shortly if the problem is not immediately recognized and treated.

Ventricular Aneurysm. The section of heart muscle affected by the heart attack can expand and thin out like a weak portion on a bald tire. This bulge (or aneurysm) leads to ineffective pumping, rhythm disorders, and difficult-to-control chest pain.

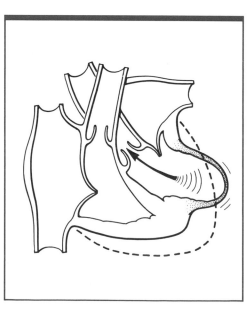

A heart attack may weaken a portion of the heart wall, producing a bulge (aneurysm). When the ventricle contracts, the aneurysm may actually bulge further out.

An aneurysm, especially early after the heart attack, is associated with a much higher risk of death, heart failure, arrhythmias, and blood clots.

Ventricular Rupture. Because the damaged heart muscle is "mushy" until it forms a firm scar, the heart wall at the site of the myocardial infarction can actually break through (rupture). This catastrophic complication is like a blowout on a worn tire. Shock and circulatory collapse suddenly develop (because in this case the blood does flow out of the heart itself). Ventricular rupture almost always results in death. Fortunately, this complication is uncommon. When it does happen, it usually occurs within a week after the heart attack itself.

Some people may have an incomplete rupture of the wall of the heart. In this case, the pericardium (the sac surrounding the heart) and blood clots may seal the site of rupture. Death is not immediate in such cases. If the person can be stabilized, surgical repair is possible.

Clot Formation. Clots can form inside the ventricle, next to the muscle affected by the heart attack, especially when it becomes dilated or develops an aneurysm. Any clot that forms in the left ventricle can break loose and travel (embolize) to the blood vessels in the brain, causing a stroke. Medications that keep blood from clotting (anticoagulants) are essential.

Recurrence of Angina. Around the zone of damaged muscle in the heart, there is usually a region of myocardial cells that survived the heart attack but are in danger of permanent damage if any further ischemia occurs. If angina recurs after a heart attack, it may indicate that the heart attack is extending into this "area at risk." Such symptoms early after a heart attack should prompt an immediate aggressive attempt to limit further damage. This might include catheterization (see page 217) to determine whether blocked vessels can or should be opened up or bypassed.

Pericarditis.   Inflammation of the pericardium (the sac surrounding the heart) develops in about 10 percent of people with heart attack. The inflammation is related to the death of the cells in the heart wall. The condition is usually brief and responds to anti-inflammatory drugs; only rarely is it a recurrent or persistent problem.

Cardiogenic Shock. Cardiogenic shock results when the heart muscle is too weak to contract with enough force to maintain the blood pressure at a level that provides a sufficient amount of blood to the body and the heart muscle itself. A vicious cycle develops. The coronary arteries do not get enough blood, which makes the heart weaker, which in turn further decreases the blood supply. This cycle is fatal in most cases.

Cardiogenic shock is a complication during the first days after a heart attack in about 7 percent to 15 percent of people. Those who die of cardiogenic shock have infarction of 40 percent or more of the left ventricle. Most have severe disease in three of their coronary arteries.

New clot-dissolving medications or special catheterization techniques may help prevent this complication or decrease its severity.

Myocardial Infarction

Possible Tests

Measurement of cardiac
    enzymes (see page 190)
Electrocardiography
    (see page 192)
Chest X-ray (see page 200)
Echocardiography
    (see page 209)
Cardiac scanning (see page 203)
Coronary angiography
    (see page 216)

Possible Treatment

Cardiac Care Unit (CCU)
    admission (see page 267)
Medications
    (see pages 266 and 301)
Percutaneous transluminal
    coronary angioplasty
    (see page 270)
Coronary artery bypass surgery
    (see page 272)

Silent Ischemia

At the age of 53 years, Ben was feeling great but was required by his company to have a medical examination before his promotion. His physical examination, chest X-ray, and blood tests were normal. His doctor told him, however, that his treadmill exercise test showed abnormalities consistent with ischemia, even though Ben had reached a good exercise level and had no symptoms other than getting normally breathless at the end.

The simple scenario presented by Ben's situation actually raises a number of complex and controversial issues. What conclusions should Ben and his doctor draw from his examination?

- Is the treadmill test incorrect? It is well recognized that it is not a perfect test and may occasionally yield a false result (see page 199).
- Is the test correct and does Ben have true ischemia even though it causes no symptoms?
- Is it necessary to do further testing to see whether the test is correct?
- If the test is correct, is treatment necessary? After all, Ben is not having any symptoms.
- Of course, the overriding question perhaps is: "Should Ben have had the screening treadmill test in the first place?"

The fact is that many of these questions cannot be answered with certainty for individual people. For now, it is important to recognize that coronary artery disease can be present and cause myocardial ischemia even in people who have no symptoms.

Causes of Silent Ischemia. Silent ischemia, like all ischemia, is caused by a blockage in a coronary artery. Silent ischemia may be caused by brief or less severe blockage. Or ischemia may be "silent" because of a difference in pain perception in different people or in different circumstances.

Unrecognized ischemia may be discovered when a person undergoes any kind of stress test (see page 198) or is monitored with electrocardiography for an extended period of time (see Ambulatory Electrocardiography Monitoring, page 199). Although silent ischemia does not cause symptoms, it may be a warning sign of future problems.

How Serious Is Silent Ischemia? Ischemia can be entirely silent (without symptoms) and still be severe enough to cause a heart attack. In fact, one large study of the population of Framingham, Massachusetts, showed that 35 percent of heart attacks in women and 28 percent in men are not recognized as heart attacks; about half were silent, and about half caused symptoms incorrectly attributed to another cause. Numerous people with typical heart attacks have had no prior "warning symptoms" despite having had coronary artery disease for some time. Even people with symptoms of angina are often found, upon examination with appropriate monitors, to also have episodes of ischemia without angina.

Growing evidence suggests that silent ischemia predicts a future course of events similar to that with typical symptoms—but this theory is hard to prove and is currently controversial. An educated guess based on several studies suggests that in the United States there are probably about 1 million men and women like Ben who have no idea that they have significant myocardial ischemia. Nevertheless, it is certainly not yet clear that "looking for" these people with expensive screening tests will have an overall benefit for them either individually or as a group.

Kawasaki Syndrome. Kawasaki syndrome is named for the Japanese doctor who, in 1967, described a newly recognized childhood illness. This syndrome is capable of producing coronary artery disease in children, and rarely it can cause heart attacks and death in this young age group. Since its discovery, the number of children affected by the illness has increased, and it is now the most common cause of acquired heart disease in children (as distinct from congenital heart disease)—a position once occupied by rheumatic fever.

Causes of Kawasaki Syndrome. No one is certain what causes Kawasaki syndrome. It is not considered contagious because no infectious agent has been identified, but it does tend to occur in outbreaks, especially in the winter and spring. Some experts suspect that an unusual virus or other germ may be the culprit, or toxic agents may be involved. Most of the hallmarks of Kawasaki syndrome are related to inflammation, and the damage that sometimes occurs in the coronary arteries or heart muscle may be due to the body's immune response.

Symptoms of Kawasaki Syndrome. Children who experience a lengthy (more than 5 days), high, spiking fever and any four of the following indicators are suspected of having Kawasaki syndrome, as long as there is nothing (such as a staphylococcal infection) to otherwise explain them.

- Conjunctival infection (swollen, watery eyes)
- Reddened, cracked, and swollen surfaces of the lips, tongue, mouth, and throat
- Swollen, reddened hands and feet, followed by peeling of the skin in these areas
- Measles-like rash
- Swollen lymph glands of the neck

The feverish stage of the disease usually lasts 1 to 2 weeks, followed by improvement. It is during the phase of improvement that the heart can be affected. In about one out of five children with Kawasaki syndrome that is not treated, heart-related problems develop. The most common is expansion (aneurysm formation) of sections of coronary arteries. In some children, the aneurysm can become obstructed by clotted blood and cause a heart attack. Fortunately this is rare, especially with treatment.

How Serious Is Kawasaki Syndrome? Although the illness can be harrowing, and despite its effect on the coronary arteries, Kawasaki syndrome is usually a self-limited illness. The death rate in treated children is well below 1 percent. Even among those in whom coronary problems develop, most have substantial resolution or improvement with time.

Treatment is designed to reduce inflammation and stave off damage to the heart and coronary arteries. This goal seems to be accomplished by relatively high doses of aspirin tablets and injections of immunoglobulin (purified human antibodies).

Who Is Affected by Kawasaki Syndrome? Four of every five people who get Kawasaki syndrome are less than 4 years old. People of Asian descent, even if they have lived in the United States for generations, are more susceptible. Some reports suggest that children with the syndrome had been exposed to recently shampooed carpets, but this finding has been inconsistent.

Palpitations and Passing Out (Arrhythmias)

Most likely you are entirely unaware of your heartbeat despite the continuous contraction and relaxation of your heart day in and day out. Like many things, your heartbeat remains unobtrusive as long as it is functioning smoothly and predictably. Unless you make some effort to detect your heartbeat by feeling the pulse at your wrist, you may never even appreciate the constant motion occurring inside you. You may become aware of the action of your heart only when normal circumstances are altered. If you lie on your left side in bed, with your ear pressed against the sheet, you may notice that you hear the sounds of your heart beating, transmitted through the mattress from your chest to your ear. Some people who notice this for the first time become concerned, but of course all they are hearing is their usual heartbeat.

The predictability of the heartbeat is what keeps the heart functioning "on schedule" and also lets you "get used to it" and ignore it. Although the normal heartbeat is predictable, it does not beat with clocklike precision. For one thing, your heart varies its rate of contraction during changes in your activities. It speeds up when you exercise, for the simple reason that by beating faster it can pump more blood to your laboring muscles. When your activity ceases, the rate of the heartbeat declines again to its normal resting level. If you exercise hard enough, your heart rate can accelerate to approximately 200 beats per minute.

The heart rate normally varies somewhat, even from one beat to the next. Heart rates from 50 to 100 beats per minute when you are inactive are normal, and you are seldom conscious of your heartbeat at those rates. This is called normal sinus rhythm. Disturbances of the heartbeat that cause it to go outside the limits of normal speeds or beyond the usual degree of variation may cause problems that range from the trivial and asymptomatic to the very abnormal and deadly. The evaluation and treatment of abnormal heartbeats (called arrhythmias, meaning abnormal rhythms) constitute a major portion of the practice of cardiology.

Recall that the conduction system of your heart can be thought of as the electrical wiring that transmits impulses throughout the heart muscle and stimulates it to contract in an organized and regular way. It assures that your heart can carry out its task of pumping blood most efficiently. Problems with the electrical function of the heart account for the occurrence of arrhythmias.

SYMPTOMS OF ARRHYTHMIAS.
The effect an arrhythmia has on you, in terms of symptoms and overall health, depends on several factors. To begin with, it depends on the specific type of arrhythmia. Sometimes, doctors can make educated guesses about what the arrhythmia is simply by observing (or hearing about) what has happened to you. Another factor is whether the arrhythmia is extremely abnormal or only a little abnormal. Not unexpectedly, the worse the arrhythmia (for example, very fast or very slow), the more severe will be the symptoms you experience.

Yet another consideration is the frequency with which an arrhythmia occurs. Does it occur daily? If so, it may cause major problems. If it occurs only once a year (or once in a lifetime), it might be considered a relatively minor problem. Of course, some arrhythmias are so serious that they need to occur only once to be devastating.

Another factor is how long the arrhythmia lasts when it occurs. Some arrhythmias last for only a single beat,

although they may occur again in the next few seconds, minutes, or hours. Others last for hours or days or even throughout a person's life. Finally, the consequences of an arrhythmia depend on whether it is the only problem with the heart or whether there are additional problems such as cardiomyopathy or a recent heart attack. Usually, arrhythmias in the setting of other heart disease are more worrisome than if they occurred in an otherwise healthy heart.

DIAGNOSIS OF ARRHYTHMIAS.
The evaluation of an arrhythmia may come about either because symptoms have occurred that might be due to a rhythm disorder or because an abnormality was discovered on an electrocardiogram (ECG; see page 192) during a routine checkup. Symptoms that may prompt a search for an arrhythmia include palpitations, fatigue, shortness of breath, light-headedness, syncope, or sudden death (and successful resuscitation, of course). You may wish to review the detailed descriptions of these symptoms (see pages 22–35). The specific arrhythmias that may cause them are discussed in the following pages.

To treat an arrhythmia effectively (or, indeed, to determine whether treatment is even advisable) and overcome the symptoms it may be causing, the type of arrhythmia must be discovered. An ECG shows the electrical component of the heartbeat most clearly. It would seem a simple matter to obtain an ECG, make a diagnosis, and start treatment.

Unfortunately, there are obstacles to this seemingly easy route. Just like clanking sounds beneath the hood of your car that go away as you drive into the mechanic's shop, arrhythmias and the symptoms they cause are notoriously hard to "catch." Several sophisticated tests have been devised to get around this obstacle (see Electrophysiology Studies, page 224), but it has not been eliminated. Once the arrhythmia is detected, other obstacles are the problems of deciding whether it is the cause of the symptoms and, if it is intermittent, whether it is likely to recur often enough or with serious enough consequences to warrant treatment.

CLASSIFICATION OF ARRHYTHMIAS. Problems with the conduction system and rhythms fall into four general categories. The first category consists of abnormalities that are seen by the doctor on your ECG but do not directly cause an arrhythmia. In other words, you would not notice any unpredictable types of heartbeats by taking your pulse, nor would you experience any symptoms. This category is called "conduction system abnormalities." Because a problem in this category is not truly a rhythm abnormality, it cannot really be called an arrhythmia. The second category is slow heartbeats (bradycardia). The third category might be termed irregular heartbeats. The final category is fast heartbeats (tachycardia). These three categories are true arrhythmias.

Some specific arrhythmias overlap into different categories, as you will see in the descriptions that follow. For example, atrial fibrillation is usually both irregular and fast. The so-called sick sinus syndrome consists of both fast rhythms and slow rhythms at different times. Thus, not all arrhythmias fit neatly into one category, but all in all such a scheme helps to make sense of a very complicated topic.

Conduction System Abnormalities

Bonnie is a 78-year-old retired credit union employee who has been entirely healthy throughout her life. A general medical examination this year disclosed a "bundle-branch block" on the ECG. Other than recommending her usual periodic physical examinations, her doctor does not recommend further action.

The heart contracts in an orderly fashion on each beat because the electrical impulse, or signal, travels over the circuit known as the conduction system. Not uncommonly, portions of the conduction system become defective and are unable to transmit the signal. Sometimes the signal is just slowed down as it travels down the defective portion of the circuit so that it is delayed in reaching its destination. In some cases the signal cannot get through that part of the conduction system at all; it is "blocked." The conduction system extends like branches out from a tree trunk. If the block occurs in just one branch, the electrical impulse will have to take a detour to reach its destination.

When the impulse detours, the rate and rhythm of the heartbeat are not affected, but the abnormal pathway the electrical impulse takes can be spotted by the doctor on the ECG. There are several patterns that indicate where the block is located: The medical names of the main patterns are right bundle-branch block and left bundle-branch block. These can be further subdivided.

Another type of block that does not actually change the speed at which the heart beats occurs at the point where the impulse travels from the atria to the

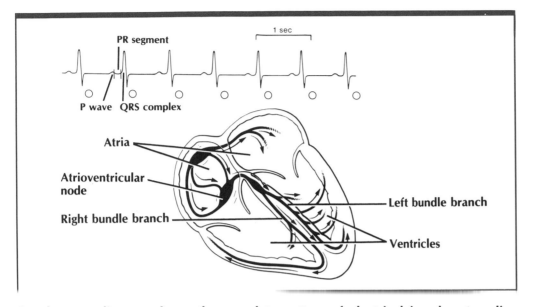

An electrocardiogram shows the complete pattern of electrical impulses traveling throughout the heart during each heartbeat. When all parts of the conduction system are working properly, the electrocardiogram typically appears like this: a small "P wave" (atrial impulse) precedes a brief "PR segment" (as the impulse travels through the atrioventricular node), which is followed by a tall, narrow "QRS complex" (ventricular impulse). The circles (which do not actually appear on an electrocardiogram) show when the pulse from each heartbeat would be felt. (See also page A12.)

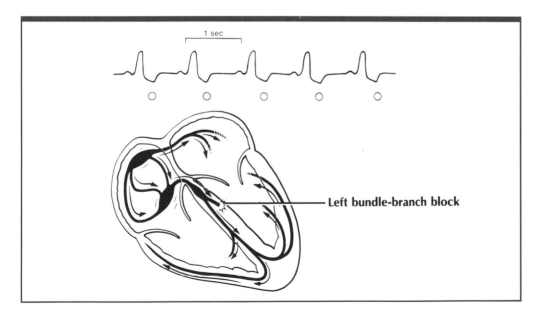

In bundle-branch block (in this case, of the left bundle), the pattern of the electrocardiogram changes in characteristic ways. Because the impulse now has to take a more time-consuming and indirect route through the ventricle, the QRS complex becomes wide and abnormally shaped. However, the P wave, PR interval, heart rate, and strength of the pulse are not affected.

ventricles (the atrioventricular node). The impulse normally slows down here in order to coordinate the beating of the atria and ventricles. This slowing may become exaggerated, a fact that is recognizable only on the ECG; the slowing does not cause symptoms. It is referred to as "first-degree atrioventricular block." (You can probably guess that there are other degrees of atrioventricular block. You're right—they belong in other categories and will be explained shortly.)

If these conduction abnormalities do not cause symptoms, are they merely curiosities? As a matter of fact, they almost never require treatment. Their significance lies in the fact that they may be a subtle sign of other heart problems that may not have been recognized as yet, or they may be a harbinger of more serious rhythm problems. For example, researchers have found that people with left bundle-branch block have a somewhat higher chance of developing coronary artery-related problems, such as heart attacks, than people without left bundle-branch block. However, most doctors believe that its value as a clue in this regard is too unreliable to warrant searching for evidence of coronary artery disease when it is the only apparent abnormality in heart function.

There are a few exceptions to the benign nature of these conduction abnormalities. If left bundle-branch block develops during a heart attack, it is usually advisable to use a pacemaker temporarily, because left bundle-branch block in this fragile situation may indicate that a very slow heart rhythm may abruptly occur. Also, if a person with syncope has no evidence of any problem except conduction system disease, even after a thorough evaluation, many doctors believe the cause of syncope is probably an intermittent, very slow heartbeat. A pacemaker might therefore be recommended (see Figure 46, page A14).

Bradycardia (Slow Heartbeats). Any time the rate of heartbeats drops below 50 per minute, the rate is considered to be slow. However, the circumstances during which the bradycardia occurred must be taken into consideration. During sleep, for example, it is not unusual for the heart rate to descend into the 40s and even 30s in healthy individuals. Indeed, a slow heart rate, as long as the ECG and heart are otherwise normal, may be regarded as a sign of general fitness. Trained athletes often have resting heart rates of about 40 to 50 beats per minute. Any slow heartbeat, regardless of cause, is referred to as bradycardia. Thus, these slow heartbeats are called sinus bradycardia because the heartbeats still originate from the sinus node, your heart's natural pacemaker.

Symptoms of Bradycardia

Megan is a 72-year-old retired professional flutist who began noticing sudden extreme fatigue about 2 weeks ago. Any of her routine activities caused her to be very tired and vaguely short of breath. She came to the doctor today because she suddenly "found herself on the kitchen floor" as she was preparing lunch. The office nurse takes her pulse: It is 32 beats per minute.

Although slow heartbeats in athletes and during sleep are nonpathologic (that is, they are abnormal in the strict sense but they do not indicate an unhealthy state), other types of bradycardia are pathologic, or potentially so. Bradycardia in this sense means either a steady slowness of the heart over an extended time or pauses between heartbeats, either of which causes symptoms or runs a significant risk of causing future symptoms.

Typically, the symptoms produced by steady, slow heartbeats are fatigue, shortness of breath, or light-headedness (although these symptoms can also be due to many other causes). These are easy to understand; when your heart beats too slowly it is not providing the rest of the body with sufficient blood supply to function efficiently. Occasional pauses between heartbeats may cause no symptoms if they are relatively brief (less than 3 seconds), especially if you are lying or sitting down when they occur. Pauses from 3 to 5 seconds will usually produce at least a passing sensation that you are about to black out; indeed, some people will abruptly lose consciousness because of the instantaneous (but short) lack of oxygen supply to the brain. Pauses longer than 5 seconds will likely make you very lightheaded or cause you to black out, unless you are lying quietly or are asleep.

Classification of Bradycardia. Bradycardia is differentiated on the basis of where the problem originates. There are three basic sites: the nerves that control the speed of the heartbeat (the autonomic nervous system), the sinus node that originates the heartbeat (it is the "spark plug" of the heart, so to speak), and the conduction system that distributes the electrical signal throughout the working muscle of the heart. Compromised function of any of these components may lead to a slow heartbeat.

Problems With Control by the Nervous System. Inappropriate function of the autonomic nervous system may cause abnormally slow heartbeats or, more often, pauses. The reflexes that automatically control the heartbeat temporarily seem to go haywire in some people. One of these reflexes seems to have its basis in evolution: in certain animals, such as walruses, the heartbeats are known to slow down abruptly to an extraordinary degree when they dive into frigid waters. This decrease reduces the rate at which they use up energy and oxygen so they can remain submerged longer.

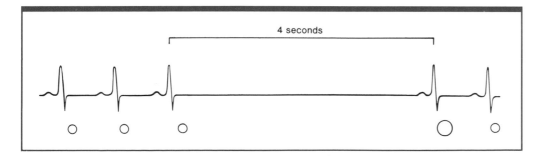

This electrocardiogram shows a sudden pause in the electrical impulses produced by the sinus node. This results in a pause in the heartbeat, as depicted by the circles. In fact, you might feel a "stronger" heartbeat after the pause. This pause could produce light-headedness or even very brief loss of consciousness if you were standing up.

Some people have pauses (and subsequent symptoms) because the part of the autonomic nervous system that promotes heart slowness suddenly does its job too well. Occasionally, this change can actually be provoked. For example, a tight necktie or collar may press on a region of the carotid artery in the neck called the carotid sinus. Nerves running through the neck at this point become activated by this pressure and may send a "slow down" message to the sinus node of the heart. (Don't confuse the carotid sinus and the sinus node—they are entirely different structures.) If you are too sensitive to the "slow down" signal, your heart may not just slow down a little (which would be normal), but it may actually stop for 5, 10, or even more seconds. The result is syncope. This type of syncope is called "carotid sinus hypersensitivity."

Other factors may activate the "slowing" part of the autonomic nervous system, such as straining at a bowel movement, urinating, gagging, or applying pressure to the eyeballs.

Doctors check for evidence of autonomic nervous system malfunction in people who report syncope by pressing (or massaging) on the carotid sinus while watching an electrocardiogram monitor. The doctor checks before-hand to make sure there is no evidence of blockage in the carotid artery, because the massage may aggravate it and precipitate a stroke.

Sometimes pain, fear, exhaustion, or low blood pressure can provoke bradycardia as well as further lowering of the blood pressure. When this happens, you may faint. "Simple fainting" (also referred to as vasovagal syncope) can usually be distinguished from other more serious causes of loss of consciousness by the circumstances and by the associated symptoms. Typically, fainting is preceded by sweatiness, nausea, a prickly sensation in the skin, pallor, and at least a few seconds of "graying out" before the actual blackout occurs. This response is different from carotid sinus hypersensitivity or other types of syncope in which the passing out is characteristically abrupt, with little or no warning.

Problems With the Sinus Node. Sometimes the sinus node fails to perform adequately in its role as your heart's pacemaker. Despite proper signals from the autonomic nervous system, it simply initiates beats too slowly, pauses too long between beats, or simply stops producing beats. If it stops producing beats, a different part of the heart must take over the pacemaker

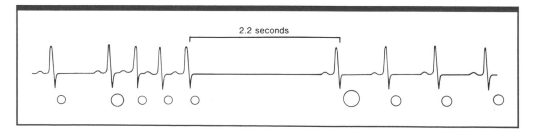

2.2 seconds

This electrocardiogram shows sick sinus syndrome. At times the heart beats rapidly and causes palpitations, and at other times there are brief pauses. The circles (which do not actually appear on an electrocardiogram) indicate that some heartbeats may feel more forceful and more rapid than normal.

function, which it usually does at a rate that is substantially slower than normal. The various ways the sinus node can malfunction are grouped under the not-so-technical term "sick sinus syndrome."

To complicate matters, sinus nodes that are "sick" also have a disconcerting tendency to beat too fast at times when they are not beating too slow. Thus, symptoms of sick sinus syndrome can be those associated with slow heartbeats (such as fatigue, light-headedness, and syncope) alternating with symptoms of fast heartbeats (such as palpitations). Either the slow or the fast rhythm can cause shortness of breath, light-headedness, syncope, or fatigue.

The fact that there is a slow and a fast component in many cases of sick sinus syndrome makes therapy complex. Sometimes a pacemaker may be required to prevent the slow heartbeats. But because a pacemaker cannot prevent fast heartbeats, additional medications to slow the heartbeat may be needed. Unfortunately, giving medications without the pacemaker may slow the heartbeats even more and lead to worse symptoms.

Problems With the Conduction System. The third type of bradycardia occurs when the electrical impulse generated by the properly functioning sinus node fails to get to the pumping chambers of the heart (the ventricles). This condition is referred to as atrioventricular block (AV block), because there is either intermittent or continuous block of the electrical signal between the atria, where the signal originates in the sinus node, and the ventricles. Again, do not confuse this "block" with coronary blockage, which is a problem with blood flow

through the coronary arteries. Also, do not confuse it with "bundle-branch block," which is blockage of the electrical signal in only a branch of the conduction system. AV block is block of the one and only thoroughfare between the atria and ventricles. AV block is occasionally simply referred to as "heart block."

AV block occurs with varying degrees of severity. First-degree AV block was already mentioned (see page 86); it does not actually cause bradycardia. "Second-degree AV block" is more serious. It occurs when there is intermittent block of impulses traveling from the atria to the ventricles. The block may be frequent (every other beat), less frequent (every third, fourth, or fifth beat), or very rare. If it is frequent, it results in an overall slowing of the heartbeat. The sinus node may be issuing signals for the heart to beat at a rate of 80 beats per minute, but if every other signal is blocked, the heart will contract at a rate of only 40 beats per minute.

However, if the block occurs infrequently, then the overall heartbeat will not be slowed all that much. Nevertheless, there will be occasional small pauses between the heartbeats when the signal does not get through. Thus, second-degree AV block can also be considered a type of irregular rhythm.

"Third-degree AV block" is the most serious type of AV block, often resulting in severe and symptomatic bradycardia. In this case, no signal from the sinus node gets through to the ventricles. Another name for third-degree AV block is "complete heart block." Fortunately, most of the time the conduction system in the ventricles or the ventricular muscle itself can initiate impulses, so the heart does not stop entirely. But these substitute pace-

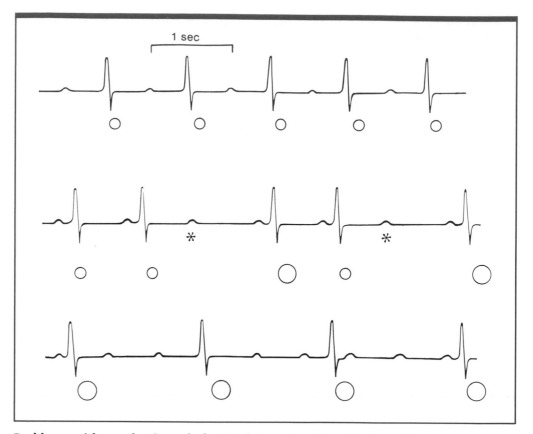

Problems with conduction of electrical impulses through the atrioventricular node range in severity.

Top, **The mildest form is first-degree atrioventricular block: the impulse is excessively slowed down as it passes through the atrioventricular node, causing a PR segment that is longer than normal. Compare the PR segment with that in the top figure on page 85.**

Middle, **Second-degree atrioventricular block occurs when some impulses originating from the sinus node do not get through the atrioventricular node. On the electrocardiogram, this is seen as some P waves (*) that are not followed by a QRS complex.**

Bottom, **The most severe form is third-degree atrioventricular block, also called complete heart block. In this situation, none of the impulses get through the atrioventricular node. On the electrocardiogram, none of the P waves are followed by a QRS complex. Instead, other parts of the conduction system may take over and produce a heartbeat, but at a much slower rate. You can see that the P waves and the QRS complexes are going at separate rates, unrelated to one another. The circles indicate that some heartbeats may feel stronger (the large circles) and more rapid (the circles that are close together) than normal.**

makers are too slow to allow the cardiovascular system to function efficiently. They are only backup systems to permit survival. However, they are not always reliable, and if they should fail the consequences could be lethal. So third-degree AV block is a medical emergency requiring treatment with a pacemaker in most cases. The only exceptions are rare individuals who are born with third-degree AV block (congenital complete heart block). They may do well until early adulthood, at which time a pacemaker is usually advisable.

Bradycardia

Possible Tests
Electrocardiography
(see page 192)
Ambulatory ECG monitoring
(see page 199)
Telephone-transmitted ECG
(see page 199)

Possible Treatment
Pacemaker (see page 280)

Irregular Heartbeats. Irregular heartbeats can take several forms. One type has already been mentioned—second-degree AV block. More common types of irregular rhythms are those related to the occurrence of extra heartbeats and those related to atrial fibrillation. Remember that even a perfectly normal heartbeat may have some irregularity to it, but this does not cause symptoms and is of no concern even when it is obvious on an electrocardiogram.

Symptoms of Irregular Heartbeats. Irregular heartbeats, if they cause any symptom at all, produce palpitations. As a result of awareness of palpitations, some people also develop anxiety and even fatigue from worry. Occasionally there may be associated unusual pains. By and large, however, irregular rhythms produce only palpitations, and many people with very irregular rhythms remain totally unaware of them.

Types of Irregular Rhythms
André is a 51-year-old corporate lawyer who has noted "thumps" in his chest for several years. These have become more frequent in the past several weeks, which he notes have also been a stressful time professionally. They do not really bother him, but he is concerned about their implications.

Extra Beats. André is likely experiencing extra beats, the most common type of irregular rhythm. In fact, everyone has occasional extra beats even if they are unaware of them. Thus, extra beats in themselves probably should not be considered abnormal because

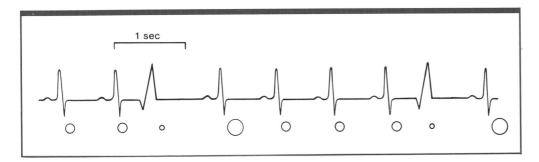

The heart can occasionally produce an early (premature) beat. The premature beats shown here originate in the ventricle. Premature beats sometimes are called "skipped beats" because it feels as if the heart is "missing" a beat. Actually, the premature beat produces only a very small pulse, as shown by the smallest circles, because the heart has not had time to fill after the previous beat. The beat after the premature beat, however, is stronger than normal to make up for the brief delay that occurs after the premature beat.

they are so common. They are abnormal when they occur frequently or in certain patterns or when they cause symptoms (palpitations). Extra beats can often increase, or be more noticeable, under stressful circumstances.

Extra beats are exactly what the name describes. (The technical term is "extrasystoles.") They are beats that are "inserted" between normal beats. In effect, they just occur too early, and therefore they beat the next normal beat to the punch. Thus, another term for them is "premature beats or contractions." Oddly enough, despite the presence of an *extra* beat, most people perceive a sensation of a small skip (thus, the term "skipped beats") between heartbeats followed by a "thud." The reason for this is that the premature beat is so early that it makes the heart contract before it has really had a chance to expand and fill with blood. So it is like firing a blank charge—no effective pulse is generated. *After* the premature beat, the heart usually has a little extra time for filling so the next normal beat enthusiastically pushes out a lot of blood with a rather big thump.

Premature beats can originate from the ventricles (ventricular premature contractions) or from above the ventricles (supraventricular premature contractions). Their only direct significance is the discomfort they may cause, especially if the palpitations are frequent. If ventricular premature beats are extremely frequent or occur in series of several in a row, *and* if they are associated with certain types of heart disease, they may be a warning sign of worse rhythms in the future. Under these circumstances, further evaluation and treatment may be appropriate.

Sara is a 54-year-old magazine editor in whom rapid pounding of her heart developed yesterday afternoon. She says her heart feels like it is racing and "out of sync." These symptoms do not seem to make her feel bad, but she is troubled by the constant "bumping around" in her chest and "fullness" in her throat. Her doctor takes her pulse: it is 128 beats per minute and irregular. The doctor makes a diagnosis of atrial fibrillation, and this is confirmed by an ECG. The findings on the rest of Sara's medical examination are satisfactory, although she tells the doctor she drinks 10 or 12 cups of regular coffee daily.

Atrial Fibrillation. A very common arrhythmia occurs when the atria cease to have effective orderly contractions and begin to quiver continuously. The activity of the sinus node is shut off, and the fibrillation takes over the rhythm of the heart. Because the atria are experiencing a continuous electrical impulse traveling through them, this impulse is also always trying to travel down through the atrioventricular node. The atrioventricular node, remember, functions like an electrical gate so it prevents a continuous flow of impulses into the pumping chambers. But many impulses get through at irregular intervals. The result is a very irregular rhythm with varying intervals between heartbeats. It also tends to be a fast heartbeat, so atrial fibrillation is also considered a form of tachycardia (see page 93). The heartbeat is so irregular that doctors refer to it as "irregularly irregular" to distinguish the cadence of the pulse from the patterned variations caused by second-degree AV block or premature beats.

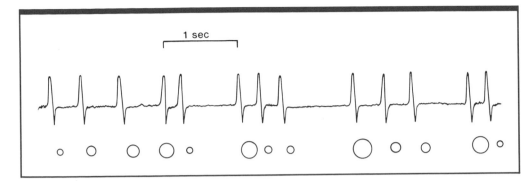

This electrocardiogram shows atrial fibrillation. The atria are twitching chaotically so no P waves are visible. Electrical impulses go through the atrioventricular node at irregular intervals and cause an irregular heart rate. As with premature contractions, the pulse (shown again by circles on the figure) caused by early heartbeats is weaker than the pulse after a longer interval.

Atrial fibrillation is prone to cause palpitations, and if it is exceedingly fast it may cause chest pain, shortness of breath, light-headedness, or fatigue. Without atrial contractions, the heart beats less efficiently; in individuals who may have weakened heart muscle to begin with, congestive heart failure may develop. Another consequence of atrial fibrillation is the risk of a blood clot forming in the atria. Because the atria are not actively contracting, blood may not swirl around as much when it passes through the atria. This lack of motion predisposes to clotting. The clot may dislodge and travel out of the heart into an artery and obstruct it (see page 99).

If you have atrial fibrillation, the initial goal of treatment is to regain normal sinus rhythm, either with medication or shock treatment (cardioversion). Caffeine and alcohol have been implicated as culprits in promoting the occurrence of fast rhythms in the atria, and they should be avoided once a normal rhythm is restored. Also, the doctor will order blood tests to determine whether the atrial fibrillation is

due to an overactive thyroid, which would require specific treatment. If cardioversion is unsuccessful, or if the atrial fibrillation recurs despite treatment with medications, the goal is to keep the rate of ventricular contractions at an acceptably slow pace, although it will still be irregular. Most people get used to the irregularity as long as the heart rate is not too fast.

Irregular Heartbeats

Possible Tests
Electrocardiography
   (see page 192)
Ambulatory ECG monitoring
   (see page 199)

Possible Treatment
Medication
   (see pages 279 and 307)

Tachycardia (Fast Heartbeats).
Tachycardia is another major problem for a large number of people. New techniques for assessing and treating tachycardia offer relief of symptoms

and better long-term outlook for people who have some of these rhythm disorders.

Symptoms of Tachycardia. Regardless of the specific type, tachycardia causes various symptoms, including palpitations, shortness of breath, angina, light-headedness, and syncope. Some types of tachycardia cause immediate symptoms (which may be bad enough) but also pose a risk of catastrophe, including death.

Classification of Tachycardia.
Tachycardia, like extra beats, can originate either from a ventricle (ventricular) or above a ventricle (supraventricular). Indeed, most types of tachycardia start from an extra beat at one of these sites. Different types of tachycardia can be present at either of these locations. In general, fast ventricular rhythms have more dire consequences because they make the heart function especially inefficiently, tend to cause more severe symptoms, and have a greater potential to result in death.

Types of Supraventricular Tachycardia. *Atrial flutter.* Like atrial fibril-

lation, atrial flutter is also a very rapid, ineffective beating of the atria, but it is somewhat more coordinated and regular. Atrial flutter causes the atria to beat about 300 times per minute. If the ventricles were also to beat at that rate, blood would not circulate efficiently. Luckily, the atrioventricular node usually performs its gating function and prevents at least every other atrial beat from being transmitted to the ventricles. Consequently, if you have atrial flutter your pulse rate is usually about 150 beats per minute. Sometimes the atrioventricular node lets only every third or every fourth beat through, in which case your heart rate would be 100 beats or 75 beats per minute, respectively.

The symptoms of atrial flutter are those of any tachycardia, namely, palpitations, chest pain, shortness of breath, or light-headedness.

Paroxysmal supraventricular tachycardia. This term applies to bursts of rapid heartbeats originating above the ventricles. They are usually all transmitted to the ventricles, but may occasionally be blocked. The bursts usually

A fast heartbeat can originate in the atria, such as shown in this electrocardiogram of a supraventricular tachycardia. Notice that about 2½ heartbeats occur every second, so this person's heart rate is 150 beats per minute.

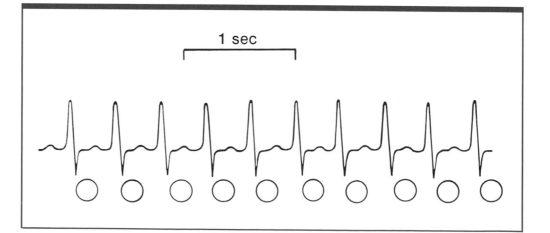

begin suddenly and end just as suddenly, sometimes with a pause that actually causes symptoms as well. The episodes can last seconds to hours or days, if not treated. The heart rate during supraventricular tachycardia can range from 140 to 240 beats per minute, and the degree of tachycardia symptoms depends in part on how fast the heart is going.

Supraventricular tachycardia is seldom life-threatening, but it can certainly produce bothersome symptoms. Conservative measures to reduce its frequency should be undertaken, such as avoiding caffeine or excess alcohol. Some people can "break" a spell of this type of rapid heartbeat by doing certain maneuvers that slow the heart rate. These include bearing down (as though straining at a bowel movement), gagging (by tickling the back of the throat), or splashing cold water on their faces. Numerous medications are available to help treat this rhythm disorder. Newer catheter techniques, as well as some operations, can cure people of some of these arrhythmias (see page 286).

Wolff-Parkinson-White syndrome.
One type of rapid heartbeat is caused by an abnormality of the conducting system. However, instead of an abnormality causing "block," it is an abnormality that consists of having an *extra* electrical pathway from the atria to the ventricles, in addition to the atrioventricular node. This is called an "accessory pathway." The accessory pathway is prone to conduct impulses rapidly, and it allows a situation to develop in which extremely rapid, and potentially dangerous, heart rhythms can occur. This is called the Wolff-Parkinson-White (or WPW) syndrome,

after the three physicians who first described it.

Although the presence of accessory pathways sometimes can be detected on an ECG, not everyone with an accessory pathway will develop tachycardias or require special treatment. While WPW is not common, it is certainly not rare either.

Types of Ventricular Tachycardia.
Ventricular tachycardia.   When used as a specific diagnosis, this term refers to a rapid, regular heartbeat originating from a site in one of the ventricles. The rate can be anywhere from about 100 to 250 beats per minute.

Many episodes of ventricular tachycardia (called VT or V tach) do not stop spontaneously, unlike paroxysmal supraventricular tachycardia. What is worse, there is a predisposition for the VT to deteriorate further into ventricular fibrillation. Thus, VT is usually a medical emergency, even if the symptoms it is causing are rather minimal. Most VT is associated with other serious heart disease, such as coronary artery blockage, cardiomyopathy, or congenital or valvular heart disease.

Treatment is directed first to ending the bout of VT. If intravenously administered medications do not produce immediate results, a shock to the chest is usually required (see Defibrillation and Cardioversion, page 283). The next step is to prevent the VT from returning; options are medications, correction of an underlying problem such as myocardial ischemia, use of an internal cardioverter-defibrillator (see page 284), or surgical or catheter techniques to eliminate the site in the ventricle that is causing the VT (see page 286).

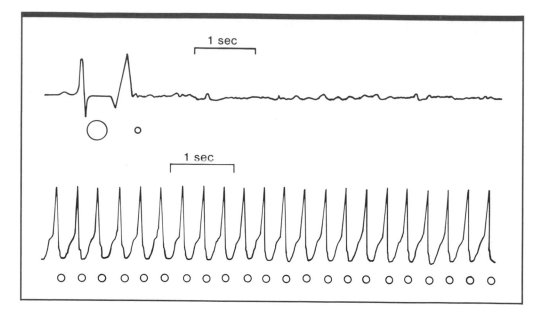

Top, Ventricular fibrillation is seen on this electrocardiogram after a normal beat and a ventricular premature beat. This chaotic twitching of the ventricles does not pump blood, so there is no pulse. Without cardiopulmonary resuscitation and defibrillation, this person would die.

Bottom, Ventricular tachycardia is a fast heartbeat originating in the ventricular muscle of the heart. In this example the heart rate is 180 beats per minute.

Tachycardia

Possible Tests
Electrocardiography
  (see page 192)
Ambulatory ECG monitoring
  (see page 199)
Stress ECG (see page 198)
Electrophysiology studies
  (see page 224)

Possible Treatment
Cardiopulmonary resuscitation
  (see page 241)
Medications (see pages 279,
  307)
Defibrillation or cardioversion
  (see page 283)
Internal cardioverter-defibrillator
  (see page 284)
Ablation (see page 286)

Ventricular fibrillation. The absolutely worst heart rhythm you can have is ventricular fibrillation (VF). In this condition there is no effective heartbeat—only useless quivering of the ventricular muscle. As far as circulation of blood is concerned, the heart is stopped. Do not confuse VF with atrial fibrillation. VF is the rhythm that is almost always the cause of "cardiac arrest" or "sudden cardiac death." Unless someone is nearby who can administer cardiopulmonary resuscitation (CPR; see page 241) when you go into VF, you will die. There are seldom second chances otherwise; this urgency underscores the importance of knowing CPR.

VF seldom occurs in the absence of other substantial problems with the heart, although rarely it may.

Diseases of the Arteries and Veins

On its journey from the heart to all the tissues in your body, your blood travels through the vascular system. The vascular system consists of the blood vessels—the arteries and veins. The vessels connected to the heart are the biggest in your body, with a diameter similar to that of a garden hose. The arteries branch into smaller vessels as they travel to your tissues, finally becoming capillaries that allow the passage of only one blood cell at a time.

In healthy persons, blood flow is regulated so that various parts of your body receive exactly the amount of blood they need. When you exercise, more blood goes to your muscles, and when you eat, more blood goes to your stomach and intestines. When you get hot, more blood flows to the outer layers of your skin to help dissipate the heat. When you are cold, blood is routed to deeper vessels away from your skin to help conserve heat.

The arteries function to carry oxygen and nutrients to the brain, other organs, and muscles. Veins function predominantly as a conduit to carry the deoxygenated blood back to the heart.

To accomplish these tasks, arteries and veins are structurally different. Arteries have muscle in their walls that enables them to expand or contract and actually helps route the blood to various parts of the body. Because veins carry blood back from the organs and body to the heart, they function under conditions of much lower pressures. Veins are thin and work more passively than arteries. They do not have the ability to squeeze or constrict as arteries do. Either the arteries or the veins can be affected by diseases but, in general, the diseases of these two different types of blood vessels are also different.

DISEASES OF THE ARTERIES.

Atherosclerosis.   The higher pressures that arteries work under make them susceptible to atherosclerosis. A degree of atherosclerosis eventually develops in almost everyone. As you age, the elastic fibers and smooth muscle cells of your arteries degenerate and are partially replaced by fibrous tissue. The arteries normally become thicker and less elastic, and the inner lining becomes abnormal.

Causes of Atherosclerosis.   In some people, the degeneration of the lining and walls of the arteries may be speeded up. The lining (endothelium) may be damaged. Blood platelets stick to the site of injury, and a chemical signal is activated that promotes an influx of cholesterol. Cholesterol and other substances such as calcium build up in the artery wall. Eventually, a plaque forms that bulges into the bloodstream and impedes blood flow through the artery.

Your risk of developing atherosclerosis increases if you smoke or have a family history of atherosclerosis. Diabetes, high blood pressure, and high levels of cholesterol in the blood increase your risk as well.

Many times the blockages are incomplete and develop over time, gradually narrowing the artery until the blood flow is nearly stopped. In some, but not all, cases the body can compensate for these narrowings by developing small branches, called collaterals, that bypass the narrowed sections or blockages. The collaterals, although helpful, are not always enough to restore circulation to an affected region of the body.

Symptoms of Atherosclerosis. Symptoms usually develop gradually with atherosclerosis. As the arteries become increasingly blocked, progressive symptoms frequently develop. The specific symptoms depend on which artery or arteries are obstructed. If the leg arteries are affected, then the symptoms are usually numbness, fatigue, or pain in the leg (claudication). Atherosclerotic obstruction of the coronary arteries may lead to symptoms of angina or even a heart attack. Other commonly affected arteries include the carotid arteries in the neck (a situation that predisposes to stroke) and the abdominal aorta (which may become partially obstructed and cause claudication or become weakened and lead to aneurysm).

Symptoms caused by progressive atherosclerotic narrowing of an artery are more likely to occur during exercise than at rest, at least initially. Early symptoms may occur only after great exertion, but as the narrowing worsens, less and less activity is required. The symptoms develop during exertion because your arteries cannot supply your muscles with enough oxygen and nutrients. The more severe the blockage, the less exertion it takes to surpass the ability of the artery to supply adequate blood. When you stop and rest, the discomfort resolves in a few minutes. However, blockages can be so severe that even resting muscle does not get enough blood flow, and you may experience symptoms, such as claudication or angina, even when sitting still.

Indeed, it is the symptoms caused by inadequate blood flow to a part of the body that may bring you to a physician, who then attempts to discover the cause. Atherosclerosis is the cause of chronic obstruction of the arteries in 95 percent of cases, but other causes are important to know about.

Atherosclerotic Blockage

Possible Tests
Measurement of blood lipids
    (see page 190)
Noninvasive vascular studies
    (for limb artery blockage)
    (see page 227)
Angiography (carotid or limb
    artery blockage)

See page 75 for possible tests
    for angina that could be
    caused by atherosclerotic
    blockage in coronary arteries

Possible Treatment
Smoking cessation
    (see page 146)
Lipid control
    (see pages 132, 148, and
    302)
Exercise (for limb artery
    blockage) (see page 99)
Balloon catheter dilation
    (see page 287)
Surgical removal of blockage
    (see page 287)
Bypass of blockage
    (see page 287)

See page 75 for possible
    treatments for angina that
    could be caused by
    atherosclerotic blockage in
    coronary arteries

Arterial Thrombosis and Arterial Embolism. Sometimes clotting of blood (thrombosis) inside an artery results in a blockage (see Figures 30 and 31, page A10). A blood clot that forms and stays at its place of origin inside a blood vessel (or the heart) is called a thrombus. A thrombus can partially or totally obstruct the artery and prevent sufficient blood flow.

When a blood clot forms in one place but breaks off and travels through the blood vessels to another point in the circulation where it lodges, the resulting problem is referred to as thromboembol*ism*. The actual blood clot is a thromboembolus. A thromboembolus is often referred to simply as an embolus. Emboli can also originate from infected cells in the circulation (septic emboli), from cancer cells that enter the circulation (tumor emboli), or from fat cells that enter the bloodstream, especially after major bone fractures (fat emboli).

A sudden blockage (occlusion) may occur when an embolus lodges in one of your arteries. Blood clots can originate from the chambers of the heart or can develop in large arteries and lodge in smaller arteries after they break loose. This process often occurs where arteries branch or divide.

Symptoms of Embolism. When arteries are suddenly blocked, there is no time for collateral arteries to develop, and the blood flow to the tissues beyond the blockage literally stops. This blockage results in pain, whiteness, weakness, tingling, numbness, or coldness below a blockage in an artery to one of your limbs. If an embolus lodges in an artery to the brain, a stroke results. A coronary artery embolus may

Living with claudication— what can help?

Although intermittent claudication does not affect your life expectancy, it may affect your life-style. Treatment options include a walking program, medication, and correction of the arterial obstruction by surgery or angioplasty.

- If it hurts to walk, why might your doctor recommend a regular walking program? The answer is that regular walking for periods of 30 minutes (stopping to rest as necessary) 5 days a week may increase your ability to walk, climb stairs, or complete other physical tasks of everyday living. Regular walking promotes the development of collateral vessels and promotes blood flow to the affected muscles. This may result in an actual improvement in blood flow and may slow progression of the disease.
- Medications that decrease blood viscosity, in a sense making it easier for the blood to flow through narrowed vessels, may improve your comfort while walking.
- Surgery or angioplasty (dilating the narrowed site of an artery with a balloon catheter) is often elective (optional); it depends on your need or desire to walk farther. If you have a nonhealing skin ulcer or pain at rest due to severe obstruction of arterial blood flow, then improving blood flow by angioplasty or surgery is recommended to relieve symptoms and lessen the risk of amputation.

produce a myocardial infarction (heart attack).

How Serious Is Embolism? If the blood supply is cut off to a limb, finger, or toe for more than a few hours, the muscle and skin in an affected limb may become gangrenous. If the blockage is not removed or dissolved promptly, the tissue below the blockage may die and require amputation.

Atherosclerosis partially blocks this carotid artery, and thrombus (clot) has also formed. If any of the blockage breaks free, it would travel up to a branch of an artery in the brain and completely block blood flow. The result would be a stroke (see also Figure 48, page A15).

Embolic or Thrombotic Blockage

Possible Tests

Electrocardiography (for coronary artery blockage) (see page 192)

Noninvasive vascular studies (for limb artery blockage) (see page 227)

Angiography (coronary, carotid, or limb artery blockage)

Possible Treatment

Medication to dissolve blood clot (see pages 266 and 301)

Surgical removal of blockage (see page 288)

Stroke: A Neurologic Condition Related to Cardiovascular Disease. Stroke refers to a brain injury that is caused by an inadequate supply of blood (ischemia) to the brain. Transient ischemic attacks (TIAs) are temporary episodes that resemble a stroke. They are regarded as serious warning signs that a stroke may occur in the future.

Because the brain is the organ affected by strokes, if you have a stroke you will be attended to by a neurologist. However, strokes are closely related to cardiovascular disease and therefore are mentioned here.

Causes of Stroke. Many strokes are caused by a small bit of clot or cholesterol debris breaking off from its site of formation in the carotid arteries in the neck. The clot travels up in the bloodstream through smaller branches of the artery until it becomes wedged into a small branch in the brain and blocks further blood flow. This is called a cerebral embolism.

Clot or debris can also form in the aorta upstream from the branches of the carotid arteries or in the left side of the heart such as the left atrium, left ventricle, and artificial valves in the aortic or mitral position. The clot can break off and travel to the brain, where it causes a stroke.

Atherosclerosis or a blood clot that forms and stays in the carotid or cerebral artery (arteries in the neck and brain) can block blood flow enough to cause TIAs or a stroke. This condition, called cerebral thrombosis, differs from cerebral embolism in that the clot has not moved from its site of origin.

A less common but important cause of stroke is formation and release of a blood clot from a vein in the legs (an

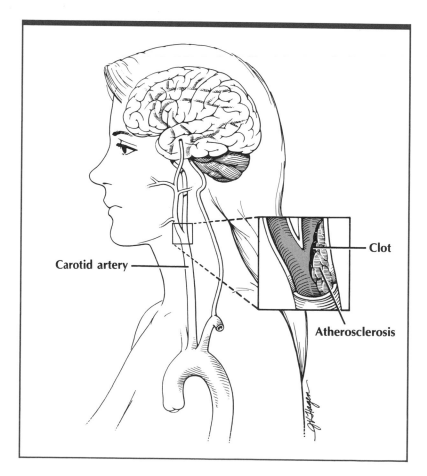

Carotid artery

Clot

Atherosclerosis

event that in itself is *not* rare) that travels to the heart. The clot crosses from the right side of the heart to the left side of the heart through an abnormal opening in the septum (partition that divides the atria and ventricles). From the left side of the heart, the clot then proceeds through the arterial circulation into the brain, where it causes a stroke. This event is occasionally the first sign that there is a hole in the wall separating the two sides of the heart (septal defect).

Not all strokes are caused by clots or obstruction. Other causes of stroke include bleeding into the brain (cerebral hemorrhage) or around the surface of the brain (subarachnoid hemorrhage).

Symptoms of Stroke. The symptoms of stroke can be extremely varied, because they depend on which area of the brain was affected. Symptoms can include paralysis or weakness of a limb, abnormalities of sensation (such as numbness of a limb), and defects of speech, comprehension, or vision.

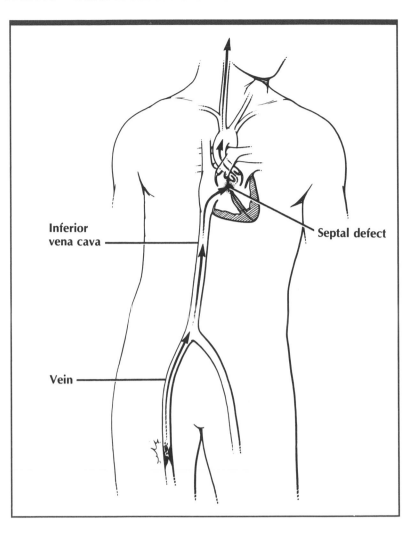

Inferior vena cava

Septal defect

Vein

TIAs or Stroke

Possible Tests

Computed tomography scanning of the head

Magnetic resonance imaging of the head

Angiography (carotid)

Oculoplethysmography (see page 229)

Duplex scanning (see page 231)

Echocardiography (see page 209)

How Serious Is Stroke? Depending on the severity and location of the stroke, it is often possible for the person to improve with physical therapy or by relearning skills that were lost, but there is a residual defect in half the people who survive. Of the 500,000 people in the United States who have a stroke each year, about one-quarter of them die.

Aneurysms. Sometimes atherosclerosis can damage the walls of blood vessels and lead to a situation in which the arteries, including the aorta, de-

Rarely, a stroke can be caused by a blood clot that forms in a leg vein, breaks away and crosses through to the left side of the heart (by way of a septal defect), and then proceeds into an artery of the brain.

velop abnormally widened areas called aneurysms (see Figure 49, page A15). Aneurysms can occur in virtually any artery, but the segment of the aorta that runs through the abdomen is the most common site of localized ballooning. Other sites of aneurysm are the aorta in the chest and the arteries in the thigh and behind the knee.

Causes of Aneurysm.   More than 90 percent of abdominal aortic aneurysms are associated with atherosclerosis.

Symptoms of Aneurysm.   Most abdominal aortic aneurysms do not produce symptoms, but some people feel a pulsating sensation in the abdomen. These silent (asymptomatic) aneurysms are often recognized by careful physical examination, chest X-ray, and ultrasonography. When aneurysms do not cause symptoms and are small, they can be safely watched and do not require surgery. It is important, however, to have periodic evaluations. When aneurysms become larger the chance of sudden rupture is greater, and these should be surgically repaired.

Who Is Affected by Aneurysm?   Abdominal aortic aneurysm is most likely to occur in people older than 60 years, and it affects men more often than women.

How Serious Is an Aneurysm?   The main risk of an abdominal aortic aneurysm is that, like a balloon that is blown up too far, it may rupture, and rupture results in life-threatening internal hemorrhage (bleeding). The larger the aneurysm gets, the more likely it is to rupture. Timely surgery prevents rupture.

Surgery usually is warranted only when the aorta (which normally has a diameter of less than 1 inch) enlarges to about 2 inches, because the likelihood of rupture increases at that point. A 2-inch-wide aneurysm has a 1 in 25 chance of rupturing within 1 year. An aneurysm that is 2¾ inches across has a 1 in 5 chance of rupturing in the next year. Aneurysms usually grow about ⅛ to ¼ inch per year, but this rate can be highly variable.

Surgical correction often involves replacing a part of the diseased artery with a graft or tube made from synthetic materials.

Abdominal Aortic Aneurysm

Possible Tests
Noninvasive vascular studies
    (ultrasound) (see Figure 49A,
    page A15)
Angiography (aortography)

Possible Treatment
Surgical repair (see page 289)

Berry Aneurysm.   Important, but less common, types of aneurysm are not related to atherosclerosis. Berry aneurysms are bulges in the walls of arteries within the brain. As the name implies, they appear like little berries attached to a blood vessel, usually at a point of branching. They usually do not cause symptoms unless they rupture, in which case they may cause stroke or coma or be fatal.

Aortic Dissection.   Dissection is a catastrophic form of arterial disease. It usually involves the aorta or a portion of it (aortic dissection). Dissection means that layers of the wall of the aorta separate. The inner layer peels off from the remainder of the vessel so that blood can be forced between the layers, extending the dissection along the involved artery.

Causes of Dissection.   Aortic dissection tends to occur in persons with high blood pressure. There is also some association with diseases that cause general defects in the structural tissue of the body such as a hereditary syndrome called Marfan's syndrome, abnormalities of the blood vessel walls such as cystic medial necrosis, certain types of atherosclerotic plaques that burrow into the heart vessel wall, certain types of arteritis (inflammation of arteries), bicuspid aortic valve (two cusps instead of the normal three), and pregnancy.

Symptoms of Dissection.   Dissection of the aorta causes sharp and tearing chest and back pain. Often the pain is focused in the back between the shoulder blades, although it may descend into the lower back as well or feel as if it is "boring" into the chest. Typically the pain is severe and comes on suddenly. It can be vague or like angina (see page 72), and it is sometimes misinterpreted at first by both patients and doctors as a heart attack.

Who Is Affected by Dissection?   Dissection of the aorta is two to three times more common in men than in women. It usually occurs between ages 40 and 70 years.

How Serious Is Dissection?   This condition is often fatal if the blood erupts outside the aorta. The dissection

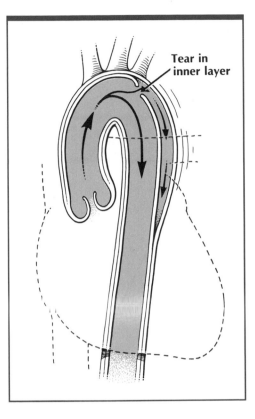

Tear in inner layer

An aortic dissection occurs when blood pushes forcefully into a tear in the inner layer of the aortic wall and splits the inner layer away from the outer layer.

can extend into or block branch vessels of the aorta, such as the carotid arteries to the brain and arteries to the arms, kidneys, legs, or spinal cord. The result is decreased or absent blood flow to these organs. Dissection of the aorta may require urgent surgery, depending on the areas of the aorta that are involved. Even before surgery, though, the first goals of management are to reduce blood pressure to the lowest acceptable level and to determine the portion of the aorta involved by the tear.

The aorta may be ruptured in crushing injuries or with sudden deceleration such as in automobile accidents or falls. With sudden deceleration, aortic rupture usually occurs in the chest and is usually fatal. Aortic injury due to penetrating wounds usually results in life-threatening hemorrhage (bleeding).

Aortic Dissection

Possible Tests
Electrocardiography
   (see page 192)
Echocardiography
   (see page 209)
Computed tomography
   (see page 231)
Angiography (aortography)

Possible Treatment
Blood pressure reduction
   (see page 289)
Surgical repair (see page 289)

Inflammation of Arteries.   In some diseases, arteries become inflamed. The inflammation can result in narrowing of the opening (bore or lumen) of the vessels. The medical term for inflammation of the artery is arteritis. If the inflammation persists, the vessel may become permanently scarred and narrow. There are many different types of arteritis. Although each type has different symptoms and can affect different arteries, the primary goal of treatment is to reduce the inflammation and prevent scarring of the arteries.

Typically, arteritis is part of a generalized illness with disease in other organs.

Examples of arteritis are the following:

- Takayasu's disease
- Temporal arteritis
- Buerger's disease
- Polyarteritis nodosa

Takayasu's Disease.   This is also called "pulseless disease," because some pulses usually present are absent. Takayasu's disease is rare and oc-curs mostly in women younger than 40 years. It occurs in women nine times more often than in men. It is an inflammatory process that most commonly produces marked thickening of the aorta and its main branches, eventually blocking the major branches of the arteries. The blockage reduces the pulse downstream, for example, at the wrist if the artery to the arm is involved.

Temporal Arteritis.   Temporal arteritis is also called cranial arteritis or giant cell arteritis. People who have temporal arteritis are almost always older than 55. It is twice as common in women as in men. In this disease, the inflammation may involve one or both temporal arteries on the side of the head. Headache and a tender, red, inflamed artery in the temple are clues to the diagnosis, which can be verified by removing a tiny sample (biopsy) of the affected artery. Treatment with corticosteroids controls this disease and prevents complications such as blindness.

Buerger's Disease.   One particularly severe form of vessel inflammation is thromboangiitis obliterans, also called Buerger's disease. In this disease, inflammation obliterates small and medium-sized arteries. It occurs most commonly in men younger than 30 years who use tobacco. Redness and tenderness of superficial veins of the feet or legs and pain in the arch of the foot or calf when walking suggest Buerger's disease.

Progression of Buerger's disease can be thwarted by abstaining from tobacco use. People in whom the disease continues are usually those who continue to smoke.

Polyarteritis Nodosa. As the name suggests, polyarteritis involves inflammation (*itis*) of many (*poly*) arteries. The areas at greatest risk are the skin, intestines, kidney, and heart, although any area of the body can suffer. Symptoms are often vague: unexplained weight loss, progressive fatigue, weakness, and fever. The diagnosis is confirmed by removing a tiny sample (biopsy) of the involved part of the body for microscopic evaluation of the arteries. Treatment is a prolonged course of corticosteroids, often supplemented by other medications.

Fibromuscular Dysplasia (Overgrowth of Muscle in Artery Walls). Another cause of obstruction in the blood vessels is overgrowth of the muscle in the wall of the artery, which is called fibromuscular dysplasia. The arteries to the kidneys are most vulnerable. Renal (kidney) arteries can also develop atherosclerotic blockages.

Regardless of cause, when blood flow is diminished to the kidneys, your blood pressure tends to increase. Here's why: when your kidneys get inadequate blood flow they react as though blood pressure were low all over the body. This response triggers the kidneys to release hormone "messengers" that increase blood pressure. This process is similar to blowing cold air on a thermostat: the thermostat responds by increasing the heat in the whole house. Artery blockage in the kidneys can also lead to a decrease in their ability to eliminate waste products.

Arterial Spasm. Spasm of the arteries is a rare cause of arterial blockage. Often it is associated with taking medications that provoke spasm, especially ergots (which are in some medications used to treat migraine headaches).

Raynaud's Phenomenon. Raynaud's phenomenon is an exaggerated response to the normal reflex mechanism which causes blood vessels in the hands and feet to narrow (spasm) in the cold or with emotion. It affects 1 in 20 Americans to some degree, mostly women.

If you experience Raynaud's phenomenon, your fingers or toes (and in some people, ears and nose) turn chalky white when you are exposed to cold, and they also sting. Your skin may turn blue or bright red upon return to a warmer environment before normal color returns.

Raynaud's Phenomenon

Possible Tests
Noninvasive vascular studies
    (see page 230)

Possible Treatment
Medications (see page 290)

DISEASES OF THE VEINS.
Venous Thrombosis. Diseases of the veins are different from those of the arteries because of the structural differences. Blockages can occur in the veins, but these are usually caused by blood clots (thrombi) and not by atherosclerosis. When a thrombus forms in a vein, blood is prevented from traveling back toward the heart. The collection of blood results in increased pressure and often leads to swelling and tenderness. For example, a blood clot in the deep vein of the calf will cause the calf and foot to become swollen and tender. This condition is referred to as deep venous thrombosis.

The leg is still getting enough oxygen and nutrients from the arteries, so it is not threatened, but the back pressure of unreturned blood and the resulting seepage of fluid into the surrounding tissues (edema) can be uncomfortable. Clotting of blood in the veins tends to occur whenever the blood flow in the vein is slow or becomes stagnant. Typically this occurs in the legs when you are still, as in a long ride in a car or plane, when you are constantly in bed because of illness or surgery, or after an injury to the leg.

The main risk of blood clots forming and causing deep venous thrombosis is that the blood clot can enlarge and extend up the vein. If a piece breaks off, it can travel upstream and lodge in the heart or lungs. Just as in the arterial circulation, this disorder is called thromboembolism. A thrombus that dislodges from a vein in the leg will travel through larger and larger veins until it reaches the right side of the heart. From there it will enter the pulmonary artery and lodge in a branch, at which point it blocks blood flow to part of the lung. A clot in the lung circulation is a pulmonary embolus.

Treatment with anticoagulants ("blood thinners") in the early stages of deep venous thrombosis can prevent enlargement of the clot and lessen the likelihood of pulmonary embolism.

Thrombophlebitis. Thrombophlebitis means clotting of blood (*thrombus*) and inflammation (*itis*) in a vein, most commonly in the legs. It is often just called phlebitis. It can affect either the deep or surface (superficial) veins.

Symptoms of Thrombophlebitis. When the deep veins are involved, your leg may become tender, painful, and swollen. You may also have a fever. When a superficial vein is involved, a red, hard, and tender bump or cord

Tips for preventing blood clots during long-distance travel

You are packed into a crowded airplane, bracing yourself for the 7-hour ride to your vacation or business destination. If you remain motionless in your seat for the duration, you increase your risk for the development of potentially dangerous blood clots.

Blood clots interfere with blood flow and can break loose and travel to an artery in one of your lungs. Clots can form while you sit for extended periods in cramped quarters. This problem can happen during any form of travel, but it is more common on long airline flights, especially if you are sitting in the coach section. Doctors therefore have coined the term "economy class syndrome."

Despite its name, "economy class syndrome" can develop regardless of whether you sit in first class or in the coach section. On long-distance flights or rides, follow these tips.

- Wear loose, comfortable clothing and shoes. Airlines often provide customers in the first-class cabin with bootie socks. It is easy to bring your own. They help keep your feet warm and are not as tight or confining as shoes.
- Stretch your legs occasionally, even while remaining in your seat.
- From time to time, tighten and loosen the muscles of your abdomen and buttocks.
- Take a few slow, deep breaths periodically.
- Get out of your seat and walk the aisle at least once an hour.
- Ask your doctor whether it is appropriate for you to use aspirin when you travel. Small doses of aspirin may help prevent clots from occurring. Remember to check with your doctor first, because aspirin is not recommended for everyone.
- If you have had problems with thrombophlebitis in the past, wear elastic support stockings when prolonged sitting is unavoidable. Elastic support stockings are available for both men and women.

may be present under the surface of the skin.

Who Is Affected by Thrombophlebitis? Your risk for thrombophlebitis increases if you are confined or immobile for prolonged periods. Thrombophlebitis commonly occurs after surgery, heart attack, hip or leg fracture, or prolonged bed rest or inactivity (such as sitting for a long time in a plane or car). Cancer patients also have a higher risk, as do people who are overweight, who use oral contraceptives, or whose blood has an abnormally high tendency to clot.

How Serious Is Thrombophlebitis? If the thrombophlebitis is in a superficial vein lying just under the skin, serious complications are rare. However, if the clotting is in a deep vein, the valves in the veins (see page 18) may be damaged, and this damage leads to future problems of swelling of the leg. If a portion of the thrombus is dislodged, it may travel to the lung and cause pulmonary embolism.

If the thrombophlebitis is in a superficial vein, your doctor may recommend applying heat to the sore area, elevating the leg, and using an anti-inflammatory drug. If your thrombophlebitis is in a deep vein, treatment will require hospitalization. Your leg will be elevated and an anticoagulant drug will be administered intravenously. Occasionally, if blood thinners have not been effective or cannot be given for some reason, it may be necessary to insert a "filter" into the inferior vena cava (the vein that carries blood back to the heart) to prevent the clot from traveling to your lungs. The filter can be inserted either with a catheter or a surgical procedure.

Venous Thrombosis or Thrombophlebitis

Possible Tests
Noninvasive vascular studies
   (see page 227)
Angiography (venography)

Possible Treatment
Anticoagulation (see pages 253, 290, 310)
Dissolving of blood clot
   (see pages 266 and 301)

Pulmonary Embolism. Sometime with thrombosis or thrombophlebitis of a deep vein, a portion of the thrombus becomes detached and travels through the veins to the right side of the heart and is then pumped into the lung circulation, where it blocks an artery in the lung. This is called pulmonary embolism.

Symptoms of Pulmonary Embolism. Depending on the size of the pulmonary embolus, it can cause chest pain, shortness of breath, or cough (that may produce blood-streaked sputum). In extreme cases, loss of consciousness or even sudden death may occur.

Pulmonary embolism may not be suspected, especially if the person has heart and lung disease already. Prompt diagnosis is critical, because about 10 percent of people with pulmonary embolism die within the first hour.

Who Is Affected by Pulmonary Embolism? Your risk of having a pulmonary embolus increases if you are confined or immobile for prolonged periods, in other words, the same conditions that are likely to cause deep venous thrombosis or thrombophlebitis. The most likely times for pulmo-

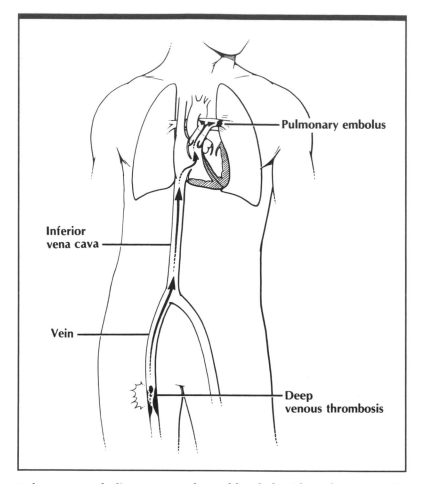

Pulmonary embolus

Inferior
vena cava

Vein

Deep
venous thrombosis

Pulmonary embolism occurs when a blood clot (thrombus) in a vein breaks loose and travels toward and through the right side of the heart, until it finally lodges in a pulmonary artery. This blocks blood flow to a portion of the lung and may result in pain, shortness of breath due to inadequate oxygenation of blood, reduced overall blood flow and blood pressure, and even death.

nary embolism to occur are after surgery, stroke, heart attack, hip or leg fracture, or prolonged bed rest or inactivity (such as sitting for a long time in a plane or car). Your risk is also higher if you are overweight or if your blood has an abnormally high tendency to clot.

How Serious Is Pulmonary Embolism? With appropriate diagnosis and treatment, the outlook is good for people who survive the immediate

event. Blood thinners (anticoagulant drugs) can keep the thrombus in the vein from enlarging and prevent further thrombus in other veins from forming. Surgery to remove the blood clot or treatment with agents to dissolve thrombi or thromboemboli (thrombolytic drugs) is sometimes necessary for massive pulmonary embolism.

Unless you have other problems, you should be back to normal within a few weeks. Typically, you will be treated with an orally administered anticoagulant (warfarin) for about 3 months after you leave the hospital. You should make a point to be as active as possible and avoid long periods of sitting without moving around. Elevating your legs and wearing specially prescribed support stockings will also help prevent the blood from pooling and clotting in your legs. Some people, particularly those at high risk or with recurring pulmonary embolism, may have to take anticoagulant drugs indefinitely.

Pulmonary Embolism

Possible Tests
Arterial blood gas tests
(see page 191)
Noninvasive vascular studies
(see page 227)
Ventilation-perfusion lung
scanning (see page 206)
Angiography (pulmonary
angiography) (see page 218)

Possible Treatment
Anticoagulation (see pages 253, 290, 310)
Medication to dissolve blood
clot (see pages 266 and 301)
Surgical removal of blood clot
(see page 291)

Destruction of Vein Valves From Thrombophlebitis (Chronic Venous Insufficiency). Another consequence of thrombophlebitis, especially in the deep veins of the legs, is damage of the valves in the affected veins. These valves prevent backward (downward) flow of blood in the veins when you stand up. Because veins do not have muscle in their walls to help "pump" the blood back to the heart, they are affected by gravity and the gentle squeezing provided by the surrounding skeletal muscle. To improve the flow of blood back to the heart, veins have valves. These valves work like safety cogs on mountain trains, which prevent them from rolling backward if they lose power while climbing up a steep mountain slope. In much the same way, the valves in the veins prevent the blood from "flowing back" as it is gradually pushed uphill toward the heart.

When the valves in the veins do not work properly, several problems can occur. The pooling of blood can lead to ballooning of the vein, resulting in varicose veins. In some cases the pooling gets so bad that the leg swells. This condition is commonly referred to as venous insufficiency. With chronic swelling and the associated increase in pressure on the skin, discoloration called stasis pigmentation can develop in some people, and in severe cases, actual skin ulceration can develop.

Venous Insufficiency

Possible Tests
Noninvasive vascular studies
   (see page 227)

Possible Treatment
Support hosiery; leg elevation

Varicose Veins. The term "varicose veins" refers to veins that are abnormally dilated. When the veins close to the surface of the legs become varicose, you can see them as soft, bluish, curving bulges under the skin.

Causes of Varicose Veins. Conditions that may lead to varicose veins include pregnancy (because the large uterus can press on veins in the abdomen and cause back pressure to build up in the leg veins), previous thrombophlebitis, or obesity. All of these problems elevate the pressure in the leg veins or damage the valves of the veins or both.

Some people are born without venous valves or without an adequate number of valves. These people frequently get large varicose veins at an early age.

Symptoms of Varicose Veins. Besides the unsightly appearance, varicose veins may cause aching and swelling in the legs.

Who Is Affected by Varicose Veins? One in 10 Americans has varicose veins. Women are twice as likely to have them as men, because of the effect of pregnancy.

How Serious Are Varicose Veins? For many people they are only a cosmetic annoyance. Still others have minor symptoms of mild swelling and a feeling of heaviness or aching in the legs at the end of the day. In some cases, varicose veins are serious enough to lead to chronic skin thickening or ulceration. For many people, support or elastic stockings to help counteract the increased pressure in the veins are extremely helpful for limiting swelling and other more serious complications.

Over time, varicose veins tend to become more prominent. You can help slow progression of your varicose veins by using elastic support stockings, by not standing for too long, or by not being too sedentary. Move around as much as possible, but periodically lie down and elevate your legs above the level of your heart ("toes above the nose") at the end of the day to help relieve swelling. Regular exercise will also decrease the pressure in the veins.

Surgery to strip or remove the varicose veins can be performed in severe cases. In one study, 85 percent of people who had surgery had no recurrence of the varicose veins during the next 10 years. If you have small and less severe varicose veins, you might be best treated with injection of the veins or with a laser.

Laser therapy may be used on very small, superficial blood vessels, but injection therapy (sclerotherapy) is usually best if the blood vessels are large enough for the procedure to be performed. Sclerotherapy may be helpful alone or in combination with surgery. Sclerotherapy is done on an outpatient basis. The physician slowly injects a solution into one or several of the visible veins while you are standing. Then, a small bandage is wrapped snugly over the veins for 24 hours. It may take more than one treatment session to achieve optimal results.

Sclerotherapy collapses the veins, and blood is then prevented from flowing into them and the discoloration is eliminated within about a month. The treatment has no significant effect on circulation in the leg. In about one-third of people who have sclerotherapy, a yellow-brown discol-

oration may appear in the area and can take weeks, months, or even longer to fade.

DISEASES OF THE PULMONARY ARTERIES.
Atherosclerosis can be present in pulmonary arteries, but it seldom if ever produces symptoms or other problems. Also, the pulmonary arteries are the "target" of emboli that may form in the deep veins of the legs, and they may also be involved in inflammatory conditions (see page 104). The pulmonary arteries, however, are subject to some problems that are different from those affecting the arteries that serve the rest of the body or from problems with the veins.

Pulmonary Hypertension. The condition that most commonly affects the pulmonary circulation is pulmonary hypertension. This general term refers to conditions that raise the blood pressure in the arteries to the lungs but not in other arteries.

Causes of Pulmonary Hypertension. In most cases of pulmonary embolism in which the initial event is survived, there are no subsequent problems with the pulmonary arteries. However, in rare cases the embolus does not dissolve and instead remains as an obstruction to blood flow through the lungs. The final result may be pulmonary hypertension.

Congenital heart conditions in which there is excessive blood flow through the pulmonary blood vessels may also lead to a condition of severe pulmonary hypertension known as Eisenmenger's complex (see page 55).

Any situation that continuously lowers the amount of oxygen getting into the bloodstream, whether it is due to constant living at a very high altitude or to emphysema, may elevate pulmonary blood pressure.

Finally, pulmonary hypertension can exist in the absence of any apparent cause. This is called primary pulmonary hypertension, to indicate that it is the main problem rather than secondary to another problem.

Symptoms of Pulmonary Hypertension. The earliest symptoms are usually tiredness and shortness of breath that become progressively worse with time. Other symptoms include angina (chest pain), passing out spells (syncope), and blueness of the skin (cyanosis). In the later stages of the disease, the right ventricle can no longer pump blood effectively, and symptoms of right ventricular failure develop: swelling of the legs, enlargement and pain in the abdomen, loss of appetite, and bulging of the jugular veins in the neck.

Who Is Affected by Pulmonary Hypertension? Individuals with previous pulmonary embolism, chronic emphysema, and certain types of congenital heart disease are at higher risk for the development of pulmonary hypertension. Primary pulmonary hypertension is rare; it occurs most often in young adults, but it can occur at any age. It affects about twice as many women as men.

How Serious Is Pulmonary Hypertension? Pulmonary hypertension is usually a very debilitating problem; however, the symptoms and life expectancy are extremely variable, even for people with the same degree of pulmonary blood pressure elevation. People with Eisenmenger's complex seem to be able to endure very severe pulmonary hypertension for years, although they may be limited in their

activities. In people with primary pulmonary hypertension, symptoms tend to develop more rapidly and life expectancy is shorter.

Pulmonary Hypertension

Possible Tests
Arterial blood gas studies
   (see page 191)
Electrocardiography
   (see page 192)
Chest X-ray (see page 200)
Ventilation-perfusion lung
   scanning (see page 206)
Echocardiography
   (see page 209)
Angiography (pulmonary
   angiography) (see page 218)
Computed tomography or
   magnetic resonance imaging
   (see page 231)
Pulmonary function (breathing)
   tests

Possible Treatment
Anticoagulation (see pages 253,
   290, 310)
Medications to reduce blood
   pressure (see page 304)
Lung transplantation

DISEASES OF BOTH THE ARTERIES AND THE VEINS. An uncommon problem with blood vessels is a malformation in which arteries and veins are directly connected, instead of being joined by capillaries. This can take two general forms: arteriovenous malformation, which is a congenital condition, and arteriovenous fistula, which is usually the result of trauma.

Arteriovenous malformations are "tangles" of small arterial vessels that are intertwined with small veins. The blood from the arteries flows directly into the veins. These malformations can be present anywhere in the body and in any organ. The consequences of having an arteriovenous malformation depend on their location and size. A small one in the brain may produce more problems than a larger one in the liver, for example.

A fistula can be thought of as a window or conduit that directly connects a large artery with a large vein. This might occur if a person receives a puncture wound that penetrates through an artery and vein that lie next to each other. Even after the healing process occurs, a connecting pathway between the two vessels may remain. Some blood from the artery may be diverted (shunted) directly into the vein before it goes to the capillaries. If a fistula (or arteriovenous malformation) is large, the blood flow through it may be very high. If so, the heart works excessively hard to keep up with the needs of the body.

Some arteriovenous malformations can be fixed by blocking the artery from which they branch. This can occasionally be done by inserting a special small balloon or other material directly into the artery with a catheter.

Arteriovenous Malformation or Fistula

Possible Tests
Noninvasive vascular studies
    (see page 227)
Angiography (venography)
Computed tomography or
    magnetic resonance imaging
    (see page 231)

Possible Treatment
Blockage with a catheter;
    surgical removal or repair

Pericardial Disease

The pericardium is the sac that surrounds the heart and portions of the great vessels (see Figure 50, page A16). It anchors the heart in place in your chest, protects it from nearby inflammation, and reduces the friction that is caused by your heart's beating.

The pericardium can be a site of disease caused by inflammation, fluid accumulation (effusion), or stiffness (constriction). These forms may occur singly or in combination.

INFLAMMATION OF THE PERICARDIUM. Inflammation of the pericardium is called pericarditis. It occurs most often in men between ages 20 and 50 years, sometimes after a respiratory infection.

Causes of Inflammation of the Pericardium. Causes of inflammation of the pericardium include infection, usually from a virus, or widespread inflammatory diseases such as lupus (systemic lupus erythematosus). Pericarditis may result from cancer or radiation to treat some types of cancer. However, in most cases the cause is unknown.

Symptoms of Inflammation of the Pericardium. Inflammation of the pericardium produces a fairly characteristic set of symptoms and findings on examination. The main symptom is chest pain, but usually it is very different from angina. Typically, it is a sharp, piercing pain over the center or left side of the chest. The pain can extend up to the left shoulder and worsen when you take a deep breath. It can be lessened somewhat by sitting up and leaning forward and worsened by lying down.

Although this is the classic pattern, the pain can also be insidious or dull. You may have a low-grade fever, and in general, you just feel sick. Some people have pain with swallowing.

How Serious Is Inflammation of the Pericardium? Acute inflammatory pericarditis usually lasts 2 to 6 weeks and does not lead to any further problems. About one in five people has a recurrence within months or rarely within years. Each recurrence tends to be less severe, until the episodes finally stop.

PERICARDIAL EFFUSION. Pericardial effusion means that there is a collection of fluid around the heart within the pericardial sac (see Figure 51, page A16). The type of fluid in the pericardial sac depends on the underlying cause. Infection may produce a collection of pus. Tumor that has extended into the pericardium or rupture of the heart after a heart attack with leakage of blood can produce bloody pericardial effusions.

Pericardial effusions may or may not press on the heart enough to limit its movement within the sac. If the fluid accumulates slowly so that the pericardial sac can distend, it may not compress the heart. However, if the fluid accumulates fast enough or reaches a large enough amount, it can compress the heart and reduce its efficiency.

In this case the heart cannot expand enough during diastole to fill sufficiently, so there is less blood to be pumped out on the next beat. When the

heart is affected in this way, the condition is called cardiac tamponade.

Causes of Pericardial Effusion. Pericardial effusion can be caused by inflammatory pericarditis as well as other factors. These include heart attacks, cancer extending into the pericardium, or kidney failure.

Cardiac tamponade may occur when there is bleeding after heart surgery, infections, tuberculosis, radiation treatments for some kinds of cancer, and trauma.

Symptoms of Pericardial Effusion. If the heart is not compressed by the collection of fluid, there may be no symptoms.

Cardiac tamponade produces symptoms of inadequate heart function, because the heart is unable to pump blood effectively to the lungs and body. People with tamponade are obviously ill. Their skin may have a bluish discoloration because of lack of oxygen. They may be short of breath, anxious, light-headed, or dizzy, and they may go into shock.

PERICARDIAL CONSTRICTION (STIFFNESS). One of the aftereffects of some cases of pericarditis is the development of a very stiff pericardium (see Figure 52, page A16). It is similar to the result of soaking your leather shoes in the rain—the leather becomes stiff. The stiff pericardium decreases the ability of the heart muscle to expand between contractions and fill with blood. It occurs in all age groups, but it is more common after age 30.

Causes of Pericardial Constriction. Pericarditis that was originally caused by infectious agents such as tuberculosis, by radiation exposure during treatment of cancers in the chest, or by inflammatory conditions is most likely to lead to pericardial constriction.

Symptoms of Pericardial Constriction. Pericardial constriction involves both ventricles, but the most prominent symptoms are usually those of right-sided heart failure such as swelling of the abdomen and legs. Shortness of breath and fatigue are also common and usually precede the swelling.

How Serious Is Pericardial Constriction? In cases of heart failure, the pericardium may need to be removed surgically. If this happens, you do not need to worry. You can get along fine without your pericardium, just as you can get along without your appendix or gallbladder.

Pericardial Disease

Possible Tests
Electrocardiography
   (see page 192)
Chest X-ray (see page 200)
Echocardiography
   (see page 209)

Possible Treatment
Pericardiocentesis
   (see page 292)
Pericardiectomy (see page 293)
Anti-inflammatory medications

PART 3

Reducing Your Risk of Coronary Artery Disease

EFFECT OF VARIOUS RISK FACTORS

You may not really want to live *forever*, but most people want to stay healthy and live as long as possible. Certainly, no one wants to be cut down in the prime of life by a heart attack or sudden death. You can affect your health by the way you live. Developing good habits and avoiding harmful ones can have positive effects not only on the length but also on the quality of your life.

Certain "risk factors" can increase your chances of developing the most common type of heart disease—coronary artery disease. Blockages in the coronary arteries can lead to angina, heart attack, and death. A risk factor is any characteristic or behavior that increases the probability for development of coronary artery disease and its complications.

Some risk factors can be controlled, so it is important to understand what they are, whether they pertain to you, and, if so, what you can do to elimi-nate or modify them. Modifiable risk factors are high blood pressure, high blood cholesterol, cigarette smoking, diabetes mellitus, excess weight, a sedentary life-style, and an aggressive response to stress. Certain drugs may also put you at higher risk for a heart attack.

Unfortunately, not all risk factors can be altered. Men seem to have a higher risk of coronary artery disease than women. Age is also a nonmodifi-able risk factor: the older you are, the higher the chances of having coronary artery disease (if all other factors are equal). Having a first-degree relative (father, mother, brother, or sister) who had coronary artery disease, especially if it occurred before age 55, also puts you at a higher risk for coronary artery disease. Although these risk factors cannot be changed, they are far from irrelevant. The presence of one or more unmodifiable risk factors pro-vides even more incentive for ad-dressing the factors that can be improved.

Risk factors interact with each other in important ways. If you have two risk factors (for example, if you have high cholesterol and smoke), the odds of getting coronary artery disease are much higher than if you had either one alone. Indeed, the total risk of multiple factors may be greater than merely adding the risks of each factor to-gether: the effect is actually magnified.

As important as risk factors are in understanding how you can have con-trol over your health, it is important to understand what "risk" means. Risk refers to "odds" or "chances," not to inevitability or guarantees. Although risk factors affect the odds of coronary

Risk factors for coronary artery disease

High blood pressure
High blood cholesterol
Cigarette smoking
Diabetes mellitus
Excess weight
Sedentary life-style
Stress and behavior
Certain drugs (cocaine, oral contraceptives for women
    who smoke)
Family history of coronary artery disease
Increased age
Male sex
Menopause

artery disease developing, having one or many risk factors does not guarantee that coronary artery disease will develop, just as the absence of risk factors does not guarantee that you will avoid it.

If you drive your car 10,000 miles a year, you are more likely to have a car accident than someone who drives only 500 miles a year. However, the high-mileage driver might never have an accident, and the low-mileage driver might get hit by a truck as he or she leaves the driveway. Similarly, occasionally someone who smokes two packs of cigarettes a day for his or her whole life lives to a ripe old age, yet a vigorous exerciser who eats right, stays in shape, does not smoke, and seems to be doing everything right may nevertheless die early. These observations probably mean that there are risk factors that have not yet been recognized but that have an influence on our health and life span.

It is all a matter of odds, and that is the essence of understanding risk factors and deciding your response to them in your life. Your decision revolves around the value you place on your health in relation to the risks that may compromise it in the future. Persons who value a long, healthy, and productive life place a high priority on increasing their chances of attaining those goals. Like many games of chance, it comes down to each individual plotting a strategy based on the odds (your risk factors) and the stakes. With coronary artery disease, the stakes are your health and your life span.

Most people, if asked to rank the importance of their health and life span, would place them at the top of their list. Yet, whether through laziness or lack of discipline, they take risks. Regardless of what the specific risks may be, it is useful to consider what might motivate persons to risk their well-being.

There are several fundamental reasons why people take risks. First, risk does not imply certainty, so you may believe or hope that the risky behavior will not actually affect you. Second, although health is a high priority, conflicting priorities certainly exist. Some risky activities may be rewarding in some other sense, such as seeming fun, glamorous, carefree, or sociable. Third, most people take their health for granted; they have only a dim idea of what it is actually like to be deprived of their health. Finally, the consequences of risk factors usually do not show up immediately; rather, they occur later in life, beyond the normal planning period of most young people. Understanding this "psychology" of risk factors is an important first step for you to deal with them constructively.

UNMODIFIABLE RISK FACTORS

Risk factors for heart disease that cannot be changed are heredity (family history), age, and sex. Your risk of coronary artery disease is higher if you have a close relative (mother, father, brother, or sister) who developed coronary artery disease before age 55. Your risk also increases as you age. Women in general have a lower risk than men, at least until menopause, but as they get older, their risk increases. Women who smoke lose much of this advantage and have a risk of coronary artery disease similar to that in men.

Heredity

If one or both of your parents or another close blood relative had a heart attack at a young age, your risk for the development of coronary artery disease is higher than someone whose family has no members with heart disease. Even if you have eliminated risks that were not so well known a generation ago, such as smoking or high blood cholesterol, the fact that your father, for example, died of a heart attack at age 50 makes your risk somewhat higher than the risk for someone who does not have this family history.

The greatest inherited risk is in people with familial hypercholesterolemia (a genetic predisposition to have dangerously high cholesterol levels). Other genetic factors passed on from parents to children may promote the development of moderately high cholesterol levels, high blood pressure, diabetes, or obesity. There is also a genetic link for a disorder known as idiopathic dilated cardiomyopathy (see page 41). A Mayo Clinic study of 59 patients with this form of cardiomyopathy and 315 of their relatives found up to 20 percent of the families had additional family members who showed signs of the disease.

Families pass on more than genes. The types of food you eat, your exercise habits, and whether you smoke are often strongly influenced by your family. Exposure to tobacco smoke in the home, even if you do not smoke, is an additional health risk.

Your genes neither doom you to nor fully protect you from the risk of heart disease. You can make a big difference by evaluating and controlling other risk factors, especially smoking, high blood pressure, and high blood cholesterol. Being aware of your family history can be an extra incentive to develop more healthful habits.

Age

Even though the risk of many health problems increases as you age, you can slow some of the natural effects of aging by watching your weight and diet, getting regular exercise, and controlling your blood pressure and cholesterol levels.

The forerunner of cardiovascular disease can begin in early childhood, and then the disease progresses gradually. Avoiding or delaying the onset of atherosclerosis in the blood vessels by minimizing risk factors at a young age likely reduces the occurrence of disease such as angina and heart attack later in life.

Sex

Coronary artery disease is the leading cause of death for both sexes. It is hard to separate the role of your sex in the development of coronary artery disease from other factors such as smoking, blood pressure, and cholesterol levels. Men and women who smoke or who have high blood pressure or high blood cholesterol levels have higher risks of heart disease than others who control these factors.

When you consider only the sex difference, men are more likely to have coronary artery disease than women—until women reach the age of menopause. Then the difference in risk between men and women shrinks.

This difference certainly does not mean that women are "immune" from heart disease. In fact, 47 percent of American victims of fatal heart attack are women. In women, coronary artery disease develops, on the average, about 10 years later than in men.

The female hormone estrogen may be one protector against heart disease. After its decline at menopause, women's risks increase. The use of estrogen after menopause seems to reduce a woman's risk of heart disease. However, it may increase her risk of cancer in the lining of the uterus (endometrial cancer) and possibly of breast cancer. There is evidence that smoking may reduce estrogen levels in women and may hasten menopause—results that add to its list of bad effects on the heart.

Until recently, much of the research relating to coronary artery disease focused mainly on men (see page 336). New studies are under way to determine whether the findings are applicable to women as well.

MODIFIABLE RISK FACTORS

You are living at a time that emphasizes healthful life-styles more than ever. You can enjoy many social and health benefits by eating right, getting enough exercise, and taking care of your body. There has been substantial publicity and education regarding risk factors. Few people can claim that they have not heard reliable information about the health concerns related to smoking, high cholesterol, and lack of exercise. In fact, some risky behaviors, such as smoking, are now frowned on by many people and are no longer considered acceptable. There has never been more support available to help you change harmful habits.

Understanding Your Risk

Some risk factors, including high blood cholesterol levels, high blood sugar levels (diabetes), and high blood pressure, can be detected only with tests done during a medical checkup. You may wonder how often you should have a general medical evaluation. Most doctors agree that you should have a checkup every 3 to 5 years until age 40 if you are apparently healthy. During your 40s you should see your doctor four times, and during the decade of your 50s you should have five general examinations. After age 60, annual examinations are advisable.

One of the main purposes of checkups is to identify risk factors or early evidence of disease of the heart and other organs so that they can be counteracted early. Of course, if your doctor finds a problem, you may need more frequent examinations.

Some risk factors are obvious without a medical examination, including smoking, excess weight, and a sedentary life-style. You may find it easier to deal with these risk factors with help from your doctor.

PRIMARY PREVENTION. Risk factors, as they pertain to coronary artery disease, are obviously different from the coronary artery disease itself.

Treating or correcting a risk factor does not cure coronary artery disease; rather, it helps prevent it from occurring. Thus, modifying your risk factors can be thought of as preventive maintenance. Taking steps to reduce your risk factors before coronary artery disease develops is called primary prevention.

Although improved treatments for heart disease are saving more lives, about half of all deaths occur before there is time to start treatment. Thus, treatment, no matter how sophisticated it may become, is not the ideal solution for reducing deaths from heart disease. Preventing heart attacks by reducing or eliminating risk factors undoubtedly can save lives.

SECONDARY PREVENTION. What if you already have coronary artery disease and are experiencing angina or have even had a heart attack? Evidence shows that you can still reduce your chances of further complications if you reduce your risk factors. Secondary prevention is the attempt to reduce risk factors after you have documented coronary artery disease or a heart attack.

When you treat risk factors aggressively, atherosclerosis can actually improve. By giving up smoking, exercising regularly, and developing healthful eating, living, and working habits, you can diminish the effects of existing cardiovascular disease.

Cardiovascular rehabilitation programs after heart attacks are an example of secondary prevention. They try to help you reduce the risk of a second heart attack, compensate for the heart damage, decrease the extent of atherosclerosis, and resume as normal a lifestyle as possible (see pages 312–319).

How Important Are Risk Factors?

The major risk factors are discussed here. To say which risk factors are the greatest predictors of coronary artery disease for a particular person is fraught with assumptions. However, most doctors would probably agree that the most important risk factors are smoking, elevated lipids (cholesterol) in the blood, high blood pressure, excess weight, diabetes, and sedentary life-style. Obviously, many of these are not independent factors. For example, many overweight people are relatively inactive and have high cholesterol levels.

Working to reduce one risk factor may have benefits for others. If you change your diet to lose weight, you may also lower your cholesterol level and blood pressure. You may also decide to start an exercise program.

Is Prevention Worth the Effort?

The whole purpose of identifying and controlling your cardiovascular risk factors is to prevent a heart attack, early disability, and death. Millions of Americans have learned about these risk factors and have tried to modify them with help from health professionals. You can control high blood pressure, stop smoking, and lower your cholesterol level. As a matter of fact, the average cholesterol level of the population has decreased during the past 20 years, most likely because many people have changed their diets and some people are getting more physical activity. These changes have probably contributed to the declining death rate from heart disease in the United States.

Most people agree that a more healthful life-style is worth the effort, but they need a little help. It is not easy to change habits that you have lived with for many years. This part of the book describes why each risk factor is

What is your risk of heart disease?

Cigarette smoking, high blood pressure, and high blood cholesterol are major risk factors for coronary artery disease. Your chances of having a heart attack or angina or dying from heart disease within the next 8 years increase with each risk factor you have. Estimate your risk by adding up the points shown in the pink-shaded areas.

If you're a man:

1. Do you smoke? No = 0   Yes = 3

2. Find your systolic blood pressure (top number in your reading) and circle the points directly below.

Blood Pressure

100	110	120	130	140	150	160	170	180	190	200
1	2	4	5	6	7	8	9	10	12	13

3. Circle the number where your approximate age and blood cholesterol level meet.

Total Cholesterol	Age 40	50	60	70
165	4	12	18	21
180	5	13	19	21
195	7	14	19	21
210	8	15	20	21
225	9	16	20	22
240	11	17	21	22
255	12	18	22	22
270	13	19	22	23
285	15	20	23	23
300	16	21	24	23
315	17	22	24	23

If you're a woman:

1. Do you smoke? No = 0   Yes = 1

2. Find your systolic blood pressure (top number in your reading) and circle the points directly below.

Blood Pressure

100	110	120	130	140	150	160	170	180	190	200
1	2	3	4	5	6	7	8	9	10	11

3. Circle the number where your approximate age and blood cholesterol level meet.

Total Cholesterol	Age 40	50	60	70
165	4	12	18	23
180	5	13	19	23
195	5	13	19	23
210	6	14	20	24
225	7	15	20	24
240	8	15	21	24
255	8	16	21	25
270	9	16	22	25
285	10	17	22	25
300	11	18	23	25
315	11	18	23	26

4. Record Your Points

___ cigarette smoking
___ systolic blood pressure
___ age/blood cholesterol
___ sex Male = 5 Female = 0
___ **TOTAL POINTS**

5. Estimate Your Risk

Find your total points to determine your chances (out of 100) of having heart disease within the next 8 years.

Total Points	Chances (out of 100)	Total Points	Chances (out of 100)
1–10	<1	35	17
11–13	1	36	19
14–17	2	37	21
18–21	3	38	24
22–23	4	39	26
24	5	40	28
25–26	6	41	31
27	7	42	34
28	8	43	36
29	9	44	39
30	10	45	42
31	11	46	46
32	13	47	49
33	14	48	52
34	16	49	55
		50	58

Note: In this table, the effect on risk from blood cholesterol is limited to total cholesterol. If the assessment also reflected a low level of high-density lipoprotein (HDL) cholesterol, the estimated risk would be higher. This assessment also omits the effects of diabetes mellitus and an abnormal electrocardiogram indicating left ventricular hypertrophy. Women who have diabetes should add 6 points to the total score, and add 4 points if an electrocardiogram shows left ventricular hypertrophy. Men who have diabetes should add 3 points to the total score, and add 2 points for an electrocardiogram that shows left ventricular hypertrophy. (Tables are based on data from the Framingham Heart Study, see page 128.)

harmful and suggests ways to decrease their harmful effects in your own life. Use the risk assessment form on page 121 to estimate your personal risk of having heart disease. Armed with both knowledge and some helpful tips for putting the knowledge into practice, you can slant the odds in your favor.

Smoking

Smoking is the leading cause of preventable illness and death in the United States. More than 400,000 deaths every year (in fact, about 1,200 per day) in the United States are attributed to smoking. At least one-third of these are related to cardiovascular disease. Smoking kills more people each year than AIDS, alcohol (including drunk driving), cocaine, other forms of drug abuse, and accidents combined. Indeed, almost 20 percent of *all* deaths in the United States are related to smoking, according to the Surgeon General.

The toll of this human tragedy is compounded by the immense expense borne by all members of society, smokers and nonsmokers alike, in terms of higher health insurance costs, lower productivity, and higher taxes. Analysis has shown that the cost to each American—every man, woman, and child, whether they smoke or not—is $221 to cover the consequences of smoking in terms of increased health care and insurance and lost productivity. A national financial burden of $37 billion to $50 billion per year suggests that the incentive to reduce tobacco use should be very high on an individual and national basis.

WHY IS SMOKING HARMFUL?

Tobacco smoke contains about 4,000 substances, and many of them, such as nicotine, tars, nitrosamines, and polycyclic aromatic hydrocarbons, are known to produce adverse effects.

The main cardiovascular risk from smoking is the development of atherosclerosis in blood vessels. The mechanisms by which this occurs remain elusive, despite the clear-cut association with tobacco use. Several potential links have been identified: smoking reduces the proportion of HDL ("good") cholesterol to LDL ("bad") cholesterol in the blood (see pages 125–133) and increases the tendency for blood to clot inside the blood vessels and obstruct blood flow. Constituents of tobacco smoke may also directly damage the internal protective lining of blood vessels (endothelium).

Inhaling cigarette smoke also produces several temporary adverse effects on your heart and blood vessels, and these may provoke serious consequences such as heart attacks. The nicotine in the smoke increases your blood pressure and heart rate. Carbon monoxide (a gas produced by smoking—the same gas in car exhaust that is lethal in an enclosed space) gets into your blood and reduces the amount of oxygen that your blood can carry to your heart and the rest of your body. It causes the arteries in your arms and legs to constrict.

Smoking may cause ischemia (lack of oxygen and blood flow to the heart muscle) by transiently decreasing the diameter of the coronary arteries. When arteries that are already narrowed by atherosclerotic deposits become narrowed even further, blood flow to the heart muscle may be reduced enough to cause angina or a heart attack. When smokers with angina exert themselves, they get chest pain sooner than they would otherwise, because smoking reduces the amount of oxygen to the heart and also makes the heart beat faster. So, ironically, the heart's demand for oxygen increases and the supply of oxygen decreases. Smoking blocks the increased blood flow that normally occurs with exercise and reduces the effectiveness of some anti-anginal drugs. Even in the absence of symptoms, studies have shown that there is evidence of myocardial ischemia during smoking. In some cases, smoking can cause coronary arteries *without* atherosclerosis to go into spasm and narrow enough to cut off blood flow to the heart muscle.

The heart and coronary arteries are not the only cardiovascular targets of smoking damage. Smoking is a major risk factor for peripheral vascular disease (atherosclerotic narrowing of the blood vessels that carry blood to your arm and leg muscles). The consequences may range from the exertion-related pain of claudication (see page 98) to the actual destruction of skin or muscle tissue supplied by blocked arteries. When severe, this condition may require operation or amputation. Women who smoke and take birth control pills place themselves at higher risk for another serious vascular problem—stroke.

Smoking is the main cause of chronic lung diseases such as chronic bronchitis and emphysema, which put an additional strain on the heart.

HOW HIGH IS THE RISK? Cigarette smokers have a risk of cardiovascular disease at least two times as high as nonsmokers. The risk increases with the number of cigarettes smoked each day. If you smoke one pack of cigarettes a day, your risk is twice as high as that of someone who never smoked. If you smoke two or more packs a day, your risk is three times as high as a person who never smoked. Cigars, pipes, and chewing tobacco also increase your risk, although to a lesser degree.

The earlier you start smoking cigarettes, the greater the risk to your health. Nine out of 10 smokers began smoking when they were younger than 21 years. Thus, the risk and damage accumulate over a major portion of their lives. Smoking-related diseases usually do not kill rapidly, but slowly rob you of your vitality over a period of years.

WHO SMOKES—AND WHY? The percentage of people in the United States who smoke has gradually declined during the past 2 decades. The probable reasons are an increasing awareness of health concerns, nonsmokers becoming more outspoken and unaccepting of smokers, and more restrictions on smoking in public places. Nevertheless, nearly a third of men and a fourth of all women smoked in 1988. If current trends continue, by the turn of the century the prevalence of smoking in this country will be about 20 percent, but by then more women than men will be smoking. Although that is an improvement in the overall number of people smoking, it still will represent a large percentage of the population and a very large number of people.

Why do people expose themselves to this risk? For many established smokers, the answer is that they have developed a repetitive behavior that is triggered by many cues—stress, meals, conversations on the telephone. Smokers also develop a physical need for the constituents of tobacco, especially nicotine, to function comfortably and to avoid withdrawal. This behavior pattern and addiction *can* be overcome.

Despite all that is known about the dangers of smoking, an estimated 3,000 children begin smoking every day. More children are likely to die ultimately from cigarettes than from drugs or alcohol. Of course, future health problems seem remote or nonexistent to young people.

When young people start smoking, underlying motives are likely to include a combination of factors such as peer group acceptance, rebelliousness against authority, and a perception that smoking imparts an image of jaunty individuality. Smoking has been considered by some to be an outward expression of exercising one's rights. All of these attitudes have been capitalized on by advertising, but they are progressively changing. Increasingly, smoking is being perceived by young people and adults as an annoying, dangerous habit.

SECONDHAND SMOKE. Not everyone who smokes does so voluntarily. Environmental tobacco smoke causes heart disease and cancer. In 1992, the American Heart Association called environmental tobacco smoke "a major preventable cause of cardiovascular disease and death." Experts estimate that 35,000 to 40,000 deaths each year from cardiovascular disease and another 3,000 to 5,000 deaths from lung cancer are directly related to exposure to environmental tobacco smoke.

Knowing this, it is reasonable to insist on a smoke-free work site and to not allow guests to smoke in your home. When you are looking for day-care facilities for your children, choose one where they will not be exposed to tobacco smoke. Children who are raised in the homes of smokers are more likely to have ear and upper respiratory infections and other problems that require them to visit the doctor and miss school more often.

The risk of secondhand (also called side-stream or passive) smoking increases as the exposure increases. There is no threshold below which there is no risk from environmental tobacco smoke.

Benefits
of quitting smoking

Immediate
- Cleaner, less smelly house, clothes, hair, breath, car
- Easier breathing, improved exercise tolerance
- Less offensive to others
- Stops exposing family and friends to risky secondhand smoke
- Food tastes better
- Eliminates smoker's cough
- Less dental staining
- Reduced fire hazard
- Reduced unnecessary expenses
- Insurance discounts
- Sets positive example for your children
- Reduced heartburn

Ultimate
- Reduced risk of cardiovascular disease
- Reduced risk of emphysema and bronchitis
- Reduced risk of lung, esophagus, and other types of cancer
- Increased life span and quality of life

DOES SMOKING LOW-TAR AND LOW-NICOTINE CIGARETTES RE-DUCE THE RISK?   No cigarettes are safe. Research has found no evidence that smoking low-tar and low-nicotine cigarettes reduces the risk of coronary artery disease, although the risk for cancer may be lower.

People who smoke low-tar and low-nicotine cigarettes often inhale more deeply, hold their breath after inhaling, and smoke more cigarettes in an unconscious effort to maintain the nicotine levels to which their bodies are addicted. Consequently, they not only do not reduce their nicotine exposure as much as they may have hoped but also inhale more of the other toxic substances contained in the smoke.

HEALTH BENEFITS OF QUITTING. From a health perspective, benefits are most obvious if you never begin smoking in the first place. If you do smoke, however, the gains from stopping are enormous. After you quit, the risk of heart disease from smoking drops dramatically within about 2 years. Although your risk probably will never be as low as if you had never smoked, it can certainly approach that level. Researchers have found that if you smoke two packs of cigarettes per day your risk of *death* from heart disease alone (not considering death from other causes or ill health not resulting in death) is double that if you never smoked. If you stop smoking (and do not resume), the risk of death from heart disease is reduced to 1.3 times what it would have been if you never smoked.

Even among relatively older individuals, there is a dramatic advantage to discontinuing cigarette use. For example, if you are older than 50 and stop smoking, the chance of dying from any cause is reduced by one-half during the next 15 years. The risk of dying of heart disease decreases by about 30 percent. Recent studies have shown that smokers older than age 60 could add 5 to 7 years to their lives by quitting. It is never too late to quit.

Smoking

Possible Tests
Pulmonary (lung) function tests
Chest X-ray (see page 200)

Possible Treatment
How to Stop Smoking (see page 146)

Elevated Cholesterol

If results of a blood test show that you have an elevated cholesterol level, you have an increased risk for the development of coronary artery disease. Thus, it makes sense to do what is necessary to keep your cholesterol in an acceptable range. In fact, the American Heart Association and the National Heart, Lung, and Blood Institute have concluded jointly that "the benefits of modifying serum cholesterol levels extend to men and women, young and old, those with high risk . . . and those with borderline high risk levels."

Cholesterol has become a household word in the past decade. Food advertising and labels focus on it. Cholesterol screening has become a nearly routine part of medical examinations, work-site wellness programs, and health fairs. But the bits and pieces of information you have probably heard from various sources may have failed to answer some basic questions, such as these: What is cholesterol in the first place? What constitutes an elevated cholesterol level? How much risk does an elevated cholesterol level pose, and when should you be concerned? What can you do to control your cholesterol level?

WHAT IS CHOLESTEROL? Cholesterol is one of several types of fats (lipids) that have important roles in your body. Despite its reputation as a risk factor for coronary disease, which tends to make people think of it only in negative terms, it is an important component of cell membranes and therefore is vital to the structure and function of all cells in your body. Cholesterol is also a building block in the formation of certain types of hormones. However, cholesterol is the predominant substance in atherosclerotic plaques, which may develop in arteries and impede the flow of blood (see pages 71 and 97). When the cholesterol level in the bloodstream becomes excessively high, the likelihood of atherosclerotic plaques developing increases.

Cholesterol is not the only lipid circulating in your bloodstream. Triglycerides are another form of fat that circulate in the blood. Triglycerides can be thought of as transportable fuel that ultimately is used for energy production by the body. Neither cholesterol nor triglycerides, being fats, dissolve in water. Therefore, to circulate through your blood, which is mainly water, they must be carried by protein packages called apoproteins. The combination of an apoprotein and a lipid is a lipoprotein. Each type of lipoprotein is defined by the type and proportion of lipid and apoprotein in its structure.

The main types of lipoproteins are low-density lipoprotein (LDL) and high-density lipoprotein (HDL). They are often referred to as LDL cholesterol and HDL cholesterol. HDL contains almost 50 percent protein and 20 percent cholesterol; LDL contains about 25 percent protein and 45 percent cholesterol. Another type of lipoprotein, very low-density lipoprotein (VLDL), contains mostly triglyceride and small amounts of protein and cholesterol.

The function of LDL is to transport cholesterol to sites throughout the

Mini-glossary of cholesterol-related terms

- *Apoproteins*: proteins that combine with lipids to make them dissolve in the blood
- *Cholesterol*: a type of lipid used by your body to build cells and certain hormones. It is found only in foods derived from animal sources
- *Fatty acids*: also called "fats," they occur in several forms in the foods you eat. Different fatty acids have different effects on your lipid profile
- *HDL cholesterol* (*high-density lipoprotein cholesterol*): a combination of about 50 percent apoproteins and 20 percent cholesterol. HDL tends to help remove excess cholesterol from your blood
- *LDL cholesterol* (*low-density lipoprotein cholesterol*): a combination of about 25 percent apoproteins and 45 percent cholesterol. LDL provides cholesterol for necessary body functions, but in excessive amounts it promotes cholesterol accumulation in artery walls
- *Lipids*: a general term referring to fats (cholesterol and triglycerides) circulating in the bloodstream
- *Lipid profile*: the amount of various lipids in your bloodstream
- *Lipoproteins*: lipids combined with apoproteins
- *Triglyceride*: a type of lipid used by your body as a source of energy. Most triglycerides are transported through your bloodstream as a very low-density lipoprotein (VLDL). Some cholesterol is also present in VLDL

body where it is used to repair the membranes of cells or is deposited. Thus, LDL tends to promote accumulation of cholesterol in the walls of your arteries, somewhat in the manner that hard water promotes a buildup of lime inside the plumbing of your house. However, cholesterol deposits are spotty, rather than an even coating throughout the "pipes."

HDL, however, mainly has the task of carrying cholesterol to the liver, where it is altered and removed from the body. In a sense, HDL is like a "clean-up" crew that sops up excess cholesterol in the system and disposes of it before it can do any damage by accumulating where it is not needed.

LDL cholesterol is mainly to blame for the risk that is associated with cholesterol. The opposite is true for HDL cholesterol: because it works to eliminate excess cholesterol, the more HDL you have, the less cholesterol will deposit in atherosclerotic plaques. Therefore, a relatively low ratio of LDL to HDL is desirable for lowering your risk for development of coronary artery disease.

The role of very low-density lipoprotein (VLDL) cholesterol in determining the risk of coronary artery disease is not well defined. A high level of VLDL seems to be an independent risk factor in women, but not in men. A high level of triglycerides corresponds to a high level of VLDL cholesterol.

MEASURING CHOLESTEROL LEVELS. Lipids are measured by analyzing a blood specimen. Eating before the blood test does not affect the level of blood cholesterol. However, it has an effect on the blood triglyceride level. Because both are usually measured from the same specimen, you should fast before the test. Do not eat

for a minimum of 12 hours before your blood is drawn. Do not drink alcohol for a full 24 hours before the test. If you follow these guidelines, your physician will have an accurate measure of your cholesterol, triglycerides, and other blood lipids, rather than depending on unreliable data that merely reflect when and what you last ate.

Fasting before a blood test for lipids does not mean that your results will be precisely the same day after day, even if you make no change in your diet, exercise, or medications. Your lipid levels may vary by about 10 percent from day to day. The importance of a blood test for lipids, therefore, is not to detect small changes in results or to make a large issue out of whether a particular value is several points "too high." Rather, it is to establish in a general sense what your risk level is, and to determine whether the response to diet, exercise, or medication is satisfactory.

CHOLESTEROL LEVELS: WHAT IS HIGH?   In a sense, it is incorrect to think of a cholesterol (or triglyceride) level as being strictly abnormal or nor-

Lipid levels and coronary risk

Item Measured	Level (mg/dl)		
	Desirable*	**Borderline**	**Too high**
Total cholesterol	< 200	200–239	> 240
LDL cholesterol	< 130	130–159	> 160
Triglycerides	< 200	250–500	> 500
LDL/HDL ratio	< 3	3–5	> 5
	Desirable*	**Borderline**	**Too low**
HDL cholesterol	> 45	35–45	< 35

*For adults without known heart disease.

Figuring out your own LDL-cholesterol level

LDL-cholesterol levels are important for determining the risk of cardiovascular disease. LDL cholesterol can be measured directly, but more commonly it is calculated based on measurements of other lipids. The calculation is usually sufficiently accurate, and it does not incur the cost of an additional blood test. The calculation is done as follows:

- Subtract your HDL-cholesterol level from your total cholesterol level.
- Then subtract one-fifth of your triglyceride level.
- The result is your LDL-cholesterol level.
- Example: Your doctor tells you that your total-cholesterol level is 226, your HDL-cholesterol level is 56, and your triglyceride level is 150. Your LDL-cholesterol level is 226 − 56 = 170, 170 − 150/5 = 140.

mal. Although ranges of cholesterol levels have been identified which are considered "too high," there is no "magic number" that separates risky levels from safe levels. Actually, the ranges for adults (see Lipid levels and coronary risk, page 127) are based on a consensus of expert investigators and physicians. They have identified levels of lipids in the blood above which the risk for development of coronary complications is high enough to warrant changes. People with cholesterol or triglyceride levels in the higher-risk zones are said to be hypercholesterolemic, hypertriglyceridemic, or simply hyperlipidemic (*hyper* means "high," *lipid* means "fat," *emic* means "in the blood").

But, as with all risk factors, being in the "high" range does not guarantee that coronary artery disease will develop, nor does being in the "low" range guarantee avoiding it.

Lipid levels are described as the number of milligrams that are present in ⅒ of a liter of blood (about ½ cup). The unit of measurement is expressed as milligrams (mg) per deciliter (dl)—mg/dl. Of course, this value can be calculated from the measurement of lipids in a much smaller blood sample.

THE SIGNIFICANCE OF CHOLESTEROL LEVELS. Research clearly shows that the amount of cholesterol in your bloodstream and the proportions of the different types of lipoproteins have a definite impact on your future risk for development of coronary blockages. This evidence has been found in extensive studies of populations whose average cholesterol levels were compared with the incidence of coronary artery disease and in studies investigating whether the tendency for development of coronary artery disease could be influenced by lowering cholesterol.

In certain circumstances, the link between lipid levels and cardiovascular risk is dramatic. Because of genes inherited from their parents, some people lack certain parts of their cells which are vital to processing cholesterol and getting rid of LDL cholesterol. In this condition, called familial hypercholesterolemia, people have extremely high levels of cholesterol, especially LDL cholesterol. This makes them very susceptible to the development of angina pectoris or heart attacks very early in their lives, even in their 20s.

In other instances, in groups whose cholesterol levels are less markedly elevated, the link still exists, although it is not as dramatic. In Framingham, Massachusetts, a careful, large-scale study of heart disease and risk factors in the general population has been ongoing for 40 years. By measuring cholesterol in a large group of townspeople (2,282 men and 2,845 women), and then waiting to determine how many of them would have coronary problems during the next 14 years, the investigators found a very straightforward trend. They observed that the higher a person's cholesterol was at the outset, the greater the chance that he or she would show signs of coronary disease during the study. In fact, among people with a total cholesterol of 300 mg/dl, coronary problems developed more than twice as often as among people with a total cholesterol of 150 mg/dl. People with cholesterol levels between these extremes had risks of coronary disease which were also in between.

Other studies have shown that the risk of dying from coronary artery disease is increased as your cholesterol level increases. One large study, called the Multiple Risk Factor Intervention Trial (its acronym, MRFIT, is pronounced "Mr. Fit"), examined what happened to more than 360,000 men whose cholesterol levels were measured. Six years later the results were clear: the likelihood of dying from coronary disease was practically four times higher in people with total cholesterol levels above 300 mg/dl compared with those whose levels were below 180 mg/dl. Numerous other studies support these conclusions.

DOES REDUCING CHOLESTEROL REDUCE RISK?

It is one thing to observe that people with relatively low cholesterol levels have less chance of getting coronary artery disease, but it is another to conclude that if you lower your cholesterol level you will also lower your risk. What if having a high cholesterol level was just a signal that you are at risk of coronary disease but

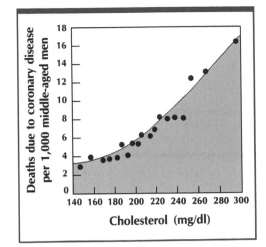

Results from the Multiple Risk Factor Intervention Trial show the relationship between total cholesterol level and the chance of dying from coronary heart disease within 6 years. The study showed that men aged 35 to 57 years with a total cholesterol of 300 mg/dl had more than four times the chance of dying as men with a cholesterol level of less than 180 mg/dl.

the cholesterol was not actually the cause of that risk? In that case, there would be very little point in doing anything to lower your cholesterol level. As a matter of fact, it has taken a great deal of effort and expense to perform studies that address that very point, but the answer now is convincing that there *is* a role for reducing your cholesterol level.

Several studies have shown a reduction in the occurrence of coronary disease by one-third to one-half in people who lower their cholesterol levels by diet or medications. In general, if your cholesterol level is high or moderately high and you lower it by 10 percent, you will lower your risk of coronary artery disease by about 20 percent. Most of these studies have also indicated that higher levels of HDL cholesterol also confer a lower risk of

The effect of lowering your cholesterol

You go to the doctor for a checkup. A blood test reveals a total cholesterol level of 260 mg/dl. You carefully and consistently adjust your diet and exercise. When your cholesterol is rechecked in 6 months, it is 208 mg/dl. Because that is a decrease of 20 percent, your predicted risk for the development of coronary disease has decreased by 40 percent if you maintain the improved level.

coronary disease. Additional research trials also indicate that a reduction of coronary disease by lowering cholesterol translates into an actual decline in deaths due to heart disease—a very important bottom line!

What about people who already have coronary problems detected by tests, or who have angina pectoris, or who have had a heart attack? Is the "horse out of the barn" as far as cho-

Discouraging and encouraging facts about cholesterol

- Approximately 55 percent of American adults have a total cholesterol level of more than 200 mg/dl.
- If your total cholesterol is 300 mg/dl, the risk for development of coronary disease is double what it would be if your total cholesterol were 150 mg/dl.
- The risk of dying from coronary disease if your total cholesterol is 300 mg/dl is four times what it would be if your total cholesterol were 180 mg/dl.
- Dietary measures alone can usually reduce the average LDL cholesterol by about 15 percent or more. Dietary measures are less likely to be effective if the triglyceride level is normal, though.
- A 10 percent reduction in cholesterol level results in a 20 percent reduction in future coronary risk.
- A 1 mg/dl increase in HDL cholesterol reduces your risk of coronary disease by 2 to 3 percent.
- Aggressive life-style modification, including cholesterol reduction, can cause at least a little reversal of coronary artery blockage in about one of three people.

lesterol is concerned for these individuals? Evidence is mounting that lowering cholesterol in this group retards the further development of coronary blockages and, most intriguingly, may even promote some regression of blockages that are already present. These changes have been observed in as little as 2 years.

Because of the possibility for regression of disease in patients with coronary artery atherosclerosis, physicians are not satisfied with levels that they consider "adequate" for people who do not have heart disease (see page 127). If you have heart disease, expect that your physician will want you to lower your cholesterol below a level that is considered adequate for someone else.

To summarize: People with relatively low LDL-cholesterol levels (and low VLDL cholesterol) or relatively high HDL-cholesterol levels experience fewer coronary artery problems and live longer, *on the average*. People included in this group are those who have lowered their LDL-cholesterol level or raised their HDL-cholesterol level by means of diet, exercise, or medications. Everyone can benefit from lowering their cholesterol level, but the people with the most to gain are those who start out with high cholesterol levels.

DOES AGE MATTER?   Middle-aged adults are the focus of most cholesterol research and recommendations. After all, they are the ones just entering the high-risk phase of life for coronary artery disease. But should lipids be a concern for children and older adults? Yes.

Children.   The process of developing atherosclerosis begins early in life, but usually it becomes severe enough to cause problems only later in life. Evidence suggests that high cholesterol levels in childhood promote an earlier development of atherosclerosis and, by extension, increase the chances for development of coronary artery disease in adulthood.

However, the evidence is not clear enough to justify recommending cholesterol tests for all children. Certainly children older than 2 who come from "high-risk" families—one parent has a cholesterol level of 240 mg/dl or higher or a parent or grandparent had evidence of coronary artery disease before age 55 should have their blood cholesterol measured. (See Cholesterol levels in children and adolescents from high-risk families, this page, for an interpretation of test results.)

If a child's cholesterol value is elevated, dietary changes are the first course of action. Actually, all children older than 2, regardless of whether a cholesterol level is known, should follow the same eating strategies that are recommended for adults. These strategies focus on reducing fat and cholesterol in the diet, maintaining a healthful weight, and encouraging physical activity. (See Recommendations for a Heart-Healthy Life-Style, pages 145–177.)

If by 10 years of age a child's cholesterol level remains elevated above 190 mg/dl (or above 170 mg/dl in children from high-risk families) despite the best dietary attempts, then one of the lipid-lowering medications may be required. Not every medication is suitable for children, however, so the pediatrician will prescribe the appropriate one.

Older Age Groups. The evidence that lowering cholesterol helps to di-

Cholesterol levels in children and adolescents from high-risk families*

Category	Total cholesterol (mg/dl)	LDL cholesterol (mg/dl)
Acceptable	< 170	< 110
Borderline	170–199	110–129
High	≥ 200	≥ 130

*One parent has a cholesterol level of 240 mg/dl or greater or a parent or grandparent had coronary artery disease before age 55.

minish, or at least slow down, the development of coronary artery disease in some people provides a strong rationale for actively aiding cholesterol control beyond middle age. People in their 60s, 70s, 80s, and 90s who have coronary artery disease or risk factors already present have the highest risk of problems if the disease progresses. Thus, many doctors believe that it is never too late to institute cholesterol-lowering measures, although at present this opinion remains unproven.

WHEN SHOULD YOU HAVE YOUR CHOLESTEROL CHECKED? The National Cholesterol Education Program recommends that all adults older than 20 years start with a blood test that measures the total cholesterol level. If your total cholesterol is more than 200 mg/dl, then have your LDL, HDL, and triglyceride values checked. Subsequent cholesterol checks should be done at regular medical checkups (see page 180 for recommended frequency). If your cholesterol is high and your doctor recommends dietary changes or other treatments, you will probably have your cholesterol rechecked in about 3 months to determine the effect of treatment. At that point, your doctor can decide whether added treatment is advisable.

Measuring only total cholesterol can be misleading

Some physicians advocate having your HDL cholesterol and triglyceride levels measured initially, in addition to total cholesterol. Why? Some people have low levels of HDL cholesterol and high levels of triglycerides but normal (or even high) LDL cholesterol. In these cases, a total cholesterol measurement might appear normal. You and your doctor would be unaware of the risk posed by the abnormalities that were not measured.

HOW TO IMPROVE YOUR CHOLESTEROL LEVEL. Three main avenues can be used to achieve and maintain cholesterol levels that minimize your risk of future coronary artery disease: diet, exercise, and medications. The first two are almost universally advisable and achievable, regardless of an individual's LDL-cholesterol, HDL-cholesterol, and triglyceride levels (the lipid profile). It appears that risk can be reduced at least somewhat even for people whose lipid profile is not very "abnormal."

On the average, dietary measures can reduce your cholesterol level by up to 15 percent. Some people may respond even more impressively. For others with a strong genetic influence on their cholesterol level, changes in diet and exercise may not be enough to improve blood cholesterol levels.

Diet. Dietary changes are the mainstay of cholesterol management (see Basic Eating Guidelines, page 153). The key concepts in making dietary changes to lower cholesterol are to reduce the total fat (especially saturated fat) and cholesterol that you eat and to lose weight (especially if your triglyceride level is elevated).

Exercise. Regular aerobic exercise often has the benefit (partly by promoting weight reduction) of reducing blood triglyceride levels and increasing the proportion of your total cholesterol that is made up of HDL cholesterol (see Improving Your Activity Level, page 168). Total and LDL cholesterol usually stay the same with exercise, but the ratio of LDL to HDL cholesterol is improved.

The appeal of dietary changes and increased activity is that although they can help improve lipid levels, they can also contribute to lowering other cardiovascular risks such as obesity and high blood pressure. Changing your diet and exercise habits does not usually require an "all-or-nothing" approach. Anyone with the knowledge of what to do and the desire to do it can make healthful changes that can rapidly become "second nature."

Medications. If periodic rechecks of lipid levels show little response to changes in diet and exercise, your doctor may recommend lipid-lowering medications (see Table 5 on page 302). Some medications have their biggest effect on LDL cholesterol, others on triglycerides, and others on HDL cholesterol. Despite their potential for being beneficial, medications are reserved for people in whom diet and activity alone have not been sufficiently successful, or people with more severe hyperlipidemia. There are several reasons to be conservative with the use of medications. All entail an expense. There is always the potential for side effects, and occasionally they can be severe. Taking medications is at least a little disruptive of daily routine activities. Nevertheless, if other measures have failed, medications are warranted.

Whether you need medications is a decision best made by you and your physician. These factors enter into the decision:

- the severity of the cholesterol or triglyceride abnormalities
- the presence of other unmodifiable risk factors (such as family history of heart attacks at a young age)
- evidence of existing coronary artery disease
- ineffectiveness of dietary and exercise changes

As a rule, if two risk factors are present (or if there is already evidence of coronary disease) and if dietary measures have not succeeded in changing your lipid profile out of the higher-risk range, then the use of medications is advisable.

One aspect of evaluating and treating high cholesterol and triglyceride levels is to determine whether they may be caused by another problem that can be treated itself. High blood lipids can be caused by low thyroid function, diabetes, kidney disease, and liver disease.

Elevated Cholesterol

Possible Tests
Measurement of blood lipid
  levels (see page 190)

Possible Treatment
Eating for better health
  (see page 148)
Improving your activity level
  (see page 168)
Medication (see Table 5, page
  302)

High Blood Pressure

High blood pressure is called the "silent killer." You can have it and not know it, because it seldom causes symptoms to warn you that there is a problem. However, it is the most common cardiovascular disease, affecting about one of every four Americans. Fifty-four percent of people older than 60 have high blood pressure. By age 70, 64 percent of all Americans have high blood pressure. High blood pressure is not a condition to take lightly, because it can damage components of the circulatory system, including blood vessels of the heart, the brain, the eyes, and the kidneys. The higher the pressure or the longer it goes undiagnosed or uncontrolled, the worse the outlook.

The medical term for high blood pressure is hypertension (*hyper* means "high," *tension* refers to the pressure inside your arteries). Hypertension killed almost 33,000 Americans in 1990 (the latest figure available) and this number does not include deaths from heart attacks and strokes caused by hypertension. The good news is that improved detection and treatment of high blood pressure have contributed to a dramatic reduction in strokes and heart attacks during the past 20 years.

WHAT IS BLOOD PRESSURE?
The pumping action of the heart pushes blood into the arteries with enough pressure to keep it flowing forward. The amount of blood pumped out of the heart (cardiac output) and the tone of the arteries (peripheral resistance) determine the amount of tension pushing against the walls of the arteries.

The standard way to measure blood pressure is in millimeters of mercury (mm Hg). This unit of measurement refers to how high the pressure inside your arteries is able to raise a column of mercury. Each blood pressure measurement has two numbers. The top number is your systolic blood pressure, or the highest pressure within your arteries that occurs during systole, when your heart is contracting. The bottom number is your diastolic blood pressure, or the lowest pressure within your arteries that occurs during diastole, when your heart is relaxing and filling with blood.

Although a typical blood pressure is considered to be 120/70 mm Hg, your blood pressure is not constant. Normal blood pressure refers to your blood pressure when you are resting comfortably. But your blood pressure varies with exercise, strong emotion, or stress. Even a change in position from lying down to sitting to standing can change your blood pressure. Therefore, it is necessary to take more than one reading to determine whether you have high blood pressure. About 35 percent of people who have high blood pressure on a single reading will not have an elevated value when the blood pressure is measured again. If your blood pressure is elevated during three separate measurements, it requires medical evaluation and treatment.

Blood pressure classifications and recommendations

Systolic (top number)
- Less than 130 mm Hg: normal blood pressure; recheck within 2 years
- 130 to 139 mm Hg: high normal; recheck within 1 year
- 140 to 159 mm Hg: mild hypertension*; confirm within 2 months
- 160 to 179 mm Hg: moderate hypertension*; see doctor within 1 month
- 180 to 209 mm Hg: severe hypertension; see doctor within 1 week
- 210 mm Hg or higher: very severe hypertension; see doctor immediately

Diastolic (bottom number)
- Less than 85 mm Hg: normal blood pressure; recheck within 2 years
- 85 to 89 mm Hg: high-normal blood pressure; recheck within 1 year
- 90 to 99 mm Hg: mild hypertension; confirm within 2 months
- 100 to 109 mm Hg: moderate hypertension; see doctor within 1 month
- 110 to 119 mm Hg: severe hypertension; see doctor within 1 week
- 120 mm Hg or higher: very severe hypertension; see doctor immediately

*Isolated systolic hypertension is defined as a normal diastolic blood pressure of less than 90 mm Hg but an elevated systolic blood pressure of 140 mm Hg or more. It often occurs in elderly people.
This information is based on the 1993 Report of the Joint National Committee on Detection, Evaluation, and Treatment of High Blood Pressure.

WHAT IS HIGH BLOOD PRESSURE?   High blood pressure is not an "all-or-nothing" problem. There are gradations in severity of high blood pressure; the significance of your blood pressure and the response you and your physician should make to alter it depend on how high it is (see Blood pressure classifications and recommendations, this page).

The diastolic pressure, the systolic pressure, or both may be elevated. Elevated diastolic pressure promotes damage to the kidneys and to blood vessels throughout the body. High systolic blood pressure is associated with a higher risk of coronary artery disease and stroke.

Diastolic blood pressure as low as 50 or 60 mm Hg may be considered normal. A diastolic blood pressure of 85 to 89 mm Hg also is normal, but it is at the high end of the normal range. It warrants a recheck in 1 year.

Mildly elevated blood pressure is important because it is more likely to progress to higher levels in the future. Thus, a systolic blood pressure of 140 to 159 mm Hg or a diastolic blood pressure of 90 to 99 mm Hg requires a recheck in just 2 months.

Systolic blood pressure of 160 to 179 mm Hg or more or diastolic blood pressure between 100 and 109 mm Hg is moderate hypertension. It should prompt a visit to the physician within 1 month for further evaluation and treatment measures if confirmed.

Severe hypertension is a systolic pressure of 180 to 209 mm Hg or a diastolic pressure of 110 mm Hg or higher. This requires urgent evaluation and treatment.

WHAT CAUSES HIGH BLOOD PRESSURE? Although increased output from the heart, such as occurs normally with exercise, may elevate blood pressure, the usual cause of abnormally high blood pressure is a persistent increase in resistance to blood flow through the small arterioles (the smaller branches of the arteries). The arterioles can be compared to a hose. It takes less pressure to push water through a hose with a large diameter than through a narrower hose.

The cause of the abnormal increase in resistance in the arterioles remains unknown in 95 percent of people, and they are said to have primary, or essential, hypertension. Hypertension runs in some families, although the problem may never develop in many relatives. Men and women are equally

"White coat" hypertension

Sometimes when people have their blood pressure measured in their doctor's office it is high, yet it is normal if measured at home. This condition, called "white coat" (or "stress" or "office") hypertension, may affect up to 20 percent of the population. In these people, blood pressure readings taken by a nonphysician may more accurately reflect the usual blood pressure. It also may be helpful to learn to take your own blood pressure at home. Portable devices that continuously monitor and record blood pressure are useful tools, because blood pressure can be recorded during the day and night. This method gives a more realistic and accurate assessment of an individual's true blood pressure.

It generally is not a good idea to have your blood pressure measured by an automated machine at a shopping mall. The machines are usually accurate when first installed, but heavy use and infrequent calibration can make them faulty. It is also difficult to be as relaxed as possible in that setting.

affected. For women who take birth control pills and smoke cigarettes, the risk of developing high blood pressure increases. High blood pressure is more common in blacks than in whites. Everyone's risk increases with age. Additional factors that promote the development of high blood pressure include lack of exercise, excess weight, and alcohol use. A high intake of sodium in the diet increases blood pressure in some people.

About 5 percent of people have high blood pressure caused by some other problem in the body (secondary hypertension). Blockage of the arteries leading to the kidneys or excess production of hormones normally involved in blood pressure control are uncommon causes of high blood pressure. Your doctor may want to determine whether one of these unusual disorders is the

Home blood pressure monitoring

Your doctor may recommend home measurement of your blood pressure as part of your treatment. You will need a device called a sphygmomanometer (pronounced "sfig-mo-ma-NOM-et-er") for measuring blood pressure. All blood pressure monitoring devices have an inflatable cuff that encircles your upper arm. It is important to check with your doctor and nurse about what cuff size is appropriate for you. When the cuff is inflated, the arteries in your arm are briefly closed.

As you gradually release the pressure with the airflow regulator and listen over an artery with a stethoscope, you will begin to hear a pulse beat (a tapping sound). The point at which you hear the first beat indicates your systolic pressure (the top number), and the point at which your pulse beat disappears indicates your diastolic pressure (the bottom number).

Mercury-column models feature an easy-to-read column of mercury that rises and falls in response to the amount of pressure exerted on the blood pressure cuff. This is the only device that actually measures your blood pressure in millimeters of mercury.

Spring-gauge models feature a round dial that is activated by a spring-pressure gauge that indicates the amount of pressure in the arm cuff. Each degree the needle moves in the measurement dial is equivalent to a millimeter of mercury.

Electronic digital models use built-in electronic sound sensors to read your blood pressure, which is displayed on a digital readout. Many models also have built-in pulse monitors that measure your pulse rate. You do not need a stethoscope for this type of device.

Multiple readings in different locations such as home or work, taken on a regular basis, can give your doctor valuable information that can help tailor your treatment. Be sure your device is calibrated periodically to ensure accurate readings.

If you have just had coffee or a cigarette or if your bladder is full, don't take a reading, because these factors increase your blood pressure. Sit quietly for 5 minutes before you take a reading. Then follow these steps:

1. Position your arm at heart level on a table or arm of your chair. Right-handed people usually find it easier

(continued on page 137)

cause of your high blood pressure so that it can be corrected.

WHY IS HIGH BLOOD PRESSURE BAD FOR YOU?   Many studies have clearly demonstrated a direct relationship between high blood pressure and stroke, heart disease, and renal (kidney) failure. People with uncontrolled high blood pressure are about three times more likely to have coronary artery disease, six times more likely to have congestive heart failure, and seven times more likely to have a stroke than people with controlled high blood pressure.

Treatment of high blood pressure can markedly decrease these risks. Untreated or inadequately treated hypertension has detrimental effects on your heart, arteries, brain, and kidneys. These are explained below.

Heart.   High blood pressure forces the heart to work harder than normal. Blood pressure is like a weight or load that the heart muscle must lift. Like any muscle, your heart gets larger with heavy weight lifting (see "Hypertrophic Cardiomyopathy," page 43). Eventually, however, the heart's pumping efficiency decreases when the muscle can no longer continue to adapt to the excessive work load. If this occurs, the heart muscle may weaken, and congestive heart failure develops.

Arteries.   High blood pressure also seems to accelerate the development of atherosclerosis in your arteries and arterioles as you age, increasing the chances of stroke or heart attack. High blood pressure can also lead to an aneurysm, or bulge, in an artery.

Brain.   Your chances of having a stroke (see page 100) are also increased if you have high blood pressure. A stroke is a form of brain injury caused by a blocked or ruptured blood vessel in the brain.

Kidneys. Mild, untreated high blood pressure caused the kidney damage in about 25 percent of the people who are now undergoing kidney dialysis. Early and adequate treatment of high blood pressure can prevent or delay the need for kidney dialysis or transplantation in some people.

EVALUATING HIGH BLOOD PRESSURE. If you have high blood pressure, your doctor will want to obtain a careful medical history, perform a physical examination, and perform a limited number of tests to answer the following three questions before deciding on the best method of treatment:

1. Is there damage to any organs?
2. Are there other cardiovascular risk factors?
3. Is the high blood pressure primary or a form of secondary (and possibly curable) hypertension?

To answer these questions, your doctor may order some laboratory tests to determine whether you have cardiovascular disease and, if so, its severity. If the physical examination and laboratory findings are normal, most people with mildly elevated blood pressure will not need further tests. However, further assessment may be needed if any of the following conditions exist:

- sudden onset or abrupt acceleration of high blood pressure
- very high diastolic pressure (greater than 110 mm Hg)

to measure the pressure in their left arm, and left-handed people in their right arm.

2. Apply the cuff to your bare upper arm. It should fit snugly, with its lower edge about 1 inch above the bend in your arm. Ask your doctor what size cuff you should use.

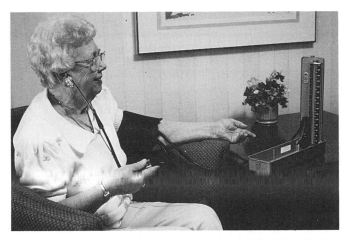

This woman is using a blood pressure cuff with a built-in stethoscope. The mercury-column measuring unit is on the table.

3. The placement of the stethoscope depends on the type of blood pressure unit you are using. If your unit has a built-in stethoscope, place the flat disk over the pulse two inches *above* the bend of your elbow. If you are using a stethoscope that is not attached to the blood pressure cuff, place the flat disk over the pulse at the bend of your elbow.
4. Squeeze the hand bulb repeatedly. When the pressure gauge reading is 30 mm Hg above your anticipated systolic blood pressure, stop pumping. You should not hear any pulse sound when you listen through the stethoscope.
5. Deflate the cuff slowly (about 2 to 3 mm Hg per second). As the pressure falls, listen for the pulse sound. Note the reading on the gauge when the beating first becomes audible. This is your systolic blood pressure.
6. Continue deflating the cuff. Note the reading when the heartbeat ceases to be audible. This is your diastolic pressure.
7. Your blood pressure is written as systolic/diastolic (for example, 140/90).

(continued on page 138)

8. Repeat the procedure at least once to confirm the accuracy of your reading.

For hearing-impaired persons, an electronic monitoring device may be best. Have your measuring device recalibrated every 6 months or so at your doctor's office, fire department, or public health service. Also check your measurement against that taken by your nurse or doctor occasionally to assess the accuracy of your results.

Your doctor will tell you how often and at what times of the day you should measure your blood pressure. Remember that blood pressure varies, so don't get too worried if a reading is unusual. Repeat the measurement in an hour.

- low blood potassium level
- evidence of kidney abnormalities
- doctor hears a bruit (pronounced "BREW-ee"), which is the sound of blood flowing through a narrowed vessel

Be sure to tell your doctor if you are taking any prescription or over-the-

---

High Blood Pressure

Possible Tests
Electrocardiogram
    (see page 192)
Determination of blood lipid
    levels (see page 190)
Urinalysis
Chest X-ray (see page 200)
Determination of electrolyte
    levels in the blood (such as
    sodium and potassium)

Possible Treatment
Eating for better health
    (see page 148)
Improving your activity level
    (see page 168)
Medications (see Table 6,
    page 304)

---

counter medications, for two reasons. First, some medications raise blood pressure. Cold, allergy, and sinus medicines, nose sprays, and diet pills can all raise blood pressure. Second, certain medications can have dangerous reactions with medications your doctor may prescribe for high blood pressure. These include certain heart medications, psychiatric medications, and diuretics ("water pills").

Excess Weight

Most people think of being overweight as a cosmetic problem. But important as appearance may be to some people, it is not the main drawback of obesity. Obesity may be a risk to your cardiovascular health. However, obesity is a bit different from other risk factors. There is little firm evidence that obesity *in itself* predisposes you to the development of coronary artery disease, the way high cholesterol or smoking does. Rather, it promotes the presence of other risk factors—such as high cholesterol, high blood pressure, and diabetes—that do increase your chances of heart disease. Also, heart disease that is already present is aggravated further by being overweight.

One of every 3 or 4 Americans is overweight, and 1 in 10 is severely overweight. Approximately 34 million adults in this country qualify as being obese.

WHAT IS A "HEALTHY" WEIGHT?
There are various ways of determining whether you are overweight—none of which are perfect. One of the easiest ways is to compare your weight with the recommended weight on the table from "Dietary Guidelines for Americans." This table and others like it have been developed based on obser-

vations of what weights correspond to the longest life spans in general. However, you must be realistic. If you have never in your adult life weighed what the table shows, the table may not be useful as a realistic goal for you.

No height-weight table can take into account individual variations in proportions of fat and lean tissue or the distribution of fat in the body. For example, a weight lifter may be overweight according to the height-weight table, and yet have a very low proportion of body fat. Men normally have a larger proportion of lean muscle and a smaller proportion of body fat than women. Conversely, an individual may not be overweight according to the tables but may have a low proportion of muscle and a high proportion of body fat.

Some overweight people have most of their excess fat deposited in their abdomens, whereas others have it deposited more in their hips and thighs. These variations may make a difference in cardiovascular risk. People shaped like apples (bigger through the abdomen and smaller in the hips and thighs—the typical male pattern of fat distribution, called truncal obesity) have a higher risk than people shaped like pears (fairly thin in the upper belly with fat accumulated in the hips and thighs—the typical female pattern of fat distribution, called gynecoid distribution). Calculating the ratio of your waist circumference to your hip circumference (divide your waist measurement by your hip measurement) can help estimate your risk. A ratio of less than 0.80 is desirable for women, and a ratio of less than 1.0 is desirable for men.

WHY IS EXCESS WEIGHT A PROBLEM? The most ominous burden

Height-weight table from "Dietary Guidelines for Americans"

Use this table for recommendations on a "healthy" weight for your height and age. Higher weights within each range generally apply to men, and lower weights to women. The table does not take into account other factors, such as your pattern of fat distribution, your bone size, or any medical problems that might influence your weight.

| Height | Weight (pounds) | |
	Ages 19–34	Ages 35 and greater
5'0"	97–128	108–138
5'1"	101–132	111–143
5'2"	104–137	115–148
5'3"	107–141	119–152
5'4"	111–146	122–157
5'5"	114–150	126–162
5'6"	118–155	130–167
5'7"	121–160	134–172
5'8"	125–164	138–178
5'9"	129–169	142–183
5'10"	132–174	146–188
5'11"	136–179	151–194
6'0"	140–184	155–199
6'1"	144–189	159–205
6'2"	148–195	164–210
6'3"	152–200	168–216
6'4"	156–205	173–222
6'5"	160–211	177–228
6'6"	164–216	182–234

From Nutrition and Your Health: Dietary Guidelines for Americans, 1990, U.S. Departments of Agriculture (USDA) and Health and Human Services (USDHHS).

The danger of excess weight

If you are this much overweight:	5%–15%	55%–60%	100%
Your risk of early death is increased by:	1.1 times	2.2 times	12 times

posed by being overweight is a shortening of your life span. The likelihood of dying early (compared with the average age of death of all people in the population) progressively increases the more overweight you are.

Some of the increased risk of early death is a result of obesity-associated problems that produce cardiac risks of their own. For example, obese people (more than 20% overweight), especially in the younger age groups, are three times as likely to have high blood pressure or diabetes and one-and-a-half times as likely to have high cholesterol. In addition, obesity increases the risk of dying from causes not related to the heart, such as pulmonary (lung) problems.

THE YO-YO SYNDROME. The risks of being overweight may not outweigh the risks of repeated weight fluctuation. Regardless of actual weight, people whose weight goes up and down because of intermittent dieting alternating with regaining the weight (the so-called yo-yo syndrome—also referred to as weight cycling) have a higher risk of coronary artery disease and death than people with more stable weights. Therefore, the best weight-loss programs look beyond a "quick fix" and help you learn a healthful way of eating throughout your lifetime.

Excess Weight

Recommendations
Eating for Better Health
(see page 148)
Improving Your Activity Level
(see page 168)

If you are not ready to make permanent changes that will keep you from ever regaining the weight, you may be better off waiting until you are more motivated. You may lose weight, but the benefit of your success may be more than undone if you simply regain it later. (Refer to the Recommendations for a Heart-Healthy Life-Style, page 145, for specific recommendations on healthful eating and exercise.)

Diabetes

People who have diabetes have at least double the risk for development of some types of heart disease compared with the risk in the general population. Unfortunately, the symptoms of heart disease in many people with diabetes are less apparent than they are in those without diabetes. In the absence of these warning symptoms, diabetic people may be unaware that they have coronary artery disease. Therefore, aggressive efforts to both *prevent* and *diagnose* coronary artery disease are all the more important for people who have diabetes.

Diabetes increases the risk for development of coronary artery disease in any of its forms (angina, heart attack, or sudden death) and for vascular disease in other parts of the body (leading to claudication, see page 98, or stroke, see page 100). People with diabetes are also more likely to have silent (or painless) myocardial ischemia or heart attacks, so significant damage to the heart can occur before treatment is initiated.

WHAT IS DIABETES? Diabetes is a disease in which too much sugar (called glucose) accumulates in the bloodstream rather than being transferred into the cells throughout the body. The full name for diabetes is diabetes mellitus (*mellitus* means "honey sweet"). The term diabetes is often used synonymously with *diabetes mellitus*, but by itself it really refers to only one of the main symptoms of the disease—frequent urination. It is derived from the Greek word for "siphon."

Diabetes is not caused by eating too much sugar. The body normally converts some of the food eaten into a type of sugar (glucose) that provides an energy source for the cells. Glucose is distributed throughout the body by the bloodstream. A hormone called insulin allows the glucose to enter the cells. In diabetes, either the pancreas stops making insulin or the body does not respond properly to the insulin that is produced. In type I, or insulin-dependent diabetes mellitus (IDDM), decreased insulin production is the main problem. In type II, or non-insulin-dependent diabetes mellitus (NIDDM), the main difficulty is a reduction in the body's response to insulin. Both types of diabetes are associated with a higher risk of cardiovascular disease.

Type I diabetes often occurs in younger people (it used to be called juvenile-onset diabetes) and affects about 1 million Americans. It is caused by decreased or no insulin production by the pancreas. The high blood levels of glucose (called hyperglycemia: *hyper* means "high," *glyc* means "sweet," *emia* means "in the blood") must be regulated by insulin injections to compensate for the deficiency of insulin production.

Type II diabetes is much more common than type I diabetes. It is known to affect at least 7 million Americans. Another 5 to 7 million people probably have type II diabetes but are unaware of it. More than 75 percent of people who have type II diabetes are over-

What is a normal blood glucose level?

- Normal blood glucose levels after an overnight fast in a person over the age of 1 year are 70 to 100 mg/dl (milligrams per deciliter). A deciliter is one-tenth of a liter, or about one-half cup
- Levels higher than 140 mg/dl measured on two separate occasions are considered indicative of diabetes

weight. Evidently, obesity is a "trigger," causing diabetes to develop in genetically vulnerable people. For them, the problem is both a deficiency of insulin and an inability of their body's cells to respond appropriately to the insulin that is there. Evidence is mounting that exercise lowers the risk

Signs and symptoms of diabetes mellitus

The American Diabetes Association estimates that 5 to 7 million Americans have diabetes but do not know it. Mild diabetes may produce no symptoms for years. People who are older than 40, are overweight or obese, and have a family history of diabetes have the greatest chance for development of type II diabetes.

Signs and symptoms of *type I* diabetes usually appear relatively suddenly:

- Increased thirst
- Increased volume and frequency of urination
- Weight loss despite increased appetite
- Fatigue

Signs and symptoms of *type II* diabetes usually develop more gradually and may be subtle. They include any of the above signs and symptoms (except weight loss) and the following:

- Frequent or slow-to-heal infections, particularly vaginitis, skin or gum infections, or bladder infections
- Blurred vision
- Tingling or numbness in the hands or feet

of type II diabetes developing, even in people who are overweight or who have a family history of diabetes. The best treatment for type II diabetes is weight loss, but if this is not achievable, then oral medications, or insulin injections, may be required.

PREVENTING CARDIOVASCULAR COMPLICATIONS OF DIABETES. Diabetes mellitus is responsible for several health complications, including an increased risk for vascular disease and coronary artery disease. Everything else being equal, the risk of heart disease is increased five times in a diabetic woman and two times in a man. The jury is still out, however, on the question of whether careful control of the blood sugar level can decrease or slow these cardiovascular risks.

Eliminating other risk factors, such as smoking, high blood cholesterol levels, high blood pressure, obesity, and lack of exercise, is especially important for people with diabetes. Any of these factors increases the risk already caused by the presence of diabetes. Refer to the detailed discussions on stopping smoking (page 146), eating for better health (page 148), and improving your activity level (page 168) for approaches to prevention.

Signs of deconditioning*

- Feeling tired most of the time
- Being unable to keep up with others of your age
- Avoiding physical activity because you know you will quickly become fatigued
- Having shortness of breath or fatigue with walking a short distance or taking a few stairs

*These symptoms can also occur because of heart problems or other diseases. If there is no medical explanation for the symptoms, gradually increasing your activity level will help you improve your physical condition.

Sedentary Life-Style

You are sedentary if you . . .

- spend most of your day sitting
- seldom walk more than a block
- have leisure-time activities that do not require you to move from place to place
- have a job that is inactive
- do not take time to exercise 20 to 30 minutes at least three times per week

Your body was built to move. It does not thrive on sitting around. Your heart and lungs perform their functions much more efficiently when you are physically active on a regular basis. The more you use your muscles, the more work they can perform before they fatigue. Regular exercise is necessary for an optimal level of health, performance, and appearance.

Maintaining a healthful activity level benefits your heart in several ways. It results in a greater capacity of the heart to pump blood. Exercise promotes weight loss. New evidence suggests that physical activity has an independent protective effect against the development of type II diabetes. Exercise may lower your total cholesterol and triglyceride levels and increase protective HDL cholesterol. It also may lower your blood pressure if you have hypertension.

All of these effects of exercise can reduce the risk for development of coronary artery disease. Exercise also may have a direct tendency to lower the risk for development of coronary artery disease independently of its effect on other risk factors.

Another way of looking at it is that *lack* of exercise, or a sedentary life-style, is a risk factor for coronary artery disease, just like smoking, a poor lipid profile, high blood pressure, a family history of coronary artery disease, and diabetes.

Most of the population of the United States is sedentary. Sedentary people have nearly twice the risk of having a fatal heart attack as active people of the same age when other factors—such as smoking and high cholesterol—are equal. The number of persons with coronary disease would decline dramatically if sedentary people would become moderately active.

Without physical activity, you will experience a gradual decline in your ability to perform activities that require physical effort. You will lose strength, endurance, and flexibility, and day-to-day activities will become harder. However, if you remain active, you can maintain or improve your fitness level. A personal exercise program is the best way to make sure that you include adequate physical activity in your daily life.

Sedentary life-style

Recommendations
Improving Your Activity Level
   (see page 168)

Stress and Personality

The question of whether psychological stress and personality cause coronary artery disease, heart attacks, and sudden cardiac death is highly controversial. A great deal of research seems to suggest that your personality, the stressful events in your life, and your body's physiological reaction to stress

What exercise can do for you

The cardiovascular benefits of an exercise program include the following:

- Increases the ability of your heart to pump blood
- Decreases your heart rate at rest and during moderate exercise
- May decrease your blood pressure if you have hypertension
- May increase your HDL cholesterol level
- May decrease LDL cholesterol and total cholesterol levels
- May decrease your triglyceride level
- Helps you control weight
- May help reduce stress
- Helps reduce elevated levels of blood sugar (glucose) in people with non-insulin-dependent diabetes

Other benefits of an exercise program include the following:

- Increases your exercise capacity, resulting in an improved ability to perform physical and mental work
- Reduces fatigue, tension, and anxiety
- May improve joint function
- Potentially reduces loss of bone mineral, therefore lessening the risk of osteoporosis
- Improves appearance and a sense of well-being
- Helps maintain bowel regularity

can increase your risk of heart disease. However, this theory is far from proven. Stress is a very difficult area to study because it is hard to measure psychological and physical responses to stress or to assess the social factors that may buffer the detrimental effects of stress.

Many different situations can be a source of stress, and the response to a given situation may vary dramatically from one person to another. These are reasons why researchers have had difficulty identifying whether or how stress contributes to the development of heart disease.

It is common for people with heart disease to report that emotional peaks cause chest pain, and it is also common for heart attacks to occur during emotionally difficult periods. The added stress of emotional upset may disrupt the balance between supply and demand of the heart for oxygen, causing chest pain.

Although in certain cases it seems possible that acute stress was a factor in precipitating a heart attack, it is not clear whether ongoing stress can cause the underlying coronary artery disease (atherosclerosis) that is usually associated with heart attacks. To try to answer that question, researchers have studied the subject of stress and heart disease in terms of people's personalities, social support systems, and their body's physiological responses to stress.

The concept of a psychological or personality component to heart disease was advanced in 1964 when two researchers, Dr. Meyer Friedman and Dr. Ray Rosenman, developed the concept of a "type A" personality. Type A people always seem to be in a hurry. They are competitive, strive intensely for achievement, and need to be productive. In many ways, these are positive characteristics in a society that emphasizes accomplishments. But type A people also are impatient, over-committed to their work, and easily provoked to hostility. They tend to have few interests outside their work. In contrast, people with type B personalities, although interested in achievement, in most instances are relaxed, unhurried, and more easily satisfied with their pace. Some researchers suggest, on the basis of one large study,

that type A people have up to twice the risk of type B people for coronary artery disease.

Research also indicates that your social situation, and your response to it, can affect your risk of disease. Stable social relationships seem to be associated with good health. Lack of social contacts or too many stressful "life events," such as divorce, death of a family member or close friend, loss or change of job, or moving to a new home, may potentially increase the risk of heart disease.

Dr. Robert Eliot proposed the concept that certain people are "hot reactors," which means that their bodies respond dramatically to stress. Hot reactors exhibit extreme increases in heart rate and blood pressure in response to the everyday stresses of life. According to this theory, these surges may gradually damage the coronary arteries and heart itself.

WHAT HAPPENS IN YOUR BODY WHEN YOU ARE UNDER STRESS?

When confronted with a difficult or threatening situation ("stressor," in the language of the stress physiologist), both animals and humans respond in a similar manner—the so-called fight or flight response. Your heart rate and blood pressure increase, blood vessels in your skin constrict, muscle tension and blood flow to muscles increase, blood sugar rises, and the tendency of your blood to clot increases. In other words, you rapidly ready yourself for vigorous action. Many of these changes are triggered by your sympathetic nervous system and by a discharge of the hormone epinephrine (adrenaline) from the adrenal gland.

The increases in heart rate and blood pressure together increase the heart's need for oxygen and may bring on angina in people with coronary artery disease. The increased tendency of the blood to clot may predispose to a coronary thrombus (clot in an artery of the heart) and a resulting heart attack.

In addition to this "alarm" type of stress reaction in the "hot reactor," Dr. Eliot proposed that there is a second type of stress reaction, which might best be termed "vigilance." The firefighter hearing the alarm exemplifies the alarm type of stress, and the air traffic controller—monitoring continuously to prevent rare but tragic problems—represents the vigilant type of stress.

Many people experience this vigilant type of stress on an ongoing basis: a patient (or parent or spouse of a patient) with a potentially recurring disease such as cancer, an employee whose company is undergoing a reorganization that may potentially eliminate his or her job, and anyone who lives or works with someone with a violent temper. Vigilance involves chronic, low-level arousal without the surges that characterize alarm.

Stress

Recommendations
Handling Stress (see page 172)

RECOMMENDATIONS FOR A HEART-HEALTHY LIFE-STYLE

There will probably never be a prescription that guarantees the health of your heart. But, waiting until heart disease strikes and then hoping for a guarantee of a failproof treatment are unrealistic expectations, too.

You can take steps to prevent or delay heart disease and to improve your outlook if it has already occurred. The impact of these steps goes beyond potential protection from heart disease—they can even improve the way you look and feel today. All of these "lifestyle" factors involve decisions you make every day. Those individual decisions—such as whether to smoke, what to eat, how to make time for exercise, how to relax—become habits.

In addition to reducing cardiovascular risks, the facets of a heart-healthy life-style complement each other. For example, if you stop smoking, your capacity for exercise will probably improve. Many people find that regular exercise relieves stress and tension and provides a feeling of accomplishment. Better eating habits and exercise work together to help you lose weight, reduce cholesterol and triglyceride levels, and improve HDL cholesterol levels. If some of your habits do not promote your health, they can be changed. Changing begins with individual decisions that become lifelong healthful habits. Many people who adopt these habits find they feel so much better that it would be worth it even if cardiovascular disease was not prevented.

Don't expect to change all your habits at once. You may find that tiny changes, over years, become more permanent. Good health habits are the work of a lifetime.

How to Stop Smoking

THE RIGHT ATTITUDE. Eighty-five percent of smokers either have tried to quit or would like to quit, but 75 to 90 percent return to smoking after any single attempt. Many are reluctant to even try because they fear failing. However, each time you try increases the chances that you will succeed. The average person takes three or four tries to quit before achieving sustained abstinence. You should think of each relapse not as a failure but as an opportunity to learn. In this way, the circumstances leading to relapse can be avoided or changed in the future.

Deciding to "tough it out" does not work well over the long term. Part of your abstinence program will be to change your patterns and thoughts associated with smoking. Start by getting rid of the cigarettes and ashtrays in your house. Make it inconvenient to respond to your urge to smoke.

It often helps to analyze when you smoke and what cues you to smoke and then to identify behaviors that you can use to replace smoking. For example, if you have the urge to smoke during telephone conversations, find something other than smoking to replace that behavior. Something as simple as doodling on a notepad that you keep by the phone might help.

Let others, especially family and friends, know how they can help and support you both in words and in action. Especially in the early weeks and months after quitting, stay away from situations in which other people smoke. If you are accustomed to smoking while having an alcoholic beverage, you may have to stop drinking for a while. Alcohol lowers your inhibitions and resolve and frequently promotes a relapse.

If you truly want to quit smoking, you have to develop a very negative image of cigarettes. You may look at cigarettes as a friend that will help you through any situation and will always "be there" for you. It is true that the cigarettes will always be there, but they will be there at a terrible cost. Think of cigarettes as the insidious killers that they are. It may also help to examine all of the positive aspects of quitting, instead of all that you are giving up. Make quitting a positive choice rather than a negative one. For some people, setting an example for their children is a strong motivator.

To quit smoking, you must develop a mental image that smoking interferes with your other lifetime goals. For many years, smokers have been in the minority. Now only 28 percent of Americans smoke, and the very act of smoking makes them less welcome in many environments and social circles.

THE RIGHT STRATEGY. Once you have decided to quit smoking and have developed an attitude that permits you to approach that effort in a positive manner, the next step is to adopt a method that has the highest possible likelihood of success. There is no single best way to stop smoking. The best way is one that you believe will work for you. No method is easy, and the focal point of every method is maintaining the commitment to quit—permanently.

Several effective techniques for quitting are available. One of the most successful techniques is to stop smoking "cold turkey." The most effective decision to stop, though, is not made in a cavalier or spontaneous fashion. Rather, the most successful stopping strategy, although sudden, is the result of planning. A specific date or event can be planned as the time for stopping. Some people find that if they tell others they intend to stop on a certain date, their commitment to quit is increased. Others turn the day of quitting into a near ceremonial occasion. Most researchers, doctors, and ex-smokers agree that the more concrete and explicit the decision and act of quitting, the more likely you will succeed. There are many different ways to quit, including nicotine-replacement therapy (gum or skin patches), self-help programs, group programs, and hypnosis.

Despite the numerous behavioral adjustments that will assist you in refraining from tobacco use, the fact that addiction to nicotine is a component of the problem means that you may need additional assistance in overcoming its effect. Nicotine withdrawal begins within hours after your last cigarette. Withdrawal symptoms can include craving, irritability, anxiety, headache, depression, restlessness, and difficulty concentrating. Although smoking behavior can and, in most cases, should be stopped abruptly, nicotine withdrawal may be most manageable if it is done more gradually.

This need for gradual withdrawal is the justification for use of nicotine gum and nicotine skin patches, both of which release low levels of nicotine into the bloodstream over extended periods to ease withdrawal symptoms. Your doctor can prescribe them for you with specific instructions on their use. Neither nicotine gum nor patches are effective unless used as part of a smoking cessation program. If your doctor prescribes nicotine gum, chew it until you feel a tingling sensation in your mouth (about 10 seconds), then ''park it'' between your cheek and gums. Then periodically re-chew and re-park for about 30 minutes. Use one piece of gum for every two cigarettes that you would have smoked. Taper off the gum until you stop using it altogether in 3 to 6 months.

Nicotine transdermal (skin) patches have also been shown to help smokers stop smoking. The major advantage the patches have over nicotine gum is the ease with which they are used. The nicotine is slowly released through the skin and enters the bloodstream. Nicotine patches are effective at reducing withdrawal symptoms and then, like the gum, their use is tapered. When the nicotine levels decrease and the addictive ''pull'' has subsided, maintenance of abstinence will depend on the behavioral adjustments you have made.

Other medications, notably a blood pressure medication called clonidine, which is available in a skin patch form, have been shown to reduce symptoms of nicotine withdrawal. They may be advisable for some people with particularly uncomfortable withdrawal symp-

General strategies for successful smoking cessation

1. Stay away from opportunities to smoke. Do not go where you are likely to be tempted.
2. Analyze when you smoke and what cues you to smoke, and then identify activities you can use to replace smoking.
3. Develop a negative image of cigarettes. They are smelly, dirty, and disgusting. They turn your fingers and teeth yellow, make your breath and clothes smell, cost you money, and offend your friends.
4. Remind yourself of all the benefits you have gained from not smoking.
5. View relapses as a learning experience.
6. Read and use helpful materials and programs from the American Cancer Society, the American Lung Association, and the American Heart Association.

Basic responses to a smoker's fears about quitting

I have failed before, and I will probably fail again.
Remember that fewer than 25 percent of smokers are able to quit on the first try. Most take three or four tries. Stopping smoking is like learning anything new: it takes several tries. Did you learn to ride a bicycle on the first try?

I will have unbearable cravings.
Most cravings last less than 20 minutes. Plan what you can do until the urge goes away.

I will get irritable and frustrated.
While you are quitting, make fewer demands on yourself. Give yourself a break.

I will be unable to concentrate.
Maybe you could quit smoking during your vacation, so the need to concentrate is not as great.

I cannot stand feeling so restless.
Take walks or other "time out" periods. Handle objects. Use your hands for other things.

I need the stimulant effect of smoking.
Increase your activity and begin an exercise program. Work on getting better sleep.

I will gain weight.
One-third of ex-smokers gain weight, one-third lose weight, and one-third stay at the same weight. Only 10 percent of those who gain weight keep the increased weight. It may help to keep a diet diary and start an exercise program while you are quitting.

I will not be able to sleep.
Do not read or watch television in bed. Go to bed only when tired. Do not nap during the day. Exercise during the day. Avoid caffeine at night. If you do not fall asleep in 30 minutes after you go to bed, get up for a while.

toms who do not tolerate nicotine gum or patches.

Of course, the problem with quitting is not the moment of stopping, but the process of never smoking again. Experts now recognize that prevention of relapse is the key to success. Again, your commitment is the mainstay, but many of the strategies to prevent relapse are designed to give your commitment a better chance.

Setting measurable, well-defined goals, recording your behavior to monitor your progress, having frequent contact with health care providers, and arranging for social support and positive reinforcement will help you succeed. Many people use token rewards to encourage their progress. It is also important to maintain this vigilance over a long time to avoid relapse.

Regardless of the specific assistance you may need in stopping smoking and maintaining abstinence, a comprehensive smoking cessation center or nicotine dependence treatment center may enhance your effort. In these settings, counseling, prescriptions, instructions, and follow-up can be focused on your specific needs.

Quitting smoking is probably the single best thing you can do to reduce your risk of heart attack. Modifying other risk factors certainly will help, but nothing can help more than getting rid of cigarettes. The combination of smoking and other risk factors greatly amplifies your risk of developing coronary artery disease.

Be a winner and quit.

Eating for Better Health

Food choices are one of the most individual parts of your life-style. Even family members who eat most meals together choose different amounts and different combinations of food. There is an almost unlimited variety of foods that fit into a heart-healthy diet.

Medical experts have identified certain nutrient components of food—fat, cholesterol, sodium, and calories—that relate to heart disease. Your doctor will probably discuss with you individual recommendations, in terms such as grams of fat, milligrams of cholesterol and sodium, etc. Sometimes it is difficult to take the next step of translating these recommendations into everyday food choices. Registered dietitians are available to help you take the next step. Your doctor can refer you to one for help. This section briefly reviews some common recommendations and then helps you pull these facts together into an overall plan for eating more healthfully.

Unfortunately, many people get discouraged by nutrition advice because they mistakenly think that they cannot eat their favorite foods. A more positive and encouraging approach is to consider that no food is forbidden. Good health comes from eating a variety of foods—meats, dairy products, and especially vegetables, fruits, and grains—in moderate amounts. You may have to change some of your routine grocery purchases, some of your cooking methods, and the amounts of some foods you are accustomed to eating, but you do not have to take the enjoyment out of eating. In fact, you will probably discover some new tastes, and your new eating habits can lead to improvement in the way you look and feel.

The following section reviews the most common recommendations about fat, cholesterol, sodium, and calories. The recommendations form the basis for practical changes in food selections you can try in your own meals.

THE CHOLESTEROL-FAT CONNECTION. Cholesterol and fat are essential nutrients in your diet, but both relate to the risk of heart disease. Cholesterol from food may affect your

Reducing cholesterol and fat one step at a time

The American Heart Association recommends a two-step approach for people trying to reduce their risk of heart disease. Step 1 may result in an improvement in blood cholesterol levels, especially for people who eat the typical high-fat American diet. When your cholesterol is rechecked after 3 to 6 months, if it has not decreased into a lower-risk range, then step 2 recommendations, which are more carefully tailored, should be considered.

	Typical American intake	Step 1 recommendations	Step 2 recommendations
Cholesterol	Men: 440 mg Women: 280 mg	< 300 mg	< 200 mg
Fat	34%–40% of total calories	< 30% of total calories*	25% to 30% of total calories
Saturated	13% of total calories	< 10% of total calories*	< 7% of total calories
Monoun-saturated	14% of total calories	< 15% of total calories	< 10% of total calories
Polyun-saturated	7% of total calories	< 10% of total calories	< 10% of total calories

*Refer to page 163 to determine how to find your 30% level of dietary fat at your individual calorie level.

blood cholesterol level, particularly when you eat it in excessive amounts. Saturated fat is another culprit in raising blood cholesterol levels. Your body converts dietary saturated fat into cholesterol and other fats that can damage your blood vessels and your heart. Therefore, it is wise to reduce your intake of both cholesterol and fat.

Cholesterol is found only in foods of animal origin, such as red meat, eggs, milk and milk products, fish, poultry, and animal fats such as lard and butter. The best way to limit the total amount of cholesterol in your diet is to go easy on animal foods and eat more grains, vegetables, and fruits.

Fat comes from both animal and plant sources. There are three types of fat, and they have different effects on blood cholesterol levels:

- Saturated fats tend to raise total blood cholesterol levels.
- Monounsaturated fats in the recommended amounts may tend to raise the "good" type of blood cholesterol, high-density lipoprotein (HDL) cholesterol, without raising total blood cholesterol.
- Polyunsaturated fats in the recommended amounts may tend to reduce total blood cholesterol, but they also lower the "good" HDL cholesterol.

All fat is made up of a mixture of saturated, monounsaturated, and polyunsaturated fats. *The most important message is to reduce the amount of all types of fat in your diet.* The foods that probably contribute most to your fat intake are fats and oils (pourable and spreadable), meat, and milk and other dairy products.

Sources of sodium

77% from sodium added to processed foods
12% from sodium naturally contained in foods
 6% salt added at the table
 5% salt added in cooking

From Mattes RD, Donnelly D: Relative contributions of dietary sodium sources. *Journal of the American College of Nutrition* 10:383–393, 1991. Copyright © and reprinted by permission of John Wiley & Sons.

Research shows that the most realistic and effective strategies to reduce fat include substituting lean meats for higher-fat selections, substituting skim milk for whole or low-fat milk, and using less "pourable" or "spreadable" fats (butter, margarine, oil, sauces, dressings, gravies).

SODIUM. The amount of sodium in the diet is important for people who have high blood pressure (see page 133) or congestive heart failure (see page 36). For some people who have high blood pressure, reducing sodium intake will help reduce blood pressure. Excess sodium encourages your body to retain fluid. Restricting sodium may therefore improve the effects of medications such as diuretics and other drugs used to treat high blood pressure or congestive heart failure.

The average American consumes about 4,000 milligrams or more of sodium a day. The new food labeling regulations establish 2,400 milligrams of sodium as the uppermost limit, even if you have no signs of heart disease. Most people with heart disease should limit their sodium intake to less than 2,000 milligrams a day.

Table salt is the most obvious source of sodium (it contains 40 percent sodium and 60 percent chloride). Just one teaspoon of salt contains 2,000 milligrams of sodium. The salt you add in cooking or at the table may be only the "tip of the iceberg" in your total sodium intake. Even many natural foods such as milk, meat, and vegetables contain sodium. But by far, sodium that is added to foods in processing is the biggest source (at least two-thirds) of sodium in your diet.

Food manufacturers are offering an expanding array of reduced-sodium products, such as luncheon meats, canned vegetables, salad dressings, and cheeses. Read nutrition labels to find the sodium content (shown in milligrams). You may need to avoid some reduced-sodium foods because they may still be high in fat. Dairy products are a natural source of sodium. Three cups of milk a day contain 375 milligrams of sodium, which is not an excessive amount. But if you drink more than 3 cups and eat yogurt, cheese, and ice cream, the amount of sodium quickly adds up.

Use fresh foods in place of processed foods so that you can control the amount of sodium that is added. And when you are cooking, go for fresh flavors instead of masking the natural flavor with salt. Use herb and spice blends for added flavor. Do not add salt to your food at the table.

It may take 6 to 8 weeks to learn to appreciate less salty flavors. You will begin to taste the other flavors after you reduce the salt.

CALORIES. Calories are a standard measure or description of the amount of energy contained in all types of food. Calories come from the nutrients fat, protein, and carbohydrates. Too many calories in your diet supply too much energy. If your body does not need the energy right away, it is stored as body fat. It takes approximately 3,500 excess calories to gain a pound. Excess body fat aggravates conditions such as diabetes, high blood pressure, and high blood cholesterol and triglyceride levels, and it puts extra stress on your heart.

High-fat foods are high in calories because fat is the most concentrated source of energy. There are 9 calories in each gram of fat but only 4 calories in each gram of protein or carbohy-

Precautions about salt substitutes

If you have been advised to reduce your sodium intake, you may wonder about using a "salt substitute." Before you try one, check with your doctor. Here's why: 1. Some salt substitutes or "lite" salts contain a mixture of sodium chloride (salt) and other compounds. To achieve that familiar salty taste, you may end up using more of the salt substitute, and the result is that you do not reduce your sodium intake at all. 2. Potassium chloride is a common ingredient in salt substitutes. Too much potassium can be harmful for people with kidney problems or people who are taking certain medications for the treatment of high blood pressure or heart failure. Some diuretics such as amiloride (Midamor), spironolactone (Aldactone), and triamterene (Dyrenium) and medications that combine hydrochlorothiazide with one of the above generic drugs (such as Moduretic, Aldactazide, Dyazide, Maxzide) cause the kidneys to retain potassium. If you take one of these medications, you may need to limit the amount of potassium you eat.

drate. (For comparison, a paperclip weighs about a gram.) Thus, small amounts of fat provide many more calories than other kinds of foods. It is

What is a reasonable calorie level?

The precise amount of calories that is best for you depends on many factors, including whether you are currently at a desirable weight or are overweight or underweight. Your level of physical activity also determines your calorie needs. The following formulas show approximate calorie requirements for maintaining your current weight.

If you are sedentary, current weight (in pounds) multiplied by 12 = daily calorie requirements.

If you are moderately physically active, current weight (in pounds) multiplied by 14 = daily calorie requirements.

If you are extremely active, current weight (in pounds) multiplied by 16 or 18 = daily calorie requirements.

easy to overeat fatty foods. Carbohydrates tend to be bulkier; therefore, you are more likely to feel full, even though the calorie content is less.

Another factor may indicate why fatty foods are so "fattening." When you eat too much fat, it is easy for your body to convert those extra calories into excess body fat. Excess calories from protein and carbohydrate can be stored as body fat, too, but your body may burn more calories in this conversion process than it does when converting fat calories into body fat.

Think of what you are getting with the calories you take in. Some foods, such as sugar and alcohol, provide calories but few other nutrients. These foods are often described as sources of "empty" calories. The ideal diet contains the right amount of calories and emphasizes foods that provide the most nutrients.

Principles of Weight Control. Perhaps it seems odd to think that the problem of being overweight is having too much energy, but that is a fact. Stored body fat (adipose tissue) is potential energy. The only way your body will use this stored energy is if you "burn" more energy than you take in. By limiting calorie intake and increasing energy use through activity, your body will have to draw from some of its stored body fat to meet your energy needs.

If you need to lose weight, a slow and steady approach is safest and more likely to be permanent. One rule of thumb for losing about a pound a week is to reduce 500 calories a day. A combination of cutting back on your calorie intake and increasing the number of calories you "burn" through exercise is an ideal way to achieve a 500-calorie deficit. (See page 173 for more information about exercise.)

It is not a good idea to consume fewer than 1,400 calories without your doctor's advice, because it is difficult to get the nutrition you need with limited quantities of food. Also, weight loss may be too rapid in some people eating fewer than 1,400 calories.

Once you are satisfied with your weight, your goal will be to maintain it by having your calorie intake evenly balance the calories you "burn."

By concentrating more on calorie balance than on pounds, you will be preparing yourself at the outset for one aspect of weight loss which is distressing to a lot of people. It is discouraging when you step on the scale after making an honest effort at restricting calories and increasing activity level, only to find that there has been negligible loss of weight. In reality, this may be a sign that you are doing it *right!* Indeed, what is occurring is that fat depots are being used up, but because of exercise you are adding muscle. Weight loss will occur if the negative calorie balance is sustained, but the key word will be "consistency."

The need for a sustained, consistent program of negative calorie balance followed by *lifelong* even-calorie balance means that the program has to mesh with the realities of your daily life. There is little to be gained by a heroic 6-week diet and exercise regimen (even if it is a nutritionally sound one, as opposed to a "crash diet") if it is so inconvenient that afterward you must eliminate it simply to get on with your life. Rather, apply the same philosophy that works for controlling your cholesterol: incorporate calorie consciousness into your daily life without letting it dominate your life. This approach will give you a head start in ensuring that the dietary principles you learn will become second nature to you.

TAKE THE NEXT STEP.   The types and variety of foods you select make a difference to your heart and your overall health. You already know the importance of controlling fat, cholesterol, sodium, and calories. Too much sugar and alcohol also are not healthful. The following section provides specific suggestions for replacing less-healthful foods with more-healthful, tasty food choices.

BASIC EATING GUIDELINES.
These recommendations for improving your diet for your heart's sake are not a "prescription" diet. Eating healthfully is something your whole family can enjoy together. The principles of good nutrition are basically the same whether you are trying to maintain your health or whether you need to reduce your level of blood cholesterol, lose weight, or control high blood pressure or diabetes. Your doctor or registered dietitian may suggest more specific changes in your diet to help you lose weight or customize the treatment of diabetes, high blood pressure, or high blood cholesterol.

The following six basic guidelines will make your diet more healthful. They start by suggesting you eat more—not less—of certain types of foods.

1. Eat five or more servings of various fruits and vegetables every day.
2. Eat six or more daily servings of grain products, preferably whole-grain breads, cereals, rice, and pasta.
3. Include two to three servings of low-fat or skim milk dairy products in your daily diet.
4. Eat no more than 5 to 7 ounces of meat a day. Occasionally substitute other high-protein, low-fat foods, such as eggs and dried beans, for meat.
5. Use fats sparingly—no more than 6 to 8 teaspoons of spreadable or pourable fat in your daily diet.
6. Eat fewer sweets and desserts and drink less alcohol.

Use these basic principles when you eat, shop for groceries, and plan meals, as well as when you eat out. You will most likely decrease fat and calories in your diet by eating more fruits, vegetables, and grains, and the temptation to eat higher-calorie processed foods that may be higher in fat and sodium will diminish.

The following pages discuss each guideline in more detail and provide specific suggestions for grocery shopping, reading labels, and cooking. With a few simple substitutions, you will be eating more healthfully.

Eat Five or More Servings of Various Fruits and Vegetables Every Day.   What do fruits and vegetables

---

Fruits and vegetables

Best Choices
Fresh, frozen, or dried fruits and vegetables

Go Easy On
Canned fruits (because of added sugar and less fiber) and canned vegetables (because of higher sodium content)
Avocados and olives (because of higher fat content)

Limit or Avoid
Coconut, fruits and vegetables in cream or creamy sauces, cheese sauce, butter, and dips, and breaded and deep-fried vegetables

Grains without guilt (lower-fat alternatives)

	Instead of these	Fat, grams	Choose these	Fat, grams
Breakfast	Donut (cake or raised yeast)	12	Toast, 2 slices with spreadable fruit	2
	Fast-food biscuit	13	English muffin	1
	Granola (about ⅓ cup)	5	Cold cereal	1
	Danish or toaster pastry	7	Cooked cereal	0–2
Snacks	Microwave popcorn (4 cups)	7–17	Air-popped popcorn	Trace
	Potato chips (1 ounce)	10	Pretzels (10 twists)	2
	Corn chips (1 ounce)	10	Rice cake, 1	Trace
	Cheese snack crackers (1 ounce)	10	Melba toast	Trace
Lunch or dinner	Croissant	12	Pita bread	1
			White hard roll	2
			Wheat roll	2
			Rye roll	2
			Bagel (plain)	2
Desserts	Carrot cake, frozen	12	Angel food cake from mix, ¹⁄₁₂ of cake	Trace
	Chocolate cake from mix, ¹⁄₁₂ of cake	11	Pound cake, frozen, fat free, ¹⁄₁₀ of cake	0
Cookies	Homemade chocolate chip, 2	5	Graham crackers, 2 squares	2
	Chocolate sandwich cookies, 2	4	Animal crackers, 15	3
			Gingersnaps, 3	1
			Fortune cookies, 2	Trace

have to do with heart disease? Most fruits and vegetables are low in fat and contain no cholesterol. Depending on how they are prepared, most fruits and vegetables are also low in sodium and calories, which is an important factor if you are trying to control your blood pressure or weight.

Eating more fruits and vegetables in place of foods that have more fat and calories is a relatively easy way to improve your diet without cutting back on the amount you eat. You will learn to enjoy the natural flavors, and the increased fiber in your diet will have added health benefits (see page 155).

Steam vegetables or cook them in a microwave oven with a small amount of water. This method will help preserve natural flavors so butter or sauces are not necessary. Experiment with different spices, herbs, and flavored vinegars to add pizzazz to vegetables.

Many vegetables are good to eat raw. Keep celery, carrots, cauliflower, broccoli, cherry tomatoes, and other raw vegetables ready to eat in your refrigerator when the urge to snack attacks. Remember not to smother them with dips that may contain a lot of fat. Commercial low-fat dips are available, or make your own with low-fat yogurt or low-fat cottage cheese mixed with various flavorings.

Fruits are another good snack food. They are rich in nutrients and high in fiber. Consider using fruit as a naturally sweet dessert. There is one precaution, however. Some people with high triglycerides may not be able to eat all the fruit they want because of its natural sugar content.

Eat Six or More Servings of Grain Products (Preferably Whole-Grain Breads, Cereals, Rice, and Pasta)

Every Day. Contrary to popular belief, foods such as bread, pasta, and some baked goods are low in fat and calories. However, you have to be selective about what you add to these foods. For example, fat-laden cream-based or cheesy sauces are often added to pasta. Likewise, not all baked goods are low in fat; croissants, many sweet breads, and even some crackers are high in fat.

Look for whole-grain breads and cereals instead of refined products. Whole grains have more protein, fiber, and trace minerals such as iron, which are stored in the kernel's bran and germ. During the refining process, the kernel's bran and germ are removed.

If you choose whole-grain products, you will automatically increase the amount of fiber you eat. Foods high in fiber are good replacements for higher-fat food choices.

Fiber comes in two forms: *soluble* and *insoluble*. Soluble fiber is most beneficial for the health of your heart. Soluble fiber seems to regulate your body's production and elimination of cholesterol. Good sources of soluble fiber are oat products, dried beans and peas, lentils, apples, and citrus fruits.

Insoluble fiber, because it travels through your digestive tract faster than soluble fiber, may prevent or relieve constipation. Some experts believe that because insoluble fiber moves through your body faster, it may reduce the time that potentially cancer-causing substances remain in your digestive tract. Insoluble fiber is found in whole-grain products and many fruits, vegetables, and cereals.

Most Americans consume only about half the amount of fiber that they should. Try to include at least 20 to 25 grams of fiber every day from various

Grains

> *Best Choices* (lowest in total fat)
> Whole-grain breads and cereals, English muffins, bagels, bread sticks, rice, pasta, macaroni, low-fat crackers (such as soda, graham, rye, plain), angel food cake, plain popcorn, pretzels, vanilla wafers, and fig bar cookies
>
> *Go Easy On* (contain moderate amounts of total fat)
> Muffins (small bran, blueberry, or apple), frozen waffles, cornbread, granola bar, gingerbread, animal crackers, quick breads, cake donuts
>
> *Limit or Avoid* (highest in total fat)
> Frosted cakes, pies, cheesecake, Danish pastries, pecan rolls, croissants, cupcake-type muffins (jumbo size, loaded with nuts, chips, coconut, or cream cheese), buttered popcorn, egg noodles, high-fat snack crackers, and chips

food sources. More than 50 grams has not been shown to be beneficial. If you include more fruits, vegetables, and grains in your diet, especially those that are fresh, raw, and whole, you will naturally increase your fiber intake.

New food labeling requirements will make it easier to determine which foods are good sources of fiber. Food manufacturers must show the total amount of dietary fiber per serving. Manufacturers have the option of providing information about the soluble and insoluble fiber content of the food.

Increase the amount of fiber in your diet gradually to let your body adjust. If you eat too much fiber when you are not accustomed to it, you may experience bloating, gas, and diarrhea.

As you increase the fiber in your diet, it is important to increase the amount of liquids you drink, because fiber absorbs fluid as it passes through your body. To maintain fluid balance, drink 8 to 10 glasses of water a day.

Include Two to Three Servings of Low-Fat or Skim Milk Dairy Products in Your Daily Diet. Dairy products do not have to be a significant source of fat in your diet. To get an idea of the differences among dairy products, consider that 8 ounces of whole milk contain about as much fat as 8 ounces of skim milk plus 2 teaspoons of butter or margarine. Skim milk has an added advantage—the calcium content is higher than that of whole milk. For women, who especially need adequate calcium to help prevent osteoporosis, dairy products are a main source of calcium. You can get the benefits without the fat by focusing on low-fat or no-fat varieties.

For example, instead of eating a slice of regular American cheese, you can cut the calories in half and reduce the fat by three-fourths by choosing reduced-fat American cheese.

Although switching to milk with less fat is a good way to reduce calories and fat in the diet for most adults, infants and children younger than age 2 may need the extra calories and fat in whole milk.

Dairy products

Best Choices
Skim milk, nonfat yogurt, 1 percent to 2 percent low-fat cheese, and 1 percent to 2 percent low-fat cottage cheese

Go Easy On
2 percent milk, ice milk, low-fat yogurt, creamed cottage cheese (4 percent fat), and part-skim-milk cheeses such as mozzarella, ricotta, and farmer cheese

Limit or Avoid
Whole milk, cheese or yogurt made from whole milk, ice cream, nondairy coffee creamers, and nondairy whipped toppings

---

Eat No More Than 5 to 7 Ounces of Meat a Day. Occasionally substitute other high-protein foods, such as eggs and dried beans, for meat.

Two modest changes—reducing the amount of meat you eat and switching from high-fat choices such as regular ground beef to lower-fat choices such as well-trimmed round steak, baked fish, or skinless chicken—can make a significant difference in the total amount of fat you eat. This is a much more effective and realistic strategy than totally giving up red meat or other foods you enjoy.

Meat servings should be about 3 ounces or less per person. A 3-ounce serving of cooked beef, pork, or lamb is about the size of a deck of cards. The meat from one chicken leg and thigh or from half of a whole breast is approximately 3 ounces.

Shift your meal planning from one of making meat the centerpiece to making meat the accompaniment. Prepare more casseroles or mixtures with meat as one of the ingredients, and limit high-fat ingredients such as sour cream or cheese. If you are increasing the amount of fruits, vegetables, and grains that you eat, reducing meat will become easier. The benefit is that you will reduce the amount of fat and cholesterol you eat, which are the most important dietary factors in reducing your blood cholesterol. It is also the most straightforward way to cut calories.

Choosing and Cooking Lean Red Meats. U.S. Department of Agriculture (USDA) meat grades tell you about the amount of fat in beef: USDA Prime beef has the highest proportion of fat, USDA Choice beef has less fat than Prime, and USDA Select grade has an even lower amount. Even if you closely trim all the fat off the edges of a piece of meat, interspersed particles of fat in the meat (called marbling) contribute to the fat content. The amount of marbling is one factor for determining the grade of beef. For example, Prime top round steak has about 9 grams of fat in a 3-ounce serving, Choice grade has about 6 grams, and Select grade has about 5 grams. The amount of cholesterol is almost the same in all three grades, because cholesterol is found in the muscle portion of the meat.

Leaner grades of meat may be less expensive, but they are often less tender. Tenderize lean cuts of meat by cooking them slowly in liquid or marinating them before cooking in marinades that contain herbs blended with vinegar, juice (such as lemon, tomato, lime), or wine. Pounding, grinding, and slicing across the grain can also help tenderize meats.

Use oven temperatures of 350° or lower to allow some of the fat inside the meat to melt so it can be drained away. Higher temperatures may seal the fat into the meat.

If you have been frying meats in oil or shortening, try using a nonstick pan and nonstick cooking spray to reduce the amount of fat. Better yet, use the broiler instead of a frying pan and oil to brown meat.

Remove fat from stews, soups, and broth by chilling them and peeling the hardened fat from the top. If you do not have time to chill liquids that contain fat, wrap ice cubes in a paper towel and quickly skim the cubes across the top of the liquid. The fat will stick to the cold surface. You can also use a baster to remove the fat.

Include Low-Fat Poultry in Your Diet. Almost all cuts of chicken and turkey are low in fat and cholesterol

Lower-fat meat choices

These meats are good choices when you are limiting fat and cholesterol in your diet. All the figures are for 3-ounce cooked servings, with all visible fat removed. No fat was added in preparing the meats. (Figures are rounded.)

Name of cut	Calories	Fat, grams	Cholesterol, milligrams
Beef (lean only, choice grade)			
Top round steak, broiled	165	6	70
Eye of round, roasted	160	6	60
Tip round, roasted	165	7	70
Sirloin, broiled	180	8	75
Tenderloin, broiled	180	8	70
Bottom round, braised	190	8	80
Chuck arm pot roast, braised	200	9	90
Pork (lean only)			
Tenderloin, roasted	140	4	80
Ham, boneless, water added, extra lean (about 5 percent fat)	110	4	40
Center loin chop, broiled	200	9	80
Poultry (roasted)			
Turkey, light meat, without skin	130	2	60
Chicken breast, meat only	140	3	70
Chicken drumstick, meat only	150	5	80
Chicken breast, meat and skin	170	7	70
Chicken drumstick, meat and skin	180	9	80
Fish, shellfish (baked or broiled)			
Cod	90	1	50
Lobster, boiled	100	1	100
Shrimp (steamed or boiled)	110	2	160
Tuna, light, canned in water	90	2	30
Halibut	120	2	30
Salmon, Atlantic/coho	150	7	50

Meats

Best Choices

Lean meats ("Select" or "Choice" grade), fish, poultry without the skin, egg whites or egg substitutes, water-packed tuna or salmon, cold cuts or frankfurters that contain no more than 5 grams of fat per 1-ounce serving, dried beans and other legumes

Go Easy On

Peanut butter, nuts, fish canned in oil, oysters, shrimp

Limit or Avoid

Organ meats, egg yolks, fatty and heavily marbled meats ("Prime" grade), spare ribs, regular cold cuts and frankfurters, sausage, bacon, fried meats, canned meats

Ideas for meatless main dishes

As you limit the amount of meat you eat, occasionally substitute other types of high-protein foods such as eggs or legumes (dried beans and peas) for meat. Although an egg contains a significant amount of cholesterol (about 210 milligrams), it is an excellent source of protein and contains only about 80 calories and less than 6 grams of fat. Most of the cholesterol is contained in the egg yolk. Eat no more than three to four egg yolks each week, including those contained in foods that contain a large number of eggs (such as custards, soufflés, quiches).

Discard half the egg yolks when you make scrambled eggs, or substitute two egg whites for each whole egg in most baked products. Use commercial egg substitutes, which have no cholesterol, in cooking or for scrambled eggs, omelets, or quiches.

Legumes are another low-fat meat alternative. They have the added advantage of containing no cholesterol, yet they are high in protein. Legumes also contain lots of fiber. Many choices of legumes are available: butter beans, kidney beans, black beans, lima beans, pinto beans, navy beans, "baked" beans, black-eyed peas (cowpeas), chickpeas (garbanzo beans), lentils, and split peas.

Combining legumes with foods from the grain group (for example, bean tacos, meatless chili and corn bread, peanut butter sandwich) provides high-quality protein.

when they are prepared without added fat. (Giblets—the liver, heart, and gizzard—have a high amount of cholesterol.) Most of the fat in poultry is in the skin. If you remove the skin before you eat poultry, you will reduce the fat by about half. The lowest amounts of total fat and saturated fat are in skinless white-meat poultry. Ground turkey can be a lower-fat alternative for ground beef if the skin is not ground with the meat.

Broil, grill, microwave, stir-fry, or bake poultry to retain the low-fat quality of the meat. Leave the skin on during cooking unless the recipe calls for a coating, because the skin or a coating helps keep the meat moist. Be sure to remove the skin and trim any remaining fat from all meats before you eat them.

Why Eat More Fish? Fish is one of the leanest sources of protein you can choose. In fact, even the fish with the highest fat content compare favorably with the leanest cuts of red meats and poultry. Seafood contains little saturated fat (the kind of fat most likely to raise blood cholesterol). Include varied types of fish and seafood in your menu at least twice a week.

People used to be advised to avoid some types of shellfish such as crab, clams, oysters, scallops, and lobster because of their supposedly high cholesterol content. However, new measuring techniques show that their cholesterol content is similar to that of lean beef and poultry. Of the shellfish, shrimp contains the most cholesterol, but it is very low in fat. A 3-ounce serving of shellfish is acceptable once a week, but avoid deep-fat fried fish or fish prepared with heavy, cream-based sauces. Instead of melted butter, serve shrimp, crab, and lobster with lemon juice or cocktail sauce. Broil, bake, poach, or grill fish to retain its low-fat quality.

Use Fats Sparingly—No More Than 6 to 8 Teaspoons of Spreadable or Pourable Fat in Your Daily Diet. The most obvious way to cut fat from your diet is to reduce the amount of pure fat—butter, margarine, shortening, and vegetable oils—you add to food during cooking or serving. Teaspoon for teaspoon, all types of spreads (except for the "diet" varieties) and oils contain about the same amount of fat.

Although they are similar in calories, there are meaningful distinctions between butter and margarine, for example. First, only animal fats such as butter or lard contain cholesterol. No vegetable fat contains cholesterol. Another distinction among fats is their degree of saturation. Saturated fats tend to raise total blood cholesterol levels. Unsaturated fats, classified as monounsaturated and polyunsaturated, do not raise total blood cholesterol levels. In fact, when you eat monounsaturated fats in limited amounts, they tend to raise the "good" type of cholesterol—high-density lipoproteins (HDLs).

No fat is 100 percent saturated, monounsaturated, or polyunsaturated. For example, olive oil is called a monounsaturated fat because it is predominantly monounsaturated, but it also has smaller proportions of saturated and polyunsaturated fatty acids.

The first strategy to keep in mind is to reduce the amount of any type of fat that you use. Then, the next strategy is to make selections that are lower in saturated fat and cholesterol. Avoid hydrogenated fats—common ingredients in commercial baked goods and

Fats

> **Best Choices** (in small amounts)
> Polyunsaturated oils (safflower, corn, sunflower, soybean, sesame, or cottonseed) and monounsaturated oils (olive, canola, or peanut). Salad dressings made with unsaturated oils, margarine made from polyunsaturated oil, or margarine whose main ingredient is "liquid" oil (listed first on the label)
>
> **Go Easy On**
> Mayonnaise, creamy salad dressings, reduced-fat sour cream or cream cheese
>
> **Limit or Avoid**
> Saturated fats, including butter, lard, and bacon. Gravy and cream sauces, cream, half-and-half, sour cream, cream cheese, hydrogenated margarine and shortening, cocoa butter (found in chocolate), coconut oil, palm oil, palm-kernel oil, most nondairy creamers, and nondairy whipped toppings

Here's how the fats compare

All fats contain a mixture of saturated and unsaturated fatty acids. This list shows the predominant type of fat in different choices.

Saturated	Monounsaturated	Polyunsaturated
Coconut oil	Olive oil	Safflower oil
Palm-kernel oil	Canola (rapeseed) oil	Walnut oil
Cocoa butter	Peanut oil	Sunflower oil
Butter		Corn oil
Palm oil		Soybean oil

other processed foods—to decrease your saturated fat intake. You can also reduce the amount of fat in your diet by selecting lower-fat alternatives to mayonnaise, salad dressing, and sauces that are made with fat and oils.

Eat Fewer Sweets and Desserts and Drink Less Alcohol. This recommendation does *not* mean you must eliminate sweets, desserts, and alcohol from your diet. However, they are a major source of calories (because they usually contain large amounts of fat or sugar) and contribute very few other beneficial nutrients to your overall diet.

People who have high levels of triglycerides (a type of fat in the blood that contributes to atherosclerosis) can usually decrease their triglyceride level by:

- Losing weight and then maintaining a desirable body weight
- Cutting back significantly on sugar and sugar-containing foods. The sugar in beverages, such as sweetened soft drinks or sweetened coffee or tea, can add up quickly. Even reducing the amount of fruit and fruit juice, because they naturally contain sugar, may help lower triglycerides
- Drinking less alcohol
- Increasing the amount of exercise (see page 168)

SHOPPING GUIDE. Many of the decisions you make about eating healthfully are made in the grocery store. With a little advance planning, you can select ingredients and prepared foods that fit into a heart-healthy life-style. Without planning, it is easy to slip back to your old way of eating or to stock up on impulse buys.

These tips will help you make wise choices in the grocery store and also will make preparing meals easier.

- Plan a week's worth of menus and include the ingredients you need on your grocery list. When you plan menus and make the grocery list, keep in mind the six basic guidelines (see page 153). You will probably need more fruits, vegetables, breads, and cereals than you previously bought. Foods you may have thought of as side dishes (such as pasta, rice, beans) will become

How to decrease your sugar intake

Best Choices
Fruit juices (unsweetened and in reasonable amounts), sugar-free carbonated beverages, sparkling water, fresh or unsweetened fruit (reasonable amounts), sugar-free hot chocolate, sugar-free gelatin or pudding, bread sticks, popcorn, or pretzels

Go Easy On
Plain donuts, plain cookies (such as vanilla wafers), plain cakes (such as angel food cake)

Limit or Avoid
Regular sweetened soft drinks, lemonade, and fruit drinks, cake, pie, donuts, pastries, ice cream, ice milk, sherbet, sorbet, sugar-sweetened gelatin, cereals with more than 5 grams of sucrose and other sugars per ounce, candy, chocolate, sugar, honey, jam, or jelly

How to decrease your alcohol intake

Best Choices
Sparkling or mineral water or club soda, non-alcoholic sparkling fruit juice, tomato or vegetable juice, unsweetened fruit juice (reasonable amounts), fruit-juice spritzers (unsweetened fruit juice and sparkling water or club soda), sugar-free carbonated beverages

Go Easy On
Low-alcohol beer, wine spritzers (wine and club soda), mixed drinks with ½ jigger of liquor

Limit or Avoid
Beer (including light beer), wine and wine coolers, liquor, liqueurs, and cordials

Changing old habits
at the grocery store

If high-fat, high-calorie, high-cholesterol items are among your standard grocery purchases, you do not have to make drastic changes in your meal plans to enjoy more healthful foods. Here is a grocery list "makeover":

Old list	New list	This change reduces fat	This change reduces cholesterol	This change reduces calories
Donuts, powdered sugar	English muffins with jam	✓	✓	
Canned corned beef	Canned chicken, canned water-packed tuna	✓	✓	✓
Ice cream	Frozen yogurt	✓	✓	✓
Mayonnaise	Fat-free, cholesterol-free mayonnaise	✓	✓	✓
Fish sticks	Fish fillets with no coating	✓		✓
Eggs	Egg substitute	✓	✓	✓
Frozen broccoli with cheese sauce	Fresh broccoli or plain frozen (sprinkled with lemon juice)	✓	✓	✓
Canned pineapple or other fruits in heavy syrup	Fresh pineapple (look for it on the salad bar to buy a small amount), or canned juice-packed fruit			✓
Macaroons	Vanilla wafers, fig bars, or ginger snaps	✓		✓
Spareribs	Well-trimmed pork chops	✓	✓	✓
Hamburger	Ground turkey or a lean cut of beef such as round steak or flank steak	✓		✓
Bologna	Reduced-fat bologna or wafer-sliced lean ham	✓		✓
Potato chips	Pretzels or popcorn	✓		✓
Carrot cake with cream cheese frosting	Angel food cake with fresh strawberries	✓	✓	✓

more prominent on your list. Keep the smaller portion sizes in mind when buying meat. In the dairy department, look for low-fat or skim milk products.

- Buy only those items on your list.
- Do not shop on an empty stomach. If you shop when you are hungry, you may be tempted to buy foods you don't need.

Quick tip

Any food that contains more than 3 grams of fat for every 100 calories contains more than 30 percent of calories from fat. As you look at food labels, this is a handy guide to keep in mind.

- Shop when you have time to read food labels.
- If possible, buy fresh foods rather than mixes or ready-to-eat foods so that you can control what ingredients are added.
- Shop the perimeter of the store. Many supermarkets place some of the most healthful foods (fresh fruits and vegetables, fresh meats, bread, and dairy products) on convenient perimeter aisles.
- If you cannot resist the temptation of impulse buys, arrange for someone else to do your grocery shopping.

HOW TO INTERPRET FOOD LABELS. As you seek out more healthful foods, labels can provide valuable information. Until now, many food labels provided incomplete or misleading nutrition information.

In May 1993, the first parts of food label reform became effective. By May 1994, manufacturers will need to be in full compliance with the new labeling requirements from the Food and Drug Administration (FDA) and the U.S. Department of Agriculture (USDA).

Before the new regulations, about half of food products had nutrition labels. Now nutrition information should be available for almost all types of packaged foods. The FDA is encouraging voluntary nutrition labeling for fresh foods also. The changes are designed to make food labels more accurate, clear, and useful.

Even with the new regulations that tighten the rules on claims such as "low fat" and "low cholesterol," the actual figures that show you the amount of calories, fat, saturated fat, cholesterol, and sodium are the most helpful. You can use that information, taking into account how much of the product you will actually eat, to plan heart-healthy meals.

Here is a sampling of the changes that pertain directly to heart health.

New labels focus on fat: Labels will be required to show the total amount of fat, saturated fat, and cholesterol in a serving. In addition, the new label shows the number of calories derived from fat (calculated by multiplying the grams of fat by 9—there are 9 calories per gram of fat). Use the information about fat to compare products and to add up the amount of fat you eat on a typical day. (See Fat math, page 163, for an estimate of your fat limit.)

Daily values: In the past, although some labels showed the amount of fat, for example, in a serving, it wasn't too meaningful unless you knew how this amount fit into a full day's allowance for fat. To some label readers, 12 grams of fat might sound like a lot; to others, 12 grams sounds insignificant. Unless you know that approximately 65 grams of fat is the limit in a 2,000-calorie diet, it's hard to judge whether this food is a good choice in an overall meal plan. New food labels will show you *Percent Daily Values* for fat, saturated fat, carbohydrate, protein, and fiber, based on a 2,000-calorie diet. The new label will show that 12 grams of fat represents 18 percent of the daily limit for fat. A 2,000-calorie diet is not appropriate for everyone, but this level was chosen as an average. Use the box on page 151 to determine a reasonable calorie level for yourself.

Fat math

The basic principles are as follows:

■ Limit your daily fat intake to 30 percent of your calorie intake. This guideline does *not* mean that every food you eat should have less than 30 percent of calories from fat. If so, you would have to eliminate foods such as margarine or peanut butter. Rather, the variety of foods you select should *average* less than 30 percent of calories from fat.

■ Limit your saturated fat intake to 10 percent of your calorie intake.

Question: How many calories should I be eating?
Answer: Recommended calorie levels are based on your age, sex, activity level, and current weight. See page 151 for some general recommendations. Your doctor may recommend a specific calorie level for you if you need to lose or gain weight.

Question: How do I know how much fat is in food?
Answer: One of the best sources of information is food labels. The label shows you the amount of fat and saturated fat in a serving. The fat measurement is given in grams.

Question: How does my daily limit of fat translate into grams?
Answer: Multiply your recommended calorie level by 30 percent (0.30). (This figure shows you how many fat calories are allowed; starting in May 1994, food labels will show you this amount.) To convert this figure into grams of fat (a common measurement shown on food labels), divide by 9 because there are 9 calories in each gram of fat. The chart below shows the grams of fat allowed each day at various calorie allowances.

Calorie level	Percentage of calories contributed by fat	Fat calorie limit	Calories per gram of fat	Grams of fat allowed
2,900	× 0.30 =	870	÷ 9	= 97
2,800	× 0.30 =	840	÷ 9	= 93
2,700	× 0.30 =	810	÷ 9	= 90
2,600	× 0.30 =	780	÷ 9	= 87
2,500	× 0.30 =	750	÷ 9	= 83
2,400	× 0.30 =	720	÷ 9	= 80
2,300	× 0.30 =	690	÷ 9	= 77
2,200	× 0.30 =	660	÷ 9	= 73
2,100	× 0.30 =	630	÷ 9	= 70
2,000	× 0.30 =	600	÷ 9	= 67
1,900	× 0.30 =	570	÷ 9	= 63
1,800	× 0.30 =	540	÷ 9	= 60
1,700	× 0.30 =	510	÷ 9	= 57
1,600	× 0.30 =	480	÷ 9	= 53

(continued on page 164)

Question: How does my limit of saturated fat translate into grams?
Answer: Ten percent of calories from saturated fat is the usual recommendation. Multiply your calories by 10 percent (0.10) and then divide by 9 to calculate the grams of saturated fat allowed. Another way of thinking of this is to limit saturated fat to one-third of your total fat allowance. Find your calorie level in the chart on page 163, then divide the grams of fat allowed (in last column of chart) by 3.

Question: It does not seem realistic to keep track of how much fat I eat every day, so why bother with these calculations?
Answer: The goal is not compulsively adding every gram of fat you eat, but knowing whether your daily total fat limit should be 60 or 100 grams is a helpful perspective to have as you are reading labels. Also, as you become more familiar with choosing low-fat foods, the figures become unnecessary.

Claims about the relationship of fat, cholesterol, and fiber to heart disease: For the first time, certain foods may qualify for stating on the label that there is a link between reduced risk of coronary artery disease and lower saturated fat and cholesterol intakes to lower blood cholesterol levels. Manufacturers will be allowed to make this claim only if the food meets the standards for "low saturated fat," "low cholesterol," and "low-fat." Foods that contain at least 0.6 gram of soluble fiber per serving and are "low-fat" will be allowed to carry a claim that links fiber consumption with a lower risk of heart disease. No other health claims regarding the link between other nutrients such as vitamins or fish oil and heart disease will be allowed.

Standardized serving sizes: Tighter regulations will make serving sizes shown on labels more realistic and consistent.

For the first time, relative terms will be defined: Until now, there have been no consistent definitions for terms such as "light," "reduced," "low," and "lean." Under the new regulations there are uniform definitions:

- *low fat*: 3 grams or less per serving
- *low saturated fat*: 1 gram or less per serving
- *low sodium*: less than 140 milligrams per serving
- *very low sodium*: less than 35 milligrams per serving
- *low cholesterol*: less than 20 milligrams per serving
- *low calorie*: 40 calories or less per serving

"Light" has been one of the most overused and confusing terms. In the past, "light" could mean anything from light in color, light in texture, to fewer calories or less sodium. The consumer was usually left guessing. Now, "light" can be used only on products that contain one-third fewer calories or half the fat of a similar product. "Light" can also mean that the sodium content of a food has been reduced by at least 50 percent. If it is used in any other way, the label must be more specific about what characteristic is

The new food label at a glance

Serving sizes are now more consistent and reflect the amounts people actually eat.

Today, most people are more concerned about getting too much of certain nutrients (fat, for example) than the vitamin and mineral deficiencies of the past. The new food label highlights amounts of fat, cholesterol, and sodium.

The label will now tell the number of calories per gram of fat, carbohydrates, and protein.

Nutrition Facts
Serving Size ½ cup (114g)
Servings Per Container 4

Amount Per Serving

Calories 90   Calories from Fat 30

% Daily Value*

Total Fat 3g	**5%**
Saturated Fat 0g	**0%**
Cholesterol 0mg	**0%**
Sodium 300mg	**13%**
Total Carbohydrate 13g	**4%**
Dietary Fiber 3g	**12%**
Sugars 3g	
Protein 3g	

Vitamin A	80%	Vitamin C	60%
Calcium	4%	Iron	4%

*Percent Daily Values are based on a 2,000 calorie diet. Your daily values may be higher or lower depending on your calorie needs:

		Calories	2,000	2,500
Total Fat	Less than	65g	80g
Sat Fat	Less than	20g	25g
Cholesterol	Less than	300mg	300mg
Sodium	Less than	2,400mg	2,400mg
Total Carbohydrate		300g	375g
Fiber		25g	30g

Calories per gram:
Fat 9   •   Carbohydrates 4   •   Protein 4

New title signals that the label contains the newly required information.

Calories from fat are now shown on the label to help you meet guidelines that recommend no more than 30 percent of your calories should come from fat.

% Daily Value shows how a food fits into the overall daily diet.

Daily values are also something new. Some are maximums, as with fat (65 grams *or less*); others are minimums, as with carbohydrates (300 grams *or more*). The daily values on the label are based on a daily diet of 2,000 or 2,500 calories. Adjust the values to fit your own calorie intake.

Source: Food and Drug Administration, 1992

"light," such as the color, the flavor, the texture.

Look beyond the one-word descriptors and eye-catching advertising hype. Actually, the most meaningful parts of a food label are the ingredient list and the figures shown for calories, fat, cholesterol, and sodium in a serving. Once you know what your limits are in terms of fat, cholesterol, calories, and sodium, you will be in a much better position to compare products and to choose those that fit your desire to eat more healthfully.

COOKING TO PRESERVE THE HEALTHFUL QUALITIES OF FOOD.
All the best intentions and plans for eating healthfully can be defeated in the kitchen unless you change some of the ways you prepare food. The most important change you can make is to learn to cook with little or no oils or other fats. Here are 10 tips to get you started.

1. Look for low-fat recipes in cookbooks or magazines that provide a nutrition analysis for each recipe.
2. Invest in nonstick cookware to be able to "fry" or brown foods in no added fat. If you would normally add a tablespoon of vegetable oil to a skillet, you save 120 calories and 14 grams of fat by using a nonstick skillet instead. Or use a 1-second spray of vegetable oil cooking spray, which adds about 1 gram of fat and few calories.
3. Add a few handy kitchen gadgets such as a garlic press, spice grater, lemon zester, egg separator, and vegetable steamer to expand or revamp your cooking habits.
4. Stock fat-free flavor enhancers such as onions, herbs and spices,

colorful fresh peppers, fresh garlic, gingerroot, Dijon mustard, fresh lemons and limes, flavored vinegars, sherry or other wines, reduced-sodium soy sauce, bouillon granules, and plain, nonfat yogurt.
5. Sauté onions, mushrooms, or celery in a small amount of wine, broth, water, soy sauce, or Worcestershire sauce instead of butter or oil.
6. Microwave or steam vegetables; then dress them up with flavored vinegars, herbs, spices, or butter-flavored powders.
7. Cook fish in parchment paper (available at many supermarkets) or foil packets. This method seals in flavor and juices.
8. Poach fish or skinless poultry in broth, vegetable juice, flavored vinegars, dry wine, herbs, and spices. A covered roasting pan is an inexpensive alternative for a fish poacher.
9. Cut the amount of meat in casseroles and stews by one-third and add more vegetables, rice, or pasta.
10. In recipes, substitute low-fat cream cheese, sour cream, or processed cheeses for their higher-fat counterparts.

A HEALTHFUL ATTITUDE ABOUT EATING.
You do not have to be rigid with your diet every minute of your life. A slipup now and then in your plan to eat more healthfully should not turn into an excuse to give up. If you overindulge once in a while, you can balance things out over the long term. What is important is that you eat right *most* of the time. Then it becomes a habit, and good habits can be as difficult to break as bad ones.

Heart-healthy food guide

This chart summarizes the basic eating guidelines covered previously. As the recommended number of servings indicate, select more grains, fruits, and vegetables and lesser amounts of meat, fat, alcohol, and sweets.

Food	Best Choices	Limit or Avoid
Recommended No. of Servings		
Vegetables 3 or more servings	Any fresh, frozen, or canned vegetable	French-fried potatoes or vegetables, vegetables in cream sauce or cheese sauce
Fruits 2 or more servings	Fresh, juice-packed, or water-packed fruit	Avocado, coconut
Grains 6 to 11 servings	Whole grain breakfast cereals. Whole-grain breads and rolls, bagels, bread-sticks, English muffins, pita bread, fat-free and low-fat crackers, rice, pasta, popcorn, pretzels	Biscuits, chow mein noodles, corn bread, crackers, egg noodles, granola, muffins, pastry, packaged stuffing, waffles
Milk 2 to 3 servings	Skim and 1% milk, buttermilk, nonfat dry milk, fat-free yogurt and cheese, fat-free or low-fat cottage cheese	2% milk, whole milk, low-fat yogurt and cottage cheese, whole milk yogurt and cheese, premium or gourmet ice cream
Meats and meat alternatives 5 to 7 ounces	Fresh and frozen fish or shellfish, water-packed tuna, poultry without skin. USDA Choice or Select beef—round, sirloin, tenderloin, flank, ground round. Pork center-cut ham, loin chop, tenderloin, Canadian bacon. Egg substitutes. Cooked beans, peas, and lentils	Fried or oil-packed fish. Fried chicken. Duck or goose. USDA Prime beef. Ribs, brisket, regular ground beef, sausages, organ meats. Regular luncheon meats. Eggs (limit to 4 a week)
Fats Sparingly—no more than 6-8 teaspoons	Margarine, reduced-fat margarine, reduced-fat salad dressing, fat-free sour cream. Oils—canola, corn, olive, peanut, safflower, soybean, sunflower	Bacon, butter, coconut oil, coffee creamer (liquid or powder), whipping cream, cream cheese, gravy, palm and palm-kernel oils, shortening, sour cream
Alcohol and sweets Use moderate amounts occasionally	Club soda; mineral water; sugar-free carbonated beverages, gelatin, and hot chocolate; sparkling fruit juices; tomato or vegetable juice; fruit for dessert; fruit spreads	Beer, wine, cordials, liqueurs, and liquor. Cake, donuts, pie, pastries, ice cream, sherbet, sugar-sweetened gelatin. Candy, chocolate, sugar, honey, jam, jelly. Sugar-sweetened carbonated beverages, lemonade, fruit drinks

Examples of aerobic activities

- Walking
- Jogging
- Cycling
- Swimming
- Rowing
- Cross-country skiing
- Stair climbing
- Dancing

Improving Your Activity Level

Your body is designed so that if you regularly exert yourself a little more than usual, it responds by improving its capacity for exercise. By gradually increasing the amount of exercise you perform, you can noticeably improve your fitness level in 8 to 12 weeks.

Very strenuous exercise is not necessary to improve fitness. The total amount of exercise is more important for health than exercising at high intensities. A moderate amount of exercise, as frequently as 3 days a week, is enough to improve your fitness level. You will probably enjoy moderate activity and stay with it more faithfully than you would with overly strenuous exercise. In fact, you can gain some benefit from short periods of exercise—perhaps as short as 10 minutes—done three or more times a day.

Aerobic exercises increase your cardiovascular fitness. Aerobic activities are those in which the demand for oxygen and nourishment by the exercising muscles does not surpass the ability of the lungs and circulatory system to supply it. It consists of continuous, rhythmic contracting of the large muscle groups.

Aerobic exercise increases the rate and depth of your breathing. Your body becomes warmer, and if you exercise long enough and vigorously enough, you will perspire. However, aerobic exercises are not so intense that the need of the muscle cells for oxygen exceeds their supply. This deficiency may occur with such activities as isometric exercise or weight-lifting, activities that may increase muscle tone and bulk but are not clearly beneficial from a cardiovascular standpoint.

BEFORE YOU START TO EXERCISE. For most people, the health advantages of regular exercise far outweigh any risks. However, if you have any chronic health conditions or several major risk factors for heart disease (such as smoking, high blood pressure, high blood cholesterol, diabetes), some special precautions may apply.

To be on the safe side, check with your doctor before you begin an exercise program if you:

- Have heart or lung disease, diabetes, arthritis, or kidney disease
- Are age 40 or older
- Are very overweight
- Have parents, brothers, or sisters who had evidence of coronary artery disease before the age of 55
- Are unsure of your health status

Your doctor may recommend that you have an exercise stress test (see Exercise Electrocardiography Test, page 196) to help determine whether exercise is likely to cause an insufficient supply of blood and oxygen to the heart or to provoke heart rhythm abnormalities. Discuss with your doctor any limitations that he or she would suggest because of your existing health conditions.

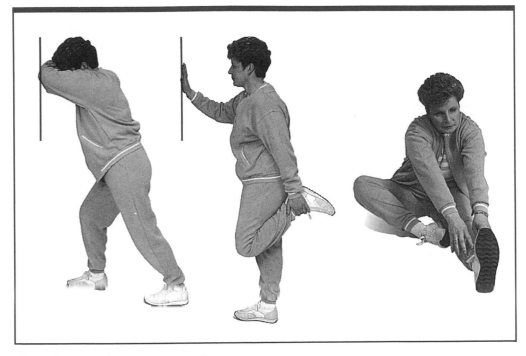

Three important warm-up exercises.
Left, Calf stretch. Starting position: **Stand an arm's length away from a wall and rest your forearms on the wall with your forehead on the back of your hands. Point your toes straight ahead. Bend your right knee and bring it toward the wall. Keep your left leg straight with the heel on the floor.** *Movement*: **Slowly move your hips forward, keeping your back straight until you feel a stretch in your left calf. Hold this position for 30 seconds and then repeat with the other leg.**

Middle, Thigh stretch. Starting position: **Stand and place your right hand on a wall or a solid piece of furniture to aid in balance. Reach behind you and grasp your left foot or ankle from the outside with your left hand.** *Movement*: **Slowly pull your left foot toward your seat until you feel muscles stretch in the front of your thigh. Hold this position for 30 seconds. Then repeat it with your right leg (and right hand). If you cannot reach your foot or ankle, grasp the hem of your pants.**

Right, Hamstring stretch. Starting position: **Sit on the floor with your left leg extended straight forward and your toes pointing toward the ceiling. Bend your right knee and place the sole of your right foot on your inner left thigh.** *Movement*: **Bend forward at the waist and slowly move both hands down your left leg until you feel a stretch in the back of your left thigh. Hold the position for 30 seconds. Repeat, using your right leg.**

A FITNESS PLAN FOR YOUR HEART.

A cardiovascular fitness program has three parts: warm-up, conditioning aerobic exercise, and cool-down. The exercise should be frequent enough, intense enough, of sufficient duration, and of the appropriate type to induce a training effect.

In general, try to set up your program so that you expend about 1,000 to 2,000 calories a week with exercise. Walking 10 to 20 miles per week accomplishes that goal for the average person. (See the chart on page 173 to compare other activities.) There is no evidence of a further reduction in cardiovascular risk by exercising to burn off more than 2,000 calories per week, unless you are trying to lose weight.

A warm-up phase develops and maintains muscle and joint flexibility and prepares the body for the conditioning phase of the program. The essential parts of the warm-up are stretching and low-intensity endurance exercises, which gradually increase your heart rate, body temperature, and blood flow to the muscles.

You may include muscle strengthening and toning exercises to improve your total fitness level. The warm-up phase should last 5 to 10 minutes.

The conditioning aerobic phase of your program may include any aerobic activity that requires continuous rhythmic muscle contraction of the legs and perhaps the arms. Walking, biking, swimming, jogging, cross-country skiing, rowing, rope skipping, dancing, and racket sports are good examples of aerobic exercises. Choose something that you enjoy and will want to continue.

Adjust the frequency, intensity, time, and type (FITT) of your exercise program so you expend the desired amount of energy to achieve your fitness goals. For example, you might walk 4 miles 5 times in 1 week, and 5 miles 4 times in another week. You may spend an hour walking 4 miles on 1 day, but jog 4 miles in 40 minutes on another day.

HOW OFTEN SHOULD YOU EXERCISE? The frequency of your exercise should be at least three times a week on nonconsecutive days to develop and maintain a good level of cardiovascular fitness. If you are exercising to lose weight as well as to im-

prove fitness, you can increase the frequency to more days or increase the duration of your exercise to burn more calories.

HOW TO JUDGE THE INTENSITY OF YOUR EXERCISE. The intensity level of your exercise should be strenuous enough that you feel you are working, but it need not be exhausting. Exercise physiologists describe exercise intensity in terms of percentage of maximal exercise capacity; they recommend an intensity of 50 to 80 percent of your maximal exercise capacity. You can determine the intensity of your exercise by counting your pulse, using a perceived exertion scale, or using the "talk test."

Many people exercising on their own use their pulse rate to determine whether their exercise is intense enough. Ask your doctor to suggest an appropriate target heart rate for you during exercise. The harder you exercise, the higher your heart rate or pulse rate climbs.

Your maximal heart rate decreases with age and is affected by cardiovascular disease and some cardiovascular medications. Regular exercise does not influence your maximal heart rate. Some people with very irregular heart rates cannot use the heart rate method to monitor their exercise intensity.

Another way to gauge the intensity of your exercise is to use the Borg Perceived Exertion Scale. It rates the intensity of exercise on a scale from 6 to 20; 6 indicates a minimal level of exertion such as sitting comfortably in a chair, and 20 corresponds to a maximal effort such as jogging up a very steep hill. Doctors usually recommend ratings between 11 and 15 on the scale. A rating of 13 usually corresponds to 70 percent of maximal exercise capacity and is considered a good intensity for most people. When you use the scale, do not become preoccupied with any one factor such as leg discomfort or labored breathing. Instead, try to concentrate on your overall feeling of exertion.

There is no real advantage to exercising at a high intensity, unless you are an athlete. You do not get major fitness benefits beyond moderate exercise, and you increase the risk of muscle or joint soreness or injury.

A moderate exercise program should not cause discomfort. You should stop exercising and call your doctor if any of the following symptoms develops:

- Chest discomfort or pressure (or arm, jaw, neck, or back discomfort)
- Severe shortness of breath
- Burst of very rapid or slow heart rate
- Irregular heart rate
- Excessive fatigue
- Marked joint or muscle pain
- Dizziness or fainting

HOW LONG SHOULD YOU EXERCISE?   The time, or duration, of exercise should generally be about 30 minutes, and the type of exercise, as mentioned before, should be aerobic. Periods of exercise shorter than 30 minutes are still beneficial. If you have not exercised for a long time, start with a conservative duration of 5 minutes or less. Gradually increase the duration as you become accustomed to exercise.

If weight loss is your goal, increase the duration of exercise sessions. If you find that you enjoy lower-intensity exercise, you can increase the duration and still get the fitness benefits.

Counting your pulse

Taking your pulse can help you determine whether the intensity of your exercise program is appropriate. To take your pulse, do the following:

1. Stop your exercise.
2. Place two fingers between the bone and the tendon over the radial artery on the thumb side of your wrist and exert gentle pressure. If your fingers are positioned properly, you will feel the pulsing of the artery.
3. Do not press so hard on the blood vessel that the flow of blood is blocked.
4. Count your pulse for 10 seconds and then multiply by 6 to determine your pulse rate per minute.

Borg Perceived Exertion Scale

6	
7	Very, very light
8	
9	Very light
10	
11	Fairly light
12	
13	Somewhat hard
14	
15	Hard
16	
17	Very hard
18	
19	Very, very hard
20	

The talk test

A very easy way to regulate the intensity of exercise is to be able to carry on a conversation with a companion. If you are too winded to talk, you are probably pushing too hard and should slow your exercise pace.

The last phase of your exercise program is the cool-down right after the conditioning exercise. The cool-down lets your heart rate return to pre-exercise levels gradually, prevents blood from pooling in the legs (which may cause dizziness), and stretches the muscles that have been used in the conditioning activity. Perform 3 to 5 minutes of low-intensity exercise such as slow walking, and then do a few stretching exercises to help relax the muscles, improve or maintain flexibility, and help prevent soreness. The cool-down period usually should last 5 to 10 minutes.

STAY MOTIVATED.   No single form of aerobic exercise is best. To be successful, choose an activity that fits your personality and life-style. Do you like to exercise alone or in groups? If you prefer solitude, walking may be your first choice. If group activities appeal to you and motivate you, enroll in an aerobic dance class or water aerobics class. Do you like being outside, or would you prefer to stay indoors? To combat boredom, watch television or listen to tapes while you use indoor exercise equipment. Help maintain your interest by changing your activity periodically. Consider using an exercise log to help record your progress.

If you have trouble finding the time to exercise, remember that all it takes is 30 minutes 3 days a week to improve your fitness level greatly. Most people do not have to exercise every day, but you may want to if you are trying to lose weight. Think of ways to fit exercise into your regular routine. Could you walk for ½ hour while the kids are taking music lessons? Could you schedule one session on the weekend and two during the week? You can be successful with a little determination, time management, and creativity.

Handling Stress

It is one thing to be aware that your personal style of approaching problems or conflicts, stressful events in your life, and your body's reaction to stress can increase your risk of heart disease, but it is another to know what to do about it. Although you cannot control some of these factors, you can control how you manage stress. A series of stressful life events does not condemn you to a heart attack or other serious illness, although it may increase your risk. Many health care professionals believe that you can raise or lower that risk by your own behavior.

Stress comes from many sources—the physical environment, other people, unexpected events, and your own thoughts and actions. It is important to recognize that it is your own behavior

---

More reasons to exercise

Your body requires a certain amount of energy to carry on its life-sustaining functions of breathing, circulation of blood, and operation of the vital organs. These needs, called the resting metabolic rate, account for 65 to 70 percent of the calories you burn in a day.

Exercise is an important variable in determining how many calories you burn. The exercise itself, because it requires your body to work harder than at a "resting" level, requires more fuel (or calories). Even after you stop exercising, your body continues to burn calories at a modestly increased rate for a few hours. The long-term effect of regular exercise is that your proportion of body fat decreases while the proportion of lean tissue (muscle, bone) increases. The more lean muscle you have, the higher your resting metabolic rate will be.

and attitudes that are the most available to change. Many people try to change the behavior of their spouse, children, boss, or co-workers if they view the behavior of those people as the cause of their own stress. Usually those efforts are in vain.

To manage your stress, you have to recognize first the symptoms of stress such as muscular tension, headache, insomnia, irritability, and changes in eating habits. Other warning signs of stress include apathy, mental or physical fatigue, and frequent illness. Once you realize you are under stress, it is possible to identify the stress factors that produce the symptoms and to develop ways to overcome them.

The next step to learning alternative behaviors is to recognize whether you may have a hostile personality. It is not easy for anyone to admit that they need to modify their behavior. It may take the terrifying ordeal of a heart attack to motivate some people to take the time to reevaluate their personal priorities and to work on changes in thinking and communicating. But you do not *have* to wait until that happens.

BEHAVIOR ADAPTATION. You will find that making simple changes in your life-style can help reduce your stress. Try walking at a more relaxed pace, driving slower, and providing ample time to complete your work. Use relaxation techniques such as muscle relaxation exercises, brisk walking, or programs of regular physical activity.

In advising people on how to modify the "hot reactor" response, experts emphasize using positive "self-talk." The messages and images that you generate in your mind and send to yourself during periods of stress can

Average number of calories burned in 10 minutes*

Activity	Weight		
	120–130 pounds	160–170 pounds	190–200 pounds
Aerobic dance	60–105	75–140	90–165
Bicycling			
Outdoors	40–145	50–195	60–230
Stationary	25–145	30–195	40–230
Calisthenics	40–105	50–140	60–165
Dancing	30–80	40–105	45–120
Gardening	30–80	40–105	45–120
Golf (carry or pull bag)	30–80	40–105	45–120
Jogging			
5 mph (12 minutes/ mile)	90	115	135
6 mph (10 minutes/ mile)	105	140	170
Skiing			
Cross-country	60–145	75–195	90–230
Downhill	40–90	50–115	60–135
Swimming	50–125	65–165	75–200
Tennis	50–95	65–130	75–150
Walking			
2 mph (30 minutes/ mile)	30	40	45
3 mph (20 minutes/ mile)	40	50	60
4 mph (15 minutes/ mile)	55	70	85

*10 minutes of continuous activity.

greatly affect your physiological responses. For example, instead of getting upset and frustrated when you have to wait for an appointment, tell yourself that waiting for some appointments is inevitable and plan for other ways to deal with the situation, such as reading a magazine, asking to reschedule, or calling work to say you may be late.

Perhaps by changing your own thoughts and actions you can interact with others more effectively, and you may even elicit new responses from them. For example, you may complain that your spouse does not do anything but watch television in the evening. Instead of complaining, find a quiet room in which to read or do other work that interests you for an hour each night, go out for evening walks with a neighbor, sign up for an adult education course, or go to a movie with a friend. You will not only enjoy yourself but also may find before long that your spouse turns off the television to join you.

View stress management techniques as options, not as strict rules about how you should act in certain situations. You can manage your stress level as *you* see fit rather than being dragged into an increasing number of commitments by an overdeveloped sense of obligation or fear of hurting others' feelings.

Finally, you cannot expect stress management to provide you with a relaxed, carefree life. Unexpected problems, even catastrophes, will still happen.

For most people, stress management can certainly be viewed as a challenge, but for some individuals more serious steps need to be taken to cope with stress. If psychological or physical symptoms are persistent, see your doctor as a first step in assessing the situation and devising a plan for gaining control of the stress in your life. Sometimes, low self-esteem or depression can undermine your motivation to make healthful positive changes. A psychiatrist or therapist may be needed for assistance with depression or other emotional difficulties. In ad-dition, there are various formal stress management programs available in many communities, ranging from work-shops for executives to public lectures and classes. Most stress management programs include an introduction to techniques such as relaxation training and problem solving.

STRESS MANAGEMENT TECHNIQUES

- *Maintain good social relationships.* By letting your friends, spouse, and family know that you love and ap-preciate them, they will be more ready to support you when times get rough. Keep in touch with a circle of friends. Many churches and social agencies offer "marriage encoun-ters," parenting classes, and self-im-provement workshops that could help you make new friends and strengthen ongoing relationships.
- *Eliminate irrational thinking.* Ac-cording to therapist Albert Ellis, much of our stress comes from irra-tional beliefs that we hold. A few examples are, "I should never make a mistake," "Everyone should like me," "It is wrong to ever get angry." Notice the occurrence of words such as "should," "always," and "never." Developing more realistic expectations for yourself and others through modifying these irrational beliefs is a powerful way to reduce stress. Use positive "self-talk" to tone down your critical or negative feelings. For example, instead of "I should never make a mistake," tell yourself "I'll try to be more careful next time," or "Not everyone likes my ideas, but many people do seem to respect my opinions." This ap-proach creates less intense negative

feelings than the more absolute statements above.

- *Improve communication skills*. Active listening is a technique that is very helpful in dealing with difficult, angry people. It helps reduce their stress—and yours—while keeping you from getting involved in arguments or becoming the target of their frustration. One way to practice active listening is to occasionally repeat or paraphrase what the other person has been saying.

Suppose a friend complains to you about what she believes are unfair demands placed on her at work. By using active listening techniques you might say, "It sounds as if things are really difficult for you at work," or "As you describe it, work seems to be really demanding." In this way, you provide support without offering advice or offending the angry person.

Assertiveness training teaches people how to get what they want through effective communication. You learn to express your needs and desires without being ignored or offending others. Assertiveness training is helpful both for the person with an overly aggressive, hostile personality who generates antagonism and arguments in conversation and for the passive person who constantly feels taken advantage of by others.

Assertiveness is based on the idea that everyone has basic rights—rights to express an opinion, to have some privacy, to make a mistake, etc. "Passive" people often give up their rights (and feel hurt and angry about it). "Aggressive" people do not respect the rights of others in trying to assert their own rights. Assertive communication involves expressing your ideas, avoiding sarcasm, and not criticizing others with whom you disagree. Here are examples of different responses to the same situation—your spouse refuses to go with you to an important, but potentially boring, social function related to your job:

Passive: "Well, if you really don't want to go, I guess I can go by myself" (but just wait until you want me to go somewhere with you...)."

Aggressive: "You're really inconsiderate. You better go to this if you expect me to . . ."

Assertive: "This is a very important meeting for me. I very much want you to be there with me."

Whether or not you pursue some additional training in communication skills, try to take a few moments to listen to others without offering your own ideas immediately. Try to avoid making conversations a win-or-lose contest, and state your opinions or feelings without criticizing others or opposing ideas at the same time.

- *Practice positive thinking* and positive "self-talk" as discussed on page 174. Avoid confusing day-to-day problems with full-blown crises. Try to practice old adages such as "Look for the silver lining in every cloud," and "Don't make mountains out of molehills."

- *Organize*. Keep a written schedule of special events so you are not faced with conflicts or last-minute rushes to get to your daughter's volleyball game. Get a desktop file or filing cabinet to keep bills straight. Use drawer and closet organizers to eliminate that frustrating 5 minutes when you cannot find your keys. Take a few minutes to plan your approach and rehearse before you go into important meetings or make important phone calls.

Organizing will take time and effort; you may have to learn some new habits and give up some youthful notions about spontaneity. The time you spend organizing will be paid back severalfold over ensuing months and years, allowing you more free time to do the things you enjoy.

- *Avoid depending on stimulants* such as excessive caffeine, alcohol, and nicotine to regulate your moods.
- *Get enough rest.* To some degree, you can catch up on sleep lost during the week by getting a little extra rest on the weekends. Do not feel guilty about an occasional nap or sleeping in a little when you can do so. Try to break late-night television habits and avoid food and beverages right before bed. Many hospitals or large clinics have sleep disorder centers you can call if you have a serious problem sleeping.
- *Have a personal hobby or activity* that gives you satisfaction outside work and family spheres. (But try to avoid letting the hobby grow into another job or a business unless you really have the time and interest for it.) Gardening, collections, crafts, and artistic activities are good choices. Reserve a little private space for yourself where you can work undisturbed.

Many of these suggestions may seem to apply primarily to married people who work outside the home or raise an active family. Single people and older persons no longer working may face different kinds of stress—loneliness, isolation, boredom, and feelings of being unproductive. Pets can be extremely valuable as companions and something to care for. Volunteerism presents various opportunities for social interaction, and for contributing to society (especially for older persons), and, for young singles, for making new friends outside the work environment. Adult continuing education has proved extremely popular, especially among older persons.

- *Exercise.* Henry David Thoreau found that chopping wood not only helped cure him of loneliness in his self-imposed isolation at Walden Pond but also helped him get over mental blocks in his writing. Exercise may improve your blood pressure, lower triglycerides and raise HDL cholesterol, improve glucose tolerance and prevent or reverse type II diabetes, help you lose weight, and, of course, make you more physically fit. Exercise also helps reduce anxiety and may help reduce mild depression and raise self-esteem. When you think of it, exercise is the appropriate action for the physiological "fight-or-flight" stress response.
- *Shift your thinking away from negative thoughts or interpersonal conflict.* In a prolonged argument, stop and write down the important points of agreement, disagreement, and irrelevancy. By shifting from talking to writing and from arguing to a cooperative effort, you can reduce

your stress and reach a compromise solution to the problem. Alternatively, if you are stuck in private thought or cannot express yourself clearly, take a break. Move around, do something. Many problems are better discussed over doing the dishes or on a walk than just sitting down across a table.

- *Practice relaxation or meditation.* Relaxation techniques need to be well learned, which means practicing them regularly when you are already somewhat relaxed. Yoga and other Eastern exercises involving defined postures and repetitive movements serve a similar purpose for persons interested in learning and practicing them. Prayer can be a form of meditation, especially when the prayer is simple, well learned, and repetitive. These quiet, repetitive exercises all serve to reverse the physiological arousal from stress. Regular practice may also provide new insights into how to reduce your stress by changing your priorities or thought patterns, because these exercises serve as another powerful form of thought shifting.

Tests to Diagnose Heart Disease

In some ways your doctor is like a detective. You describe your symptoms, which provide clues to what may be wrong. The doctor conducts a medical interview and performs a physical examination and then calls on his or her training and experience to decide which tests will help diagnose the problem.

The medical interview and physical examination are broad screening tests that give the doctor the first hint of whether you have any medical problems and what they might be. Other tests used in the early phases of evaluation can also be considered screening tests. Tests performed later in the process are more specific and are intended to define the problem precisely.

Instead of screening all people with complicated and expensive tests, doctors begin with a medical interview to find out your family history and other risk factors and whether you have any symptoms, including any that suggest heart disease. After the interview, doctors perform a physical examination to gain more information by listening, palpating, and observing specific areas of the body. If the medical interview and physical examination do not indicate any problems, the doctor may recommend that you undergo only a few screening tests. The results of these tests will help the doctor decide whether any further tests are needed, or whether treatment should be considered.

Screening tests are usually simple procedures that can single out people who might have a medical problem. However, because many people who undergo screening tests do not necessarily have any medical problems, screening tests must be safe, convenient, and cost-effective.

Cardiologists would love to know the exact condition of the coronary arteries of each of their patients, but of course they cannot have every person go to a hospital and undergo angiography, which is an expensive, invasive test (see Angiography, page 216). Although they might find some people who have blocked coronary arteries, many people would be found to have normal arteries. It would not be logical or cost-effective to subject all the people with normal arteries to such a complicated procedure.

After taking the medical history and performing a physical examination, a doctor may be confident about whether a person's chest pain is due to coronary artery blockage. If the person has coronary angiography, the doctor in most cases can be almost 100 percent sure whether or not there is a coronary problem. However, to have coronary angiography, the person must go into the hospital for this invasive procedure, which is associated with a small but definite amount of risk and discomfort and a fair amount of expense and inconvenience.

The doctor's other option is to order an exercise stress test (see Variety of stress tests, page 198). If it shows no signs of inadequate coronary blood

How often should you see your doctor?*

Twice in your 20s (every 5 years)
Three times in your 30s (every 3 to 4 years)
Four times in your 40s (every 2 to 3 years)
Five times in your 50s (every 2 years)
Every year if you are 60 or older

*If you are apparently healthy.

flow, the doctor can be very confident that the person does not have a significant coronary problem. The doctor will not be 100 percent sure, however, because there is a chance that the exercise stress test will show normal results even though there is a heart problem. However, this small chance would not warrant the risk and expense of further testing.

If the results of an exercise stress test are abnormal, however, there is a reasonable chance that the person has coronary artery disease. Coronary angiography may be necessary to settle the issue and to help determine appropriate treatment. Doctors reserve the more complicated tests for people who have a higher chance of having heart disease or for those in whom the results of screening tests do not give a clearcut or logical answer.

Although very sophisticated tests are available to help diagnose heart disease, no test is perfect. There is always a chance that a test will give incorrect information, no matter how carefully it is done or analyzed.

Occasionally, a test may indicate that there is no problem when there really is one. This is called a false-negative result. Sometimes, a test may indicate that there is a problem when there really is not. This is called a false-positive result.

When evaluating a patient's problem, the physician must consider the likelihood of a test being accurate and whether the test result fits with other information about the patient.

Why would a doctor ever use tests that are not completely accurate? To begin with, no test is 100 percent accurate, and all tests are open to interpretation. Furthermore, as just discussed, doctors usually try to gain as much information as possible from tests that

Is more testing necessary?

From the various diagnostic tests that are available, doctors make decisions about which tests are needed, and in what order, on the basis of physical examination, medical history, and prior test results. Three common scenarios follow.

Situation	Action
Doctor has the impression, and early test results suggest, that there is a problem	No further tests required, begin treatment, or Do advanced testing to make specific diagnosis and select treatment
Doctor has the impression, and early test results suggest, that no problem exists	Avoid further testing, no treatment
Doctor's impression is, and early test results are, unclear	Advanced tests are needed to make specific diagnosis

have the least risk, expense, and inconvenience. The screening tests are used to identify whether you may need to have more extensive (and definitive) testing.

In addition, even tests with incomplete accuracy can give important information. For example, a chest X-ray cannot directly show the coronary arteries, valves, and other complex structures of the heart, but it can show the size and shape of the heart, which may be very useful information to the doctor. Chest X-rays are generally quick, safe, and relatively inexpensive. Using the information from the chest X-ray, the doctor may be satisfied that all is well, or he or she may decide more precise tests are needed to determine the problem exactly.

THE MEDICAL HISTORY

You can help your doctor choose the best diagnostic tests by providing an accurate medical history. The medical history is a report to the doctor of your "medical biography," or a history of all the significant medical events in your life. The questions asked about your medical history will be more extensive during your first visit with a doctor than on subsequent visits. Also, during a general examination the history that is obtained is broader than during an examination for a specific problem. When you are seeing the doctor for a specific problem, the history can be limited to features pertinent to that problem.

The medical interview is often conducted by the doctor, but it may be conducted by a nurse or physician's assistant. Sometimes the information is collected with a questionnaire. Regardless of the format, it is helpful if you have thought about and organized this information before coming to the doctor.

The medical history that you provide will help your doctor decide where and how to focus the subsequent evaluation. The more you can help your doctor pinpoint the problem, the better the doctor will be able to avoid unnecessary testing and focus on finding the problem. If you feel that something is worth mentioning, say it. Your doctor is more likely to make an efficient and correct diagnosis if you focus on the symptoms that are relevant to the problem at hand.

The medical history should consist of the following parts: chief complaint, medical history, family medical history, social history, and review of organ systems.

Chief Complaint

Completely, but concisely, describe the problem that brought you to your doctor. Be as precise as possible and cover all aspects of the symptoms: Where is the problem? How does it feel? How often does it happen? How long does it last? What provokes the problem? What makes it better? Is it associated with any other symptoms?

During the first visit, it is especially important to relate information in a logical order and to use specific dates and durations of events. It is always a good idea to bring notes to the doctor's office to help get the story across accurately.

Medical History

Your medical history is a review of your health throughout your life. This information not only helps sort out possible causes for the present problem but also may indicate whether there are any constraints on possible treatments. For example, a person's chief complaint may be chest pain that turns out to be angina related to coronary artery disease. However, if the person also has asthma, certain medications used for the treatment of angina are not advised because they worsen asthma.

In relating your medical history, tell your doctor about all prior illnesses, hospitalizations, accidents, operations, and allergies. In addition, discuss symptoms that concern you, medications you are taking, and questions you have. It may be helpful to jot down a brief list of the things you want to cover.

If you are giving your medical history to a specialist after you have had examinations with other doctors, it is important to give the specialist copies of the earlier evaluations and X-ray films or other tests that have been done. In many cases it is a good idea to have these sent ahead of the appointment so that the specialist can review them before the actual medical interview.

Family Medical History

Your family medical history is useful for determining possible hereditary aspects of disease or identifying risk factors. For example, if a close family member had a heart attack at a young age, you may have a higher risk of coronary artery disease.

Make a list of any chronic diseases affecting your parents, grandparents, brothers, sisters, and children.

Social History

Your social history includes information about your life-style or living habits that may have an impact on disease, such as smoking and alcohol use, recreational activities that may influence general fitness, or job-related factors such as toxic exposures.

Review of Organ Systems

Your doctor will review potential symptoms related to each organ system during the medical interview. This review is a checklist for you and the doctor to go through to make sure that nothing is overlooked. For example, someone who complains of chest pain may neglect to mention that he or she experiences calf tiredness when walking a short distance. This information is important to the doctor, because both chest pain and calf discomfort or tiredness can be related to blockage in the coronary and leg arteries, respectively. Items such as this should be brought out during the course of systematically reviewing other organ systems.

THE PHYSICAL EXAMINATION

The main parts of a cardiovascular physical examination include measuring the blood pressure and the heart rate and rhythm, checking all the pulses, inspecting the veins of the neck (jugular veins), determining whether there is swelling (edema), and listening to the breath and heart sounds.

Blood Pressure

You have probably had your blood pressure checked many times. Measuring blood pressure is safe, simple, and a standard way to detect one problem that can lead to heart disease. This test also can give your doctor clues about the pumping ability of your heart and the resistance offered by your arteries.

In general, the harder the heart pumps and the narrower the arteries, the higher the blood pressure. A practical example of this principle is pushing water through a hose with a ½-inch diameter compared with pushing the same amount of water through a hose

120/70 mm Hg—
What does that mean?

Having your blood pressure checked is a painless, routine procedure. Here is how it works: To check your blood pressure, the doctor or other health care professional wraps a blood pressure cuff around your upper arm, pumps it with air so the blood flow in your arm is stopped temporarily, and then listens for the pulse (called Korotkoff sounds) with a stethoscope as the cuff is gradually deflated.

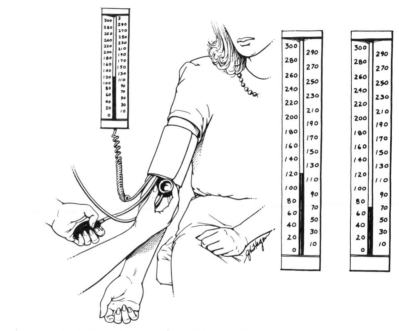

Measurement of blood pressure with a sphygmomanometer. After the cuff is pumped up, air is slowly released to reduce the pressure constricting the arm. The doctor or nurse notes the pressure on the mercury-column gauge at which the heartbeat can first be heard. This is the systolic pressure—120 mm Hg (millimeters of mercury) in the illustration. The pressure at which the sounds disappear is the diastolic pressure—70 mm Hg.

The top number in a blood pressure reading (which normally averages about 120 mm Hg) is called the systolic blood pressure. It is the point at which the person taking the measurement hears the pulse in the arm as the pressure is deflated in the cuff. This number represents the pressure in the arteries of the arm at the time the heart is squeezing blood out into the circulation.

The bottom number in the blood pressure reading (which normally averages about 70 mm Hg) is called the diastolic blood pressure. It is the point at which the heart sounds disappear as the pressure continues to be deflated in the cuff. This number represents the pressure in the arteries of the arm at the time the heart is relaxing between beats.

with a 1-inch diameter. The pressure will be higher in the hose with the smaller diameter.

Your blood pressure should be measured when you are resting quietly. Changes in blood pressure may be detected when you are lying down, sitting, and standing. A drop in blood pressure when you stand up could explain some types of positional lightheadedness. Your doctor may also measure your blood pressure in both arms, because a difference between the arm pressures may indicate a partial blockage in the aorta or either of the arteries going to the arms. Blood pressure downstream from a blockage is lower than the pressure upstream from a blockage.

Nervousness and anxiety increase blood pressure. The anxiety that some people have during medical examinations can lead to a phenomenon known as "white-coat" hypertension. People who have "white-coat" hypertension really may have normal blood pressure, but it is high when it is measured by a doctor.

Doctors do not rely on just one measurement of blood pressure to diagnose high blood pressure. Some variation in blood pressure measurements is normal. For an accurate diagnosis of high blood pressure, the blood pressure should be elevated on three separate occasions.

Heart Rate and Rhythm

Doctors can quickly assess the heart rate and rhythm by feeling (palpating) the pulse at the wrist, the carotid arteries in the neck, or the femoral arteries in the groin. Doctors can also tell whether the pulse is regular, has skipped or extra beats, or is irregular, as in atrial fibrillation (see page 92).

Health professionals usually count the pulse for 15 seconds and multiply that number by 4 (4 × 15 seconds = 1 minute) to calculate the heart rate in beats per minute. A thorough examination includes palpation of the pulses at both wrists, the pulses at the inner part of both elbows (brachial pulse), the carotid pulses in the neck, the aortic pulse in the abdomen, the femoral pulses in the groin, the popliteal pulse behind each knee, the dorsalis pedis pulse on the top of each foot, and the posterior tibialis pulse (on the inside of each leg, next to the ankle) (see figure on page 186). An absent or reduced pulse at any of these sites may indicate a blockage upstream from that site.

Venous Pulses

Doctors examine venous pulses by looking rather than by listening or palpation. They carefully look at your neck when you are lying down with your head partially raised or when you are sitting up. They observe the slight expansion made by the jugular vein in the neck as the heart beats. The jugular vein is a reliable indicator of the pressure on the right side of the heart. When the pressure on the right side of the heart is high, the blood flowing from the jugular vein into the heart backs up a bit, causing the top of the expansion to be at a higher point on the neck (see figure on page 187). Doctors can estimate the approximate pressure in the right side of the heart and also get an idea of how much extra fluid there is in the cardiovascular system by observing the jugular vein.

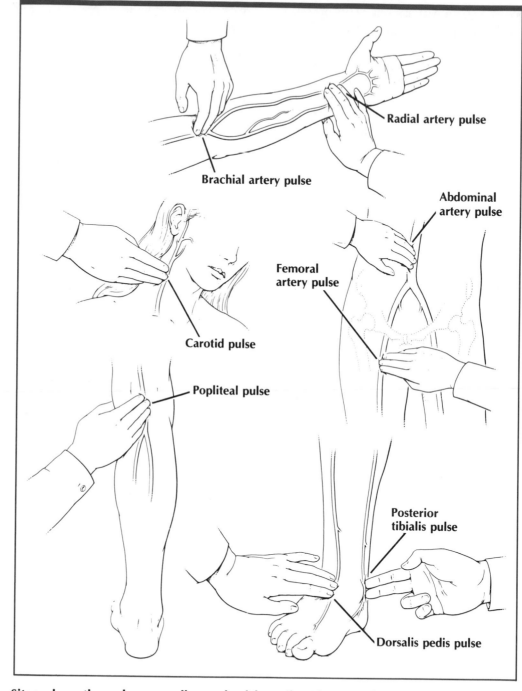

Sites where the pulse normally can be felt easily. Absence of a pulse at any of these points may signal a blockage in the artery upstream.
Radial (wrist) and brachial (elbow) pulses.
Carotid pulse.
Abdominal aortic pulse and femoral (groin) pulse.
Popliteal (behind the knee) pulse.
Dorsalis pedis (top of foot) and posterior tibialis (behind inner ankle) pulses.

Checking for Swelling (Edema)

Doctors routinely look for excess fluid by examining parts of the body that are prone to swelling. When people spend most of their time upright during the day, swelling can occur in the ankles and legs.

To gauge fluid retention, the doctor presses on the skin (for example, over the ankle) and watches how far it can be indented. If there is indentation, this is called pitting edema. Pitting edema can occur in the ankles and the area over the shin, the thighs, the lower back and abdomen, or the hands, depending on the severity of the fluid retention (see figure on page 188).

Edema can also occur if there is a blockage of a vein carrying blood back from an arm or leg. In kidney failure or if the main vein that carries blood from the head (superior vena cava) is obstructed, the person may have edema in the face, causing a puffy, rounded appearance.

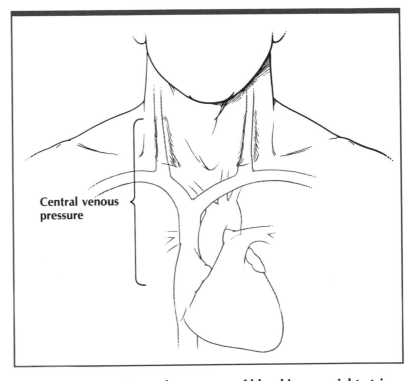

Central venous pressure

Your doctor can estimate the pressure of blood in your right atrium by observing the level of expansion of the jugular vein. Normally, the vein's bulge would not be visible above the collarbone in a sitting person. The higher it is seen to bulge above the collarbone, the higher the pressure in the right atrium. This finding, in turn, gives a good indication of the volume of blood in your circulation. The volume might be increased in conditions that cause congestive heart failure (see also figure on page 38).

Listening to Breath Sounds

Doctors spend a lot of time listening through their stethoscopes. They do this because they can get a wealth of information from listening to breathing, heart, and blood vessel sounds. They listen to your lungs by placing the stethoscope on several areas of your chest while you breathe in and out.

In addition to listening with the stethoscope, your doctor may thump on your chest (percussion). Percussion provides clues about where fluid may have accumulated between the lungs and the chest wall or about areas of the lungs that may have collapsed or become dense because of infection or inflammation. Tapping over these areas sounds dull, instead of producing a normal "hollow" sound.

From a cardiac standpoint, the doctor is mainly trying to tell whether excessive fluid has leaked into the air sacs of the lungs. This fluid makes a crackling sound in the stethoscope when the person breathes in. These abnormal sounds (referred to as crackles or rales) provide clues to different types of disease. Crackles associated with increased fluid sound "wet," like many little bubbles popping. Other

Swelling of the foot, ankle, and leg can be severe enough to leave an indentation, or "pit," when you press on the area. This swelling is caused by excessive fluid due to congestive heart failure or blockage in a leg vein.

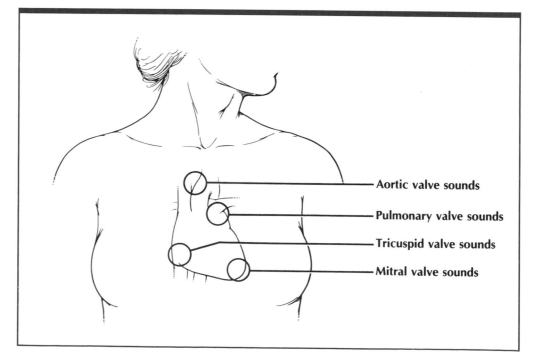

crackles sound like Velcro being pulled apart. These sounds raise a suspicion of scarring (fibrosis) in the lungs.

Listening to the Heart

When doctors listen to the heart with a stethoscope, they listen in at least four standard spots. Doctors listen to the quality of the valve sounds when they snap closed and for sounds of turbulent blood flow through the valves or other heart structures (murmurs). Murmurs can occur when blood is forced to flow through an abnormally tight valve, when it leaks back (regurgitates) through a defective valve (see page 57), or when it follows an abnormal course through the heart (for example, through a hole in the ventricular septum or around an obstructing bulge caused by hypertrophic cardiomyopathy) (see page 43).

Sometimes the cause of a murmur is not apparent, but most causes can be determined by having the person perform certain maneuvers. You may be asked to stand up, squat, or lie down as the doctor listens to your heart, because murmurs change in characteristic ways when your position changes. Murmurs also change during different types of breathing, so the doctor may ask you to breathe in and out deeply or to hold your breath and bear down

When doctors listen to your heart they focus especially on areas that give information about the flow of blood through the heart valves. They listen for murmurs, which may indicate turbulent blood flow caused by stenosis or regurgitation of a valve. Other sounds, such as gallops, clicks, rubs, or knocks, may indicate other types of heart problems.

Aortic valve sounds

Pulmonary valve sounds

Tricuspid valve sounds

Mitral valve sounds

as though you were straining during a bowel movement. Some murmurs can be heard more clearly in one position or another, so the doctor may ask you to roll onto your left side or to sit up and lean forward.

In special circumstances, the doctor may have you inhale a medication (amyl nitrite). This briefly alters your blood pressure and heart rate so that certain murmurs can be characterized more completely.

Besides murmurs, doctors also listen for "gallops," which are extra sounds in the heart that can give a galloping cadence to heart sounds. The type of gallop that is heard may help differentiate abnormalities in the relaxing phase from those in the contracting phase of the heartbeat.

Doctors also listen for various other sounds, including whoops, clicks, snaps, knocks, and rubs, all of which provide vital information about possible underlying heart and pericardial disease. Some murmurs and sounds are "innocent," meaning they may be present even though the person has no heart problems.

During the physical examination the doctor also watches and touches the chest wall to inspect the visible and palpable aspects of the heartbeat. From these observations your doctor may find clues as to whether the heart is enlarged, whether it is squeezing forcibly, and whether any blood flow abnormalities are producing vibrations (thrills) in the chest.

Listening to the Blood Vessels

The doctor may also place a stethoscope over the carotid arteries in your neck, the abdominal aorta in the torso, and both femoral arteries in the groin to listen for bruits (pronounced BRU-ees), which are whispering sounds made by turbulence of blood flow. Like a river flowing over rocky rapids, your blood might make more noise as it flows through areas with atherosclerotic deposits that obstruct its flow. Thus, the presence of a bruit may indicate a degree of blockage (stenosis) at those sites.

BLOOD TESTS

Routine blood tests are used to rule out or help diagnose a wide variety of conditions. In most general examinations, blood testing includes a complete blood cell count (CBC) to look for problems such as anemias (too few red blood cells), a chemistry group analysis, and measurement of blood lipids. Many other blood tests can be done, depending on the circumstances, including thyroid studies to assess the function of the thyroid gland

and coagulation studies to determine the rate at which the blood clots.

How Are Blood Samples Collected?

It usually takes only a few seconds to draw a small amount of blood into a vial for testing. Sometimes special preparations such as overnight fasting may be necessary. Blood may be drawn from a tiny cut made in a fingertip and placed in a small container called a capillary pipette if only a drop or two is needed. If more blood is needed, the person drawing it (the venipuncturist) places a tourniquet around the upper arm. This makes the veins bulge so they are easier to see and blood can be obtained more easily. The venipuncturist then selects a vein, cleans the skin over it with alcohol, and gently inserts a thin needle. Blood passes through the needle into an attached sterile syringe. When enough blood has been drawn, the tourniquet is released, the needle withdrawn, and the puncture site wiped again with an antiseptic. If blood is needed from an artery, a slightly different procedure is used (see page 191).

What Do Blood Tests Show?

The most common blood tests specifically relating to heart disease measure blood lipid levels (cholesterol and triglycerides), cardiac enzymes, oxygen content, and prothrombin time.

LIPID LEVELS. The usual lipids that are measured are total cholesterol, high-density lipoprotein (HDL) cholesterol, and triglycerides (see page 126). Low-density lipoprotein (LDL) cholesterol values can be calculated from the three other cholesterol values by the formula: LDL cholesterol = total cholesterol − HDL cholesterol − (triglycerides/5). This formula provides a good estimate of the LDL cholesterol value. If a precise measurement is needed, a blood test that specifically determines the LDL value is more accurate.

The lipids in the blood vary according to recent food intake, so you should have fasted since midnight before the blood is drawn in the morning. Even with fasting, the level of lipids in the blood may vary because of fluctuation in the body's processing of fats.

The laboratory test used to measure lipids is not totally precise. It is accurate to within 2 to 5 percent of the actual value. Thus, two different analyses of the same sample of blood may give two slightly different values for lipids. Thus, there is little reason to split hairs about small differences in measurements between two people or between two measurements from the same person.

Measurements from blood obtained from a vein in your arm are more likely to be accurate than measurements from a few drops of blood from your finger. A single measurement is no guarantee that your cholesterol level is normal or abnormal. At least two sets of measurements that agree are needed before any conclusions can be made. If two measurements are widely different, a third measurement is needed. (See Lipid levels and coronary risk, page 127, for a more detailed discussion on desirable and high levels of cholesterol and triglycerides.)

Currently, your doctor will probably concentrate on your total cholesterol, LDL, HDL, and triglyceride measurements. In the future, measurements of just the protein portions of lipoproteins, called apoproteins, may become important in assessing your risk of heart disease.

CARDIAC ENZYMES. Your blood can be tested for levels of enzymes (creatine kinase [CK], lactate dehydrogenase [LDH]) that may indicate damage to the heart. Enzymes usually found in the heart may leak into the blood from damaged heart cells after a heart attack. If you experience chest pain, your doctor may recommend testing your blood for these enzymes. These tests give an index of whether there has been irreversible damage to heart muscle cells.

Enzyme levels are not usually elevated immediately after the heart damage occurs. But blood tests during the day or two after a suspicious episode of chest pain can help confirm whether the heart has been damaged.

Even when a heart attack has been confirmed, cardiac enzymes may continue to be measured to be sure that enzyme levels are decreasing. Enzyme levels that increase again may be an indication of ongoing or recurrent heart damage.

The results of cardiac enzyme tests may at times be inaccurate if the amount of heart muscle damage is too small to result in an elevation of the enzymes, or if there is another source of the enzymes. Some of the enzymes may also come from damaged skeletal muscle, liver tissue, blood cells, or the brain. In most people, further specialized analysis of the enzymes can distinguish the sources.

OXYGEN LEVEL. The measurement of oxygen in the circulation at various sites helps your doctor determine whether the overall circulation is sufficient, whether the lungs are providing enough oxygen to the bloodstream, and whether there is evidence of shunting of blood in the heart which prevents some blood from traveling through the lungs to pick up oxygen.

The amount of oxygen in the blood can be measured in several ways. You can think of these measurements as a determination of how saturated the blood is with oxygen. If the blood has passed through the lungs and picked up oxygen, its oxygen saturation is high. Thus, the oxygen saturation of blood in the arteries leaving the left ventricle is high. Once the blood releases oxygen to the tissues, its oxygen saturation is lower. The oxygen saturation of blood in the veins returning to the heart from the body is therefore low.

Oxygen can be measured in the arterial blood, which carries oxygen to the tissues of the body, or in the venous blood, which returns to the heart and lungs. If the doctor wants to know the oxygen level in blood after it has received oxygen from the lungs, the blood is drawn from an artery rather than a vein.

The procedure for tests on arterial blood differs somewhat from a standard blood test. The person drawing the blood cleans the skin over the artery with an antiseptic and may inject a local anesthetic to numb the area. The typical sites are where the pulses of the following arteries can be felt: the radial artery in the wrist, the brachial artery in the elbow, or the femoral artery at the groin. The artery is punctured with a sterile needle attached to a disposable syringe that has been coated on the interior with oil to prevent room air from contaminating the blood sample. After the blood sample is drawn, the needle is removed from the artery and the sample is transferred from the syringe into sterile tubes that are placed in a blood gas analyzer. You will be asked to apply pressure to the puncture site and to rest quietly for 15 minutes before resuming normal activities.

The oxygen saturation of your blood can now be analyzed with a clip (which resembles a small clothespin) that is placed on your finger or toe. A light is passed through your skin, and it measures the oxygen saturation by assessing the redness of the blood. This clip is used during procedures such as angiography and surgery, or during monitoring in an intensive care unit, to give the doctors a constant measurement of the oxygen in your blood.

If frequent measurements of blood oxygen are needed, blood also may be obtained through a catheter that is left in place.

PROTHROMBIN TIME.   Medications that prevent the blood from clotting are called anticoagulants. Although they are often referred to as "blood thinners," they do not actually "thin" the blood. They alter the proteins in the blood which are responsible for clotting and so make it less likely to clot. They are beneficial for people with a predisposition for abnormal blood clots or for people who already have blood clots. These are people with deep vein thrombosis or pulmonary embolism (see page 107), dilated cardiomyopathy (see page 39), or mechanical artificial heart valves.

The most common anticoagulant is warfarin, which prevents the liver from using vitamin K to make certain proteins needed for blood clotting. Enough warfarin must be given to prevent abnormal clotting, but not so much that abnormal bleeding or bruising results. Excessive warfarin can cause bleeding; in fact, warfarin is the main ingredient in some kinds of rat poison.

Because individual responses to warfarin are not entirely predictable, people taking this medication must have their blood clotting monitored with a blood test that determines the prothrombin time. The longer the prothrombin time, the more anticoagulated the blood is. Your prothrombin time is compared with the value that is considered normal in the particular laboratory where it was measured. Usually, the desired prothrombin time in people taking warfarin is 1.3 to 1.5 times the normal prothrombin time. Prothrombin times should be checked at least once a month, and sometimes more frequently, especially when warfarin treatment is started.

ELECTROCARDIOGRAPHY (ECG)

Electrocardiography (ECG) is indispensable for evaluating many heart diseases. The technique of ECG has advanced remarkably since its introduction more than 80 years ago. By interpreting an ECG tracing (also called an ECG), your doctor can diagnose several abnormal conditions that can affect your heart, including rhythm disturbances, heart attack, and abnormalities of the heart's structure.

What Is Electrocardiography (ECG)?

An electrocardiogram (ECG) is a recording of the electrical activity of your heart. The so-called tracing can be displayed either on a strip of paper or on a monitor. It also can be recorded on tape or even transmitted over telephone wires. The equipment used to record an ECG is an electrocardiograph—the terminology is the same as for telegram and telegraph.

Electrical activity of the heart is detected by electrodes attached to your skin. Typically, the electrical impulses are recorded in the form of waves that are displayed on graph paper that moves out of the electrocardiograph at a set speed. Horizontally the graph corresponds to time, and vertically the graph corresponds to the voltage or strength of the electrical impulses. The recordings from each electrode represent the electrical forces from various areas of your heart. Each electrode is like a "watching post" that records the impulses from its particular location.

Different waves represent the different areas of your heart through which tiny electrical currents are flowing and causing it to contract and relax (see Figure 44, page A12). Briefly, the P wave represents the current in the atria, the QRS complex represents the current in the ventricles, and the T wave represents the electrical recovery period of the ventricles. These components of the ECG can impart an enormous amount of information about your heart.

What Does Electrocardiography (ECG) Show?

The components of the ECG tracing— the P waves, the QRS complexes, and the T waves—can occur in a seemingly endless variety of patterns, shapes, and speeds. Each variation

ECG or EKG?

Much of the development of ECG was done in the Netherlands. As a result, many doctors still say "EKG"—a historical reference to the electrokardiogram.

provides your physician with a wealth of clues about the state of your heart. The ECG gives information about the heart rate, the rhythm of the heart, the presence of heart damage or inadequate blood and oxygen supply to the heart muscle, and abnormalities of heart structure.

HEART RATE. The simplest piece of information the ECG can provide is

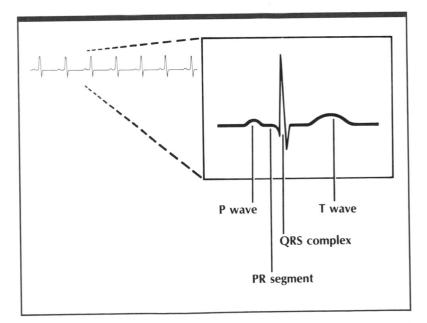

P wave   T wave

QRS complex

PR segment

The electrocardiogram of one heartbeat consists of a series of "waves" that tell about the electrical impulse in different parts of your heart. The *P wave* shows the impulse as it travels through the atrium. Following the P wave is the *PR segment*, a flat portion that represents the time the impulse travels through the atrioventricular node. The *QRS complex* occurs as the impulse travels throughout the ventricles. The *T wave* is formed during the time the heart muscle recovers electrically in preparation for the next beat (see also Figures 42, 43, and 44, page A12).

the rate of your heartbeat at the time the ECG was obtained. If 10 QRS complexes are recorded on the ECG paper or ECG monitor in 10 seconds, then your heart rate is 60 beats per minute. The ECG is seldom needed just for information about your heart rate. A check of your pulse will suffice. An ECG may be helpful, though, when the pulse is difficult to feel or is too fast or too irregular to count accurately.

HEART RHYTHM. The ECG is the most direct way to assess the rhythm of your heart. It can distinguish normal sinus rhythm from all types of tachycardia (abnormal fast rhythms) (see page 93) and bradycardia (abnormal slow rhythms) (see page 86). Your heart normally beats in sequence: the atria first and then the ventricles shortly afterward at a speed usually between 60 and 100 beats per minute. Arrhythmias (see page 82) deviate from this pattern.

For example, complete heart block exists when the atria are stimulated normally but the electrical impulse is blocked from passing through the atrioventricular node to the ventricles. Therefore, the ventricles beat at a slow "backup" rate that is different from the rate of the atrial beats. On the ECG, this condition appears as P waves going at one rate and QRS complexes going at a slower rate with no relationship to one another. All of the other heart rhythm abnormalities discussed on pages 82–96 also have their characteristic patterns, and a doctor experienced in interpreting ECGs can readily discern them.

HEART ATTACK. The ECG may provide crucially important information about whether a heart attack has occurred. It can often distinguish between a heart attack that occurred in the past and one that is in progress at the time the ECG is taken. The patterns on the ECG can indicate which part of the heart (front, back, lower, or sides) has been damaged, roughly estimate the extent of the damage, and suggest whether the heart wall was damaged throughout the full thickness.

The ECG is able to do this because injured heart muscle and scar tissue in the heart do not conduct electrical impulses normally. Consequently, the shapes of the QRS complexes and the T waves are altered in characteristic ways that lead to the diagnosis. Obviously, this early warning system is in-

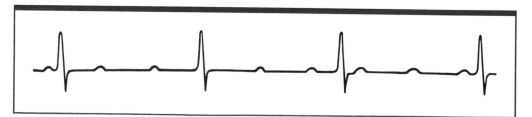

Complete heart block, also called third-degree atrioventricular block, is the most severe form of heart block. None of the impulses from the sinus node get through the atrioventricular node to the ventricles.
On the electrocardiogram, none of the P waves are followed by a QRS complex. Instead, other parts of the conduction system may take over the task of producing a heartbeat, but at a much slower rate. You can see that the P waves and the QRS complexes are going at separate rates, unrelated to one another.

valuable for getting appropriate, rapid treatment started for people with chest pain.

INADEQUATE BLOOD AND OXYGEN SUPPLY TO THE HEART MUSCLE. People with bouts of chest pain or discomfort may be having angina, or the pain may be entirely unrelated to the heart. An ECG that is obtained *during* the symptoms may be able to make the distinction (see figure at right). Inadequate blood and oxygen supply to a region of heart muscle often changes the shape of the ECG tracing, particularly the segment between the end of the QRS complex and the end of the T wave. Such an observation can be useful for deciding on further testing or treatment. Between episodes of inadequate blood supply to the heart, the ECG may be perfectly normal.

STRUCTURAL ABNORMALITIES OF THE HEART. The ECG can provide clues to the presence of thickening (hypertrophy) of the heart muscle, to congenital abnormalities, or to enlargement of the heart chambers. In most cases, other tests are required to confirm that the diagnosis is correct and to get necessary further information.

ADDITIONAL USES OF ELECTROCARDIOGRAPHY (ECG). The ECG can give information about potential health problems that are not specifically heart-related. Changes in the ECG tracing can indicate high or low potassium or calcium levels. This possibility may in turn lead to a search for kidney problems, hormonal abnormalities, or side effects of medications. The ECG is useful for assessing the effect (or even toxicity) of certain medi-

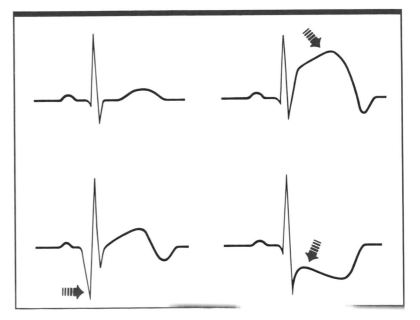

The appearance of the electrocardiogram gives important clues about certain heart problems.
Top left, A normal heartbeat.

Top right, The elevated portion (*arrow*) between the QRS complex and the T wave is a strong indication that heart muscle injury, such as a heart attack, is occurring.

Bottom left, The deep early portion of the QRS complex (*arrow*) is evidence that a heart attack may have occurred at some time in the past.

Bottom right, The lowered ST segment (*arrow*) suggests that an area of the heart is receiving insufficient blood supply. This might be observed during an episode of angina or during an abnormal exercise stress test.

cations because they alter the tracing in specific ways.

Like any other test result, the results on ECG may not always be 100 percent accurate. Some rhythm disorders are so complex that the correct explanation may not be diagnosed with certainty until further testing is done. The ECG may occasionally show signs suggestive of coronary artery disease even when further testing shows that there is no coronary artery disease. The ECG also may appear normal when coronary artery disease *does* exist, particularly if you are not having any symptoms at the time the ECG is obtained. Nevertheless, because the ECG provides so much information at such a low cost and at no risk to you, it is considered vital to the understanding of your cardiac health in most cases.

How Is Electrocardiography (ECG) Done?

The ECG test is a simple one. Usually 12 to 15 electrodes are attached to various parts of your body, including 1 on each arm and leg, 6 across the left side of the chest, and often 1 or more at other sites on the chest, neck, and back.

The electrodes are sticky patches that are attached to the skin while you are lying down. Because the electrodes are trying to detect very small electrical currents, good contact must be maintained with the skin. A conductive gel is used to improve this connection. The hair may be shaved off the chest in men, and the skin may be roughened with very fine sandpaper to ensure that the patch makes good contact and sticks well.

After the leads are attached, the person performing the ECG test will record the information from the various leads. You do not feel anything during the testing procedure. The actual ECG recording usually takes 30 to 60 seconds to complete. The test can be done in a hospital room or in the doctor's office.

Many hospitals and offices now have computerized interpretations of ECGs. Although this method increases the efficiency of performing the test, computer programs raise a further possibility of error, no matter how sophisticated they are. Thus, ECGs should be reviewed by a doctor for accurate and confident conclusions to be drawn.

Are There Risks?

There is no pain or risk from ECG. The machine is only reading your heart's electrical impulses; it does not send any electrical impulses to your body, and there is no danger of electrical shock.

Other Varieties of Electrocardiography (ECG)

One of the problems with traditional ECGs is that because they are performed over only a minute or so, some sporadic rhythm abnormalities or other problems may be missed. Thus, techniques have been developed to increase the likelihood of an ECG detecting an abnormality.

EXERCISE ELECTROCARDIOGRAPHY (ECG) TEST. One technique is the exercise ECG test, which

Undergoing electrocardiography is an easy procedure. Adhesive skin electrodes are attached to your chest and limbs to record the electrical activity of your heart while you rest.

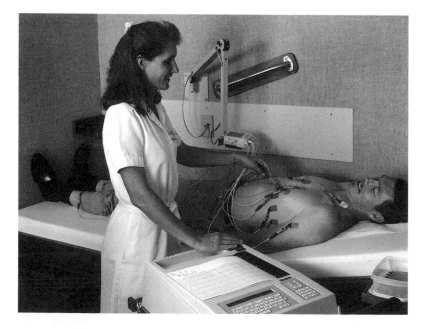

is an ECG that is obtained while you walk on a treadmill or pedal a stationary cycle. Because inadequate coronary circulation is more evident during higher heart rates, abnormalities related to ischemia (insufficient blood and oxygen supply) are more likely to occur and to show up on the ECG during exercise. Also, some rhythm abnormalities are provoked by exercise, and these too are more likely to be detected. The exercise ECG test may also be used to follow the progress of people who have had heart attacks to assess the effects of various drugs or procedures.

In this test, the electrodes are attached to your chest and back and ECG recordings are taken before, during, and after you exercise. In most exercise ECG tests, you exercise on a treadmill, but if that is not possible, you may exercise on a stationary cycle. In both instances, the exercise starts at a very relaxed pace. Every few minutes, the speed and the steepness of the incline of the treadmill (or the resistance on the cycle) are increased, and you will then have to work a little harder. The doctor or nurses monitoring the test will ask you to rate how hard you are working according to a Perceived Exertion Scale (see box on right). They will encourage you to exercise until you are too tired to continue or until you experience any symptoms such as chest pain or shortness of breath. They may simply stop the test once sufficient information is obtained.

If your heart's activity is normal during the exercise ECG test, there is a good chance that your heart will function normally when you work out. The results will be useful for establishing exercise limits and developing a special fitness program. If the ECG shows

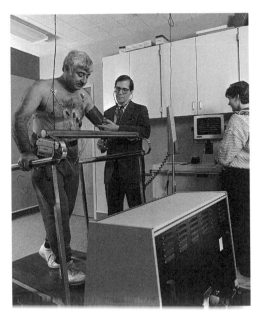

An exercise electrocardiogram ("stress test") is obtained during some form of activity—such as walking on a treadmill as shown here, or stationary cycling.

Perceived Exertion Scale

During most types of exercise stress tests you will be asked to describe how hard you are working. One standard way of describing the amount of physical effort you are experiencing is to use the Borg Perceived Exertion Scale shown below. This scale takes into account exertion, physical stress, and fatigue. When you use the scale, think about your *total* feeling of exertion, not just one factor such as a sensation that your legs are getting heavier or that you are becoming short of breath.

Borg Perceived Exertion Scale

6		14	
7	Very, very light	15	Hard
8		16	
9	Very light	17	Very hard
10		18	
11	Fairly light	19	Very, very hard
12		20	
13	Somewhat hard		

The scale ranges from "6," which indicates minimal exertion such as sitting comfortably in a chair, to "20," which corresponds to maximal exertion such as walking briskly or jogging up a very steep hill.

any abnormalities, your doctor may recommend other tests that more accurately determine whether there are coronary blockages and where they are located.

Exercise ECG tests have a small risk, because they are stressing the heart. The danger of suffering a heart attack during the test is remote—only 3.5 in 10,000. The risk of a serious rhythm problem occurring during the test is about 48 in 10,000. However, experienced personnel and equipment are available to monitor your symptoms and blood pressure continually and to handle any emergency. The technicians, nurses, and doctors are trained to handle any situation that may come up, including the need for cardiopulmonary resuscitation if necessary. In fact, a medical facility is probably the safest possible place to experience your symptoms, because the problem can be diagnosed and treated appro-

Variety of stress tests

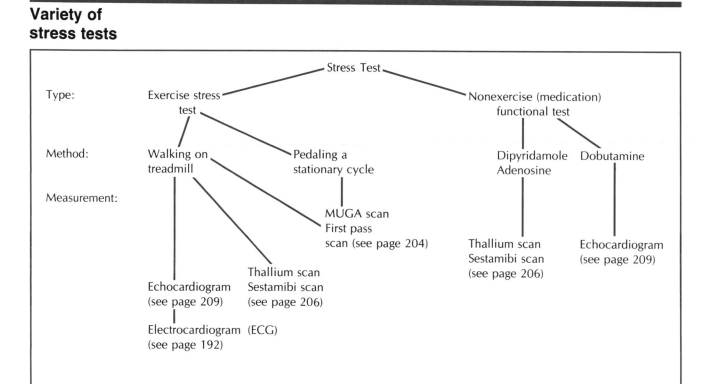

Stress tests are designed to examine the function of the heart muscle, the adequacy of the coronary blood supply, or both. Various stress tests are available. The type that is used depends on the questions that need to be answered and the capabilities of the patient. For example, an exercise test in which you walk on a treadmill while the *ECG* is monitored is a useful screening test for people suspected of having coronary artery disease. A treadmill *thallium* scan shows the actual distribution of blood flow in the heart muscle. A person who is unable to use his or her legs well (for example, because of arthritis) can undergo an *adenosine* (or *dipyridamole*) *thallium* scan (see page 206). This is not really a "stress" test, although the effect of stress on the heart is "mimicked" and similar information is obtained. Other stress tests, in addition to those listed, are occasionally done (for example, arm exercise can replace walking or cycling).

priately. However, problems rarely occur, because doctors recommend these tests only for people in whom they believe the testing will be safe.

Even exercise ECG tests are not perfect and can yield either a false-positive or a false-negative result. It is always important to interpret the results of this and any test in light of all the other information about the person. However, an ECG performed during exercise will correctly identify the presence of coronary artery disease in about 70 percent of people with the disease. In addition, the test accurately identifies people without coronary artery disease more than 90 percent of the time.

AMBULATORY ELECTROCARDIOGRAPHY (ECG) MONITORING.

Another technique that has been used to detect abnormalities that are intermittent is prolonged ambulatory monitoring of the ECG. This is also called Holter monitoring (after the man who designed it in 1961).

Patch electrodes are attached to your chest and the ECG is recorded on tape or computer chip in a recorder that you wear for an entire day or two. You keep the recorder, which is about the size of a paperback novel, with you at all times during this test, including when you are asleep. In most cases, you will be asked to keep a diary of symptoms and activities so that the doctor can correlate your experiences with the ECG obtained at that time. The recorded information can be played back and rapidly scanned by computer, specially trained technicians, and physicians to look for abnormalities of rhythm. The test can also occasionally reveal evidence of inadequate blood supply in the coronary arteries.

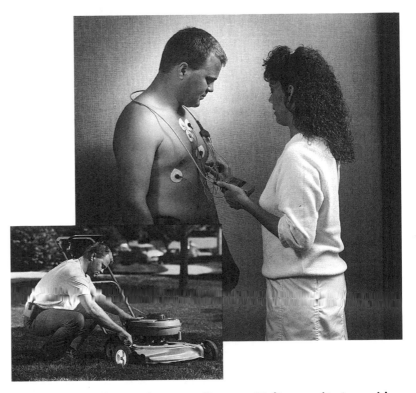

A 24-hour ambulatory electrocardiogram (Holter monitor) provides important information about the electrical activity of your heart as you perform your everyday routine. Small electrodes stick to your skin and connect to a portable recording device worn on your belt (see photo inset). Every heartbeat is recorded for analysis later.

Holter monitoring, like a regular ECG, is painless and there is no risk from the procedure. There is minimal inconvenience from keeping the recording device with you. It is important that you keep an accurate diary to help relate your symptoms to the recording obtained at the time they occurred.

TELEPHONE-TRANSMITTED ELECTROCARDIOGRAPHY

(ECG). Another technique is transmitting ECGs across telephone lines. You may receive a telephone transmitter device and be instructed in its use. When a symptom develops, you dial a telephone number and transmit the

ECG to a monitor in the hospital or doctor's office. In this way, relatively infrequent symptoms can be correlated with the ECG. However, for this test to be effective, your symptoms must last long enough for you to dial the telephone and make a transmission, and of course the transmitter and a telephone must be handy when the symptoms occur.

EVENT RECORDERS. To help diagnose symptoms that are infrequent, sporadic, or otherwise hard to "capture" over the telephone lines, another device has been developed called an event recorder. This is like a Holter monitor that is worn over a longer time, usually about a month (though it can be removed briefly to permit bathing and so on). When a symptom occurs, you push a button that tells the event recorder to remember what it recorded for several minutes before and after the button was pushed. Unless the button is pushed, the recorder simply monitors the heart rhythm. The signal from the recorder can be transmitted over the telephone or taken to the doctor's office at your convenience.

SIGNAL-AVERAGED ELECTRO-CARDIOGRAPHY (ECG). Signal-averaged ECG is a noninvasive technique used to help identify people at high risk for ventricular tachycardia or ventricular fibrillation (see page 96). A heart in ventricular fibrillation cannot effectively pump blood to the body. It is the most common cause of sudden cardiac death outside the hospital.

Signal-averaged ECG uses a computer program that can identify very low or weak electrical impulses in your heart that are not detected on a regular ECG. The computer program amplifies the magnitude of these impulses and then filters the recordings to eliminate other "noise" that may be detected from other sources such as skeletal muscle or even machines that are nearby. The computer program averages 200 or more beats to filter out these random events. The presence of characteristic tiny waves in the signal-averaged ECG, which would not be visible on a regular ECG, suggests that an individual may be at high risk of a future heart rhythm abnormality and sudden death, so that further testing and preventive treatment may be warranted.

THE CHEST X-RAY EXAMINATION

X-rays are a form of radiation (energy that moves from one place to another). Some radiation cannot pass through body structures. Light, for example, is one form of radiation that does not pass through the body; rather, it bounces off (reflects) so that your eyes see an image formed by the reflected light. In medical practice it is often necessary to see inside the body, rather

than to see the body surface alone. X-rays can penetrate the body. Because of this ability, they can create a picture of internal body structures on film, which allows doctors to see inside the body without a surgical procedure.

For many years, doctors had to rely on the clinical examination, ECG, and chest X-ray for all diagnostic efforts in heart disease. Although many complex

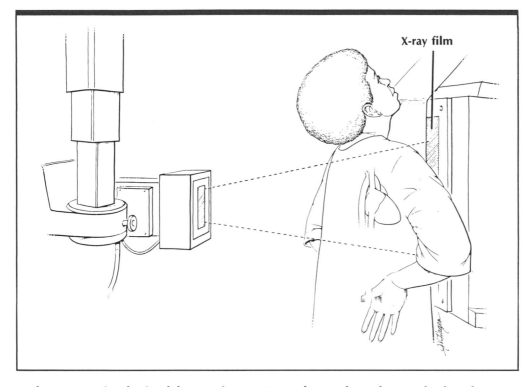

X-ray film

A chest X-ray is obtained by passing an X-ray beam through your body. The rays penetrate different tissues of the body to different extents before they reach a piece of film. Parts of your body that let most of the beams through (such as your lungs) cause the X-ray film to turn dark when it is developed. Other areas, such as your heart (or especially your bones), block many of the X-rays, preventing them from reaching the film. These areas appear light on the developed film.

imaging tests have been developed in recent decades, the chest X-ray is still a fundamental and important test in the evaluation and screening of heart disease.

What Is a Chest X-Ray?

A chest X-ray produces an image on film that outlines your heart, lungs, and other structures in your chest. An X-ray image is created by aiming X-rays at a region of the body (in this case the chest) and positioning a large piece of photographic film on the other side of the body. Just like any film, once the X-ray film is developed an image will show up. Parts of the film that received

a large exposure to the X-rays will be dark; those that received less will be lighter. This is like the negative in a picture taken by a regular camera: the parts of the film that received a lot of light rays (like a sunbeam reflected off pond water) appear dark; the parts that received little light (like a shadow) appear light.

The amount of X-rays that pass through your body and reach the film depends on the amount and type of tissues between the X-ray camera and the film. Because your muscular blood-filled heart is located between the two lungs filled with air, the silhouette of your heart is very conspicuous in the center of your chest. The heart

One important piece of information provided by the chest X-ray is the size of your heart. The X-ray on the left shows a normal-sized heart. The X-ray on the right shows a heart that is conspicuously enlarged, a sign that it is not pumping efficiently.

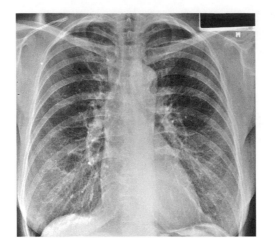 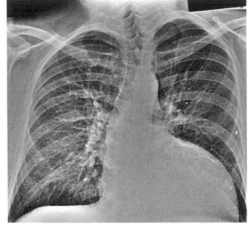

will appear light on the film because fewer X-rays were able to pass through fluid or blood and reach the film. The lungs will appear very dark because they are almost transparent to X-rays, so the film behind the lungs gets a large exposure to the X-rays.

What Does a Chest X-Ray Show?

The chest X-ray reveals several general types of information that are important in assessing the cardiovascular system: the size and shape of the heart, the presence of abnormal calcium deposits, and the condition of the lungs.

HEART SIZE AND SHAPE. Both the size and the shape of the heart can be judged on the chest X-ray, although individual parts of the heart can be distinguished only hazily and partially. Normally, the width of the heart on a chest X-ray occupies no more than about one-third to one-half the width of the whole chest. If the heart occupies half or more of the chest width, it is considered to be enlarged. As the heart enlarges, it may assume different

shapes that are related to the cause of the enlargement. Thus, a heart that is enlarged because of mitral regurgitation usually looks different from one that is enlarged from mitral stenosis or aortic stenosis.

CALCIUM DEPOSITS. Calcium is the main substance in bones. It does not allow many X-rays to pass through, so bones appear very light on X-ray films. Calcium also deposits in certain areas of diseased or injured tissue, thus drawing attention to these areas on an X-ray film. In the heart, calcium can deposit in diseased valves, coronary arteries with atherosclerosis, and damaged heart muscle or pericardium. Calcium deposits within the heart image can be distinguished from soft tissue on the chest X-ray, and they may be the first indication of a problem that requires further investigation.

THE CONDITION OF THE LUNGS. Abnormalities of heart function can affect the lungs in ways that chest X-rays can detect. A weakly pumping heart results in back pressure in the pulmonary (lung) blood vessels, causing them to become engorged and leak fluid into the air sacs (pulmonary edema; see Heart Failure, page 36). Chest X-rays can detect pulmonary veins that are swollen. X-rays do not pass through fluid as easily as they pass through air, so doctors can see fluid that has leaked into lung tissue.

How Is a Chest X-Ray Test Done?

The chest X-ray procedure is simple and painless. Before it is taken, you will probably remove your clothes and jewelry from the waist up and put on a hospital gown. (Jewelry, zippers, and other items show up on the X-ray and could obscure parts of the image.) In most cases, you will be asked to stand against the plate that contains the X-ray film, roll your shoulders forward, and hold your arms up or to the side so that they do not interfere with the picture. The radiologist or technician will ask you to take a deep breath and hold it as the X-ray picture is being taken. Holding your breath fills your lungs with air and your heart and lungs are thus more easily seen on the X-ray, and it also stops you from moving. It is often useful to see the chest from the side, so a second picture will be obtained with you turned with one side against the X-ray plate.

Are There Risks?

There is virtually no risk to you when a chest X-ray is obtained, although a small amount of radiation is involved. For most X-ray examinations, the risk of harm is very low and is greatly outweighed by the benefits of the examination. Great care is taken to use the lowest possible dose to produce the best possible image. No radiation remains after the X-ray examination.

The risk of X-rays can be put in perspective if you know that medical X-rays of all types account for only a little more than 10 percent of the total radiation exposure for the U.S. population. Other sources of radiation include radon, outer space, rocks, and soil. The amount of radiation from a chest X-ray is about the same as the amount of excess radiation you might receive during a transcontinental airplane trip.

Women who have any chance of being pregnant at the time of the X-ray examination should tell their doctors. Although the risk of causing harm to an unborn child by having an X-ray is very low, doctors take special precautions to minimize the exposure for the child.

NUCLEAR SCANNING

Nuclear scanning techniques add a new dimension to the assessment of your heart and circulation. Whereas a chest X-ray provides your doctor with an image of some of the structural aspects of your heart, nuclear scans show features of your heart's function and blood flow.

What Are Nuclear Scans?

In X-ray procedures, radiation passes *through* the body in order to produce useful images; in nuclear scanning procedures, a tiny amount of radiation is introduced *inside* the body and produces images as it radiates *outward*.

Nuclear scanning procedures operate according to the following principle: Trace amounts of radioactive material (radionuclides) are injected into the bloodstream. These "tracers" give off small amounts of energy (radiation) that are detected by special cameras, similar to Geiger counters. The radiation "counts" are processed by a computer, and an image is produced showing how the material is distributed in the body. Depending on the tracer material and the specific type of scan, information can be learned about the heart muscle and blood flow.

What Do Nuclear Scans Show?

Various nuclear scans have been developed to provide your doctor with specific types of information. Nuclear scans can show the size of your heart chambers, how effectively your heart pumps (ventricular function), how well your coronary arteries supply the heart muscle with blood (myocardial perfusion), whether there is scarring of the heart muscle from previous heart attacks, and the status of the lung circulation. Additional information can often be obtained from nuclear scanning by performing it in combination with an exercise stress test.

SIZE OF HEART CHAMBERS. A weakened heart enlarges (see page 40), so one important index of the strength of your heart muscle is an accurate measurement of the size of the pumping chambers (ventricles). One type of nuclear scanning can provide this information reliably. This test is called radionuclide ventriculography. There are two versions of radionuclide ventriculography: one is "MUGA" scanning (for *MU*ltiGated *A*cquisition), and the other is a "first-pass study." A tracer is injected into the bloodstream and it is scanned as it passes through the heart. For the MUGA, the tracer stays in the bloodstream for several hours; for the first-pass study, it remains in the bloodstream only long enough to circulate through the heart once before it is eliminated. In both tests, a special scanner camera detects the radiation that the tracer gives off as it passes through the heart.

A computer then uses this information to calculate the size and shape of your ventricles on the basis of the amount and distribution of radiation emitted from them. An image is produced that can be studied by the doctor, and numerical measurements are made of the volume of blood in the ventricles (see Figure 13, page A4).

VENTRICULAR FUNCTION. The same two forms of radionuclide ven-

How well does a ventricle do its job?

The overall efficiency with which a heart contracts can be assessed in several ways:

- *Ejection fraction*: the percentage (or fraction) of blood in the ventricle at the end of diastole (the phase of relaxation when the ventricle fills with blood) that is pumped out during systole (contraction of the ventricle). Normal is more than 50 percent.
- *Stroke volume*: the amount of blood the ventricle squeezes out with each systolic contraction. Normal is about 90 milliliters (about 3 ounces) for the average adult.
- *Cardiac output*: the amount of blood the heart pumps in 1 minute. Normal is about 5 liters (or about 5 quarts) per minute.

triculography can provide accurate and useful knowledge about the pumping function of the ventricles. For this, the computer takes the information from the scan and calculates the size and shape of the ventricles during systole (contraction) and diastole (relaxation). The difference between the size of the heart at these two points of time indicates how well the ventricles are squeezing.

A radionuclide ventriculogram can also determine whether all portions of the ventricular wall contribute equally to the pumping activity. Parts that move weakly may have been damaged by a heart attack or may receive reduced blood flow (because of coronary blockages).

BLOOD FLOW TO HEART MUSCLE. When performed in combination with exercise or another form of stress, nuclear scanning tests can provide vital information about the flow of blood through your coronary arteries. Radionuclide ventriculography can show this when your heart is scanned before and during increasing stages of exercise. The pumping functions of all parts of your ventricle are compared at each level of exercise. A normal heart will contract more vigorously during exertion. A heart in which one or more regions beat poorer than expected during exercise is likely to be receiving inadequate oxygen-rich blood to keep up with the muscle's increased need for energy. When the scan shows a region with poor function, the doctor can conclude that the coronary artery supplying that portion of your heart muscle is at least partially blocked.

Another very useful nuclear scanning procedure for evaluating your coronary blood flow is *perfusion scanning*. This is usually performed in con-

What do the results of a perfusion scan mean?

Basically, the results fall into one of three categories, although they may vary by location in your heart and by severity.

- *No perfusion defect at rest or after exercise*: Your myocardium and coronary arteries are normal.
- *Perfusion defect after exercise, but not at rest*: There are one or more coronary blockages that do not allow sufficient blood to reach hard-working myocardium. After a rest period, the tracer eventually reaches the myocardium and enters the cells, so there is at least some blood flow to the region and there are living myocardial cells present.
- *Perfusion defect after exercise and at rest*: There is an area of heart muscle which has become scar tissue because of a previous myocardial infarction (heart attack). The perfusion defect shows up because there is a blocked coronary artery and because there are no living myocardial cells at that site for the tracer to enter.

junction with exercise. Unlike the radionuclide tracer used in radionuclide ventriculography, the tracer used for perfusion scanning does not remain in the bloodstream. Rather, it enters the cells of your myocardium (heart muscle) after it is carried there through the coronary arteries. During the scanning, an image is made of your myocardium itself, not of the blood in your ventricle. If a portion of your myocardium receives less blood than the rest of your heart, it will receive less tracer and show up on the scan as a lighter area (perfusion defect) (see Figures 32B and C, page A10).

A common tracer used for perfusion scans is radioactive thallium; the term "thallium scan" is therefore often used synonymously with "perfusion scan." Other tracers are also used for some perfusion scans in special situations. The radioisotope technetium is available in a form called sestamibi, which can provide better images than thallium in large individuals.

The perfusion scanning is done after exercise and again after a rest period. Comparison of how your blood flows into (perfuses) the myocardium under these two conditions permits a diagnosis of the state of your heart muscle and coronary arteries.

Although exercise scanning with radionuclides is generally more accurate and provides more information than exercise ECG, it is also more expensive and time-consuming and requires special equipment and personnel. Thus, it is generally reserved for people in whom there is a special need to know the type of information that can be obtained only by these tests or for people in whom exercise ECG has not been as informative as hoped or would be expected to give inaccurate or ambiguous results.

Some individuals are unable to exercise because of leg or other problems.

However, similar information can be obtained about their hearts by using a medication that "mimics" stress on the heart in conjunction with perfusion scanning. Medications used for this purpose include dipyridamole and adenosine. Although these tests are very useful, an exercise test is best if it can be done.

Neither the perfusion scan nor the radionuclide ventriculogram shows coronary blockages directly; they show only the effects of coronary blockages on the myocardium. Further testing (coronary angiography, see page 216) must be done to actually see the location, number, and severity of the blockages.

LUNG CIRCULATION. Blockages in the arteries to the lungs, usually caused by blood clots (pulmonary emboli; see page 107), can be detected by a nuclear technique called *ventilation/perfusion scanning*—or, more simply, lung scanning. This is a scanning procedure that is designed to assess circulation through the lungs. As in heart scanning, a radioactive tracer is injected into the veins, and the chest is scanned. If there is a blood clot (pulmonary embolus) blocking blood flow through one or more branches of the pulmonary arteries (arteries to the lungs), the radioactive tracer will not distribute to that area.

This procedure is usually coupled with another scanning technique in which you breathe a radioactive gas and the lungs are scanned again. The adequacy of blood flow to all parts of the lung can be compared with the adequacy of air flow through the bronchi (airways). A pulmonary embolus would cause problems only with blood flow and the air flow would be relatively unaffected.

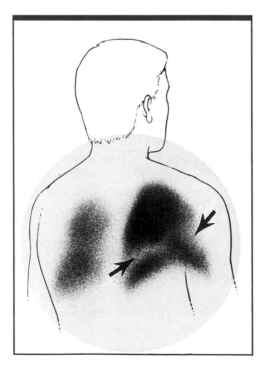

A lung perfusion scan provides an overall picture of blood circulation throughout your lungs. The light patches in the lung images (*arrows*) are areas where the tracer did not reach because of blockages in the pulmonary artery branches caused by clots (pulmonary emboli).

Ventilation/perfusion scans are useful for assessing whether certain symptoms such as chest pain or shortness of breath might be due to pulmonary embolism. A normal lung scan is reassuring because it means it is unlikely that a pulmonary embolism has occurred. People who have a positive test result, however, may need further investigation with pulmonary angiography before treatment is undertaken. This test would confirm that a pulmonary embolus is present.

How Is Nuclear Scanning Done?

EXERCISE PERFUSION SCAN.   A small dose of the tracer material is injected into a vein in your arm while you exercise on a treadmill or stationary cycle. You may be asked not to eat or drink for several hours before the test to reduce the possibility of nausea, which may accompany vigorous exercise after eating. Your doctor may tell you to stop taking certain medications before the test, because some drugs can impair the test's accuracy. Be sure to follow your doctor's instructions; stop taking medications only if you are specifically told to do so. People with diabetes may be told to maintain their regular eating patterns.

Because you will be exercising vigorously during the test, wear comfortable clothing and shoes appropriate for brisk exercise on a treadmill or cycle. The personnel of the nuclear cardiovascular laboratory may ask you to wear a hospital gown.

Before the test, you will be connected to an ECG machine. An intravenous (IV) line will be inserted into a vein in your arm, and tracer will be injected into your bloodstream at peak exercise.

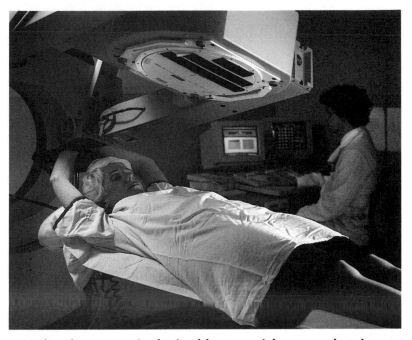

A nuclear heart scan is obtained by a special camera that detects the radiation given off by the tracer material that was injected and carried to your heart. During the scanning, the camera moves at different angles while you remain still. The signals are used by a computer to construct an image of the heart and its overall circulation (see Figures 32B and C, page A10).

Usually you will exercise on a treadmill or a stationary cycle, just as for an exercise ECG. Your heart rate and blood pressure will be monitored, and it is normal for them to increase during exercise. If you have any symptoms such as chest or arm pain, shortness of breath, or light-headedness, inform the person monitoring the test. Adjustments can be made to the exercise test depending on your symptoms, blood pressure, ECG, or degree of fatigue.

It is important to exercise for as long as you can because it increases the accuracy of the test. After you exercise nearly to your limit, the tracer material is injected, and it is carried to your heart by the blood. You then continue to exercise for another 60 to 90 seconds after the injection.

You then will lie under a camera that "takes pictures" of your heart from various angles. The camera detects the radiation being emitted by the radioactive tracer and reconstructs this into a computerized image. It is important to stay as still as possible while the pictures are being taken. It may take up to 25 minutes.

After the scanning is done, you can relax for several hours (typically 4 hours) and leave the nuclear cardiology laboratory. When you return, a second scan is obtained (without repeating the exercise) and compared with the first. (Because the size of a meal consumed before the second set of images may affect the quality of the images, ask the doctor what you are allowed to eat.) In some cases your doctor may want a third set of images taken the next day.

RADIONUCLIDE VENTRICULO-GRAM. This can be obtained while you are at rest to get a rapid and accurate assessment of heart size and function, or it can be done before and during progressively harder exercise. For a MUGA scan (see page 204), the exercise is usually done while you are lying on your back and pedaling a bicycle wheel; for a first-pass study (see page 204), you perform the exercise while upright.

Your doctor may ask you to stop taking any heart medications for a day or two before the test; but do not stop taking them unless you are specifically told to do so. You may be told not to eat a big meal within several hours before the test.

For a MUGA scan, a small amount of your blood is withdrawn into a syringe containing technetium. In the syringe, the technetium attaches to the red blood cells; this coupling ensures that the technetium stays within the bloodstream (instead of entering tissue cells) when it is reinjected. A short time later (about 10 minutes), the blood is reinjected and the first scan is taken while you are at rest. (For first-pass studies, the tracer is simply injected directly into a vein.) Then you perform easy pedaling for 3 minutes, and during the last 2 minutes another scan is taken. Then the exercise is made harder by increasing the resistance on the pedals. Again, you exercise for 3 minutes and another scan is taken while you exercise. There is no break between the stages of exercise; the test continues until you can no longer exercise. During the scanning, your ECG is recorded and your blood pressure is measured at each stage of exercise. Once the procedure is finished, special care or precautions are not necessary.

Are There Risks?

The radiation exposure during radionuclide heart scanning is comparable to that of having a bowel X-ray taken after swallowing barium. The benefits of these tests far outweigh the risks of radiation exposure, and the doses used are safe. However, for women who are pregnant or breastfeeding, radionuclide scanning will not be used unless the information is vital and cannot be obtained by other means.

Adverse reactions to thallium are very rare. About a third of people receiving dipyridamole experience headache, nausea, flushing, or dizziness, and the drug can bring on chest pain and ECG changes. The risk of heart attack with dipyridamole is extremely low. People with asthma should not receive dipyridamole. A drug called aminophylline can be given to counteract the symptoms, but it is usually not necessary because the side effects often are gone by the time the scanning is finished. Adenosine produces similar side effects in most patients, but they are even briefer than with dipyridamole.

The exercise portions of these tests involve the same precautions that apply to the exercise ECG (see page 198). The risk of heart attack or rhythm abnormalities is small. Trained personnel are equipped to deal with emergencies.

ECHOCARDIOGRAPHY

Echocardiography, a procedure developed and refined during the past 20 years, makes it possible to "look" directly at your heart without penetrating your skin. This unique procedure is reducing the need for invasive, potentially risky tests such as cardiac catheterization.

What Is Echocardiography?

Echocardiography is a special application of diagnostic ultrasound (sound that is too high-pitched to be heard). The concept behind the use of ultrasound is the same as that used in depth finders or fish locators on boats. In the case of echocardiography, ultrasound waves are sent out to and reflected (echoed) back from internal structures. The sound waves are sent into your body by a special microphone-like device called a transducer. The transducer also detects the echoes bouncing back from the surfaces of internal structures, such as your myocardium (heart muscle) and heart valves. A machine (the echocardiograph) analyzes the waves to determine how far away the structures are from the transducer.

A computer calculates the time it takes the sound waves to travel to and from your heart and then reconstructs the shape of the heart on the basis of

that information. The image (echocardiogram) of your heart is displayed on a video or television screen, and it can be recorded on videotape or printed on paper.

The echocardiogram can be obtained in various ways and can be displayed in different forms depending on the precise type of information about your heart that is required. One type of display—called an *M-mode echocardiogram*—is very abstract and looks nothing like an actual heart. However, it is very useful for measuring the exact size of various heart structures, such as the thickness of the heart muscle or the size of a heart chamber.

A second type is the *2-dimensional (2-D) echocardiogram*. As its name im-

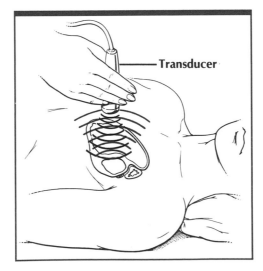

Transducer

Echocardiography is done with ultrasound waves (which are too high-pitched to hear) that reflect (or "echo") off the surfaces of your heart's structure. A computer uses this information to construct an image of the heart or analyze blood flow.

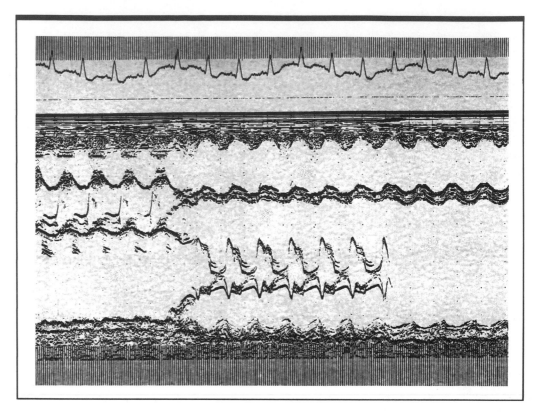

One type of echocardiogram, called the M-mode, is an image that does not really look anything like a heart. However, it is useful for making careful measurements of the dimensions of the heart. This M-mode echocardiogram is of a greatly enlarged heart that is not pumping vigorously. The patient has dilated cardiomyopathy.

plies, it shows an image of your heart in two dimensions, as though your heart were sliced like a loaf of bread so that each slice could be individually examined. By changing the position of the transducer, doctors can see most parts of your heart and get a good impression of how all of its parts function.

A third type of echocardiographic display uses the principle of *Doppler ultrasound*. When sound waves bounce off blood cells moving through the heart and blood vessels, they change pitch in a characteristic way, called a Doppler shift. (Doppler was an Austrian physicist and mathematician who lived in the early 1800s.) This effect is similar to a train whistle that sounds different when the train is mov-

ing toward you (sounds high-pitched), passes you, and then moves away (sounds lower-pitched). The change in pitch of the ultrasound waves bouncing off red blood cells can be measured, and the speed and direction of the flowing blood can be calculated. Using Doppler signals, the echocardiogram can display both the sound and the visual information about blood flow through the heart. You may hear a pulsatile whooshing sound during your echocardiographic examination—that sound is the echocardiograph's "interpretation" of blood flowing past the structures of your heart. Doppler is particularly useful for determining whether heart valves are functioning properly.

A fourth form of echocardiographic display is called *color Doppler*. The echocardiographic computer does complex calculations of blood flow through the heart based on the Doppler shift. Then it displays the blood flow

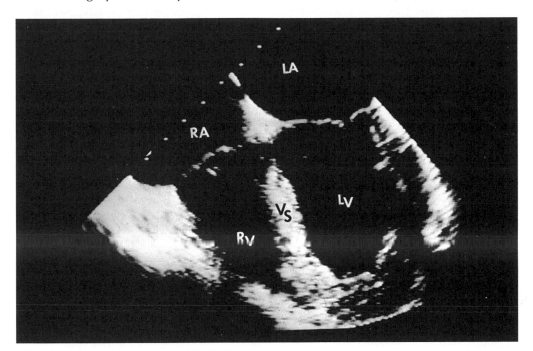

This type of echocardiogram shows the structure of the heart in two dimensions, as though we were looking at a "slice" of the heart. This appears on a TV monitor and is recorded on videotape so that it can be observed in motion. It gives an accurate view of the structure and action of the heart. (RA = right atrium, LA = left atrium, RV = right ventricle, LV = left ventricle, VS = ventricular septum)

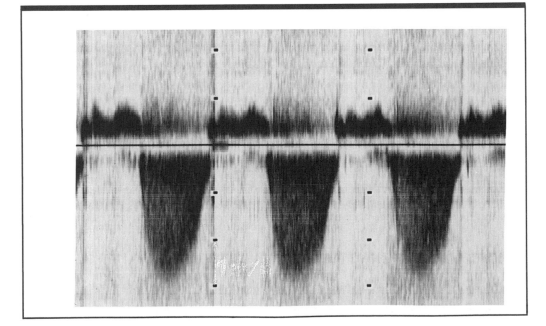

These are Doppler signals. They indicate the velocity of blood flow through a valve—information that is useful in determining whether the valve is functioning normally. Doppler signals can also be processed by the computer to make color images of blood flow in the heart (see Figures 16A and 17A, page A6).

as colors on the 2-D image (see Figures 16 and 17, page A6). Each color represents a direction and speed of blood flow. This technique is able to characterize further the way blood flows through valves, and it is useful for detecting abnormal blood flow—such as through a small hole in the atrial or ventricular septum.

What Does Echocardiography Show?

Using echocardiographic techniques, doctors accurately measure your heart's dimensions, see its overall shape and pumping action, determine the structure and function of the valves, and assess blood flow through the heart. With this information, numerous aspects of your heart's health can be observed: size, pumping strength, location and extent of damaged heart muscle, severity and type of heart valve problems, site and degree of abnormal blood flow patterns in the heart, abnormalities of the heart structures, and blood pressure in the lung (pulmonary) arteries.

SIZE OF HEART. A weakened or damaged heart, defective heart valves, and high blood pressure or other diseases can cause the heart chambers to enlarge (see page 39). The echocardiogram can reveal these abnormalities. Measurements can be made of the pertinent dimensions. Because the test is noninvasive, it can be safely repeated to follow the stability or progression of a problem and assist in determining the need for treatment. After treatment, echocardiography can be used to determine the extent of benefit.

PUMPING STRENGTH. The echocardiogram permits direct observation of the moving heart muscle. An experienced echocardiographer can tell at a glance whether the muscle is pumping at full strength and whether it is slightly, moderately, or severely reduced in function. Measurements can be made to determine ejection fraction, stroke volume, and cardiac output (see How well does a ventricle do its job?, page 204).

DAMAGED HEART MUSCLE. An echocardiogram can also show whether all portions of the ventricular wall contribute equally to the pumping activity of the heart. Parts that move weakly may have been damaged by a heart attack, or they may be receiving too little oxygen (because of coronary blockages). Also, because the echocardiogram can show the myocardium (heart muscle), the doctor can see areas that may be thinner than neighboring areas, and which do not thicken as expected during contraction of the ventricle. These are further signs of damaged myocardium.

VALVE PROBLEMS. Echocardiography is usually the best test for examining your heart valves. This study can show the anatomy of your valves and also how they move during relaxation and contraction of the pumping chambers. Do they open wide to let blood flow through? Do they close fully to prevent back leakage of blood? Are they misshapen by congenital defects, infection, deposits of calcium, or wear and tear? The basic echocardiogram can answer these questions. Does blood actually leak back through a valve? Is the flow of blood impeded by a narrowed valve outlet? The Doppler and color Doppler tests address these questions and also grade the severity of the problem.

The Doppler tests are so sensitive that doctors now realize that even most normal people have a tiny amount of back leakage through some of their valves, even though it causes no problems and cannot be heard with a stethoscope.

ABNORMAL BLOOD FLOW PATTERNS. In addition to showing blood flow problems through valves, Doppler techniques are very useful for revealing other blood flow abnormalities. For example, holes in the walls of the heart separating the two atria or the two ventricles can be detected by a "jet" of blood flow seen on a color Doppler examination. Careful examination by 2-dimensional echocardiography of the region of the "jet" may reveal the actual defect in the heart wall.

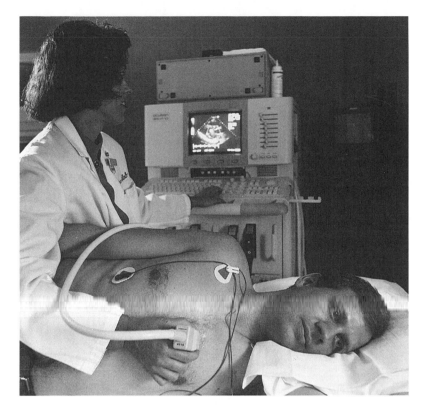

HEART STRUCTURE. Clearly, any test that can show the shape and position of the heart structures and the pattern of blood flow in the heart will be particularly useful for evaluating conditions that produce structural heart problems. Congenital heart defects can be very thoroughly examined by echocardiography—revealing abnormalities in the heart chambers, valves, and connections between the heart and major blood vessels (see pages 48–57).

Other structural abnormalities are also detectable by echocardiography. Overgrowth of the myocardium, as occurs in hypertrophic cardiomyopathy (see page 43), can be directly visualized. Furthermore, Doppler techniques can disclose the effect of the hypertrophy on blood flow. Does the overgrowth of muscle block the flow of blood out of the left ventricle? Doppler can provide the answer.

Echocardiography can also determine whether a blood clot has formed in one of the heart chambers. Such a diagnosis may be important in establishing the cause of a stroke or blockage of an artery in the leg or elsewhere. Similarly, this technique is capable of showing accumulations of infected tissue clustered on heart valves—consistent with a diagnosis of infective endocarditis (see page 58).

The pericardium, particularly if it is diseased, can be seen and evaluated with echocardiography. This technique also can detect either small or large amounts of fluid between the heart and pericardial sac (pericardial effusion; see page 113). This capability not only is important for making the diagnosis but also is helpful for accurately placing a needle or catheter through the chest wall and into the pericardial sac for draining the effusion.

When you have an echocardiogram, the technician or doctor "views" your heart with a transducer held over your chest wall. By moving the transducer, different views of the heart are obtained. An electrocardiogram is monitored at the same time.

PULMONARY BLOOD PRESSURE. For many years, the only reliable way to determine the pressure in the pulmonary arteries was to thread a catheter through a vein and into a pulmonary artery. With the advent of Doppler techniques, accurate noninvasive estimation of pressure became possible by calculating the pressures that would be required to make blood flow at a particular measured velocity.

How Is Echocardiography Done?

Echocardiography usually is done in a cardiologist's office or laboratory, although the procedure can also be done at the hospital bedside with portable machines. Echocardiography also can be performed in the emergency room, critical care unit, or operating room. No special preparations are necessary before arriving for the test. In the laboratory, you remove your clothes from the waist up, and a gown or robe is provided.

You usually are asked to lie on your back or on your left side. Special gel or oil is applied to your chest to improve the transmission of the ultrasound waves. A technician or doctor maneuvers a microphone-shaped transducer over the area of the heart in various positions to give a full picture of the heart. Although the test is noninvasive and usually painless, the transducer occasionally must be held firmly against your chest. This pressure can be uncomfortable, especially over the rib prominences. The transducer is linked by a cord to the monitor screen and other electronic components.

You will be asked to exhale and to hold your breath, because the air in your lungs can interfere with the image produced. The transducer will be moved to several sites on your chest to view your heart from various angles. A thorough echocardiographic examination may take from 15 minutes to more than an hour, depending on the nature of your problem.

If you are having a Doppler echocardiographic test to examine the flow of blood, you may hear a whooshing or pulsating sound. This is not the actual sound of your heart, but an amplified computerized audio reconstruction of the sound waves.

Factors that may limit capabilities of standard echocardiography

- Pulmonary (lung) disease
  Overinflated lungs (emphysema) from smoking
  Other causes of emphysema
- Various body shapes
  Obesity
  Emaciated/tall, thin patients
  Spinal or chest wall abnormality
  Breast implants or large breasts
- Medical situations
  Prior heart or chest surgery
  Chest injury
  Patient on ventilator

Special Echocardiographic Studies

TRANSESOPHAGEAL ECHOCARDIOGRAPHY. The latest development in echocardiography is transesophageal echocardiography. Transesophageal means "through (*trans*) the esophagus" (the tube that goes from your throat to your stomach). Traditional echocardiographic techniques view the heart through the chest wall. However, the body shape of some individuals, and other technical factors, may limit the capabilities of this approach.

Techniques have been developed in which an ultrasound transducer is attached to a tube and inserted down the esophagus, which is close to the heart. This test allows very clear images of many parts of the heart structure and blood flow.

Transesophageal echocardiography requires some preparation. You will be asked to not take anything by mouth except medication for 4 to 6 hours before the procedure to prevent nausea and vomiting. An intravenous (IV) line will be used to deliver a short-acting sedative. To help insert the transducer, the cardiologist or nurse will spray your throat with a numbing agent. If you are at high risk for endocarditis (see page 58), you may be given antibiotics before the procedure.

You swallow the end of the tube that has the transducer on it (which is easier to do than it sounds), and the cardiologist manipulates the instrument to obtain the images that are needed. The examination is extremely well tolerated by more than 90 percent of people.

The IV catheter may also be used to inject a small amount of saline (saltwater) solution into your vein. After the fluid is injected into the bloodstream and circulates to the heart, it highlights the pattern of blood flow in the heart.

You must be partially awake during this procedure, because the doctor may ask you to hold your breath or to strain as if you were having a bowel movement. Straining alters the pressures in your heart chambers, and certain problems may show up during that maneuver which did not show up under normal conditions.

When the test is over, do not eat or

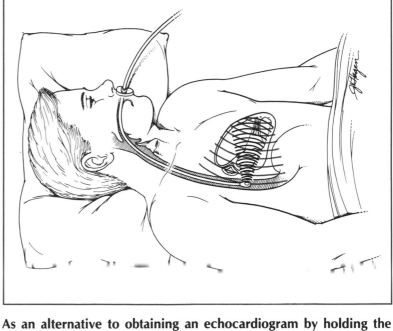

As an alternative to obtaining an echocardiogram by holding the transducer on the surface of your chest, sometimes a clearer echocardiogram image can be obtained by inserting the transducer into the esophagus. This approach positions the transducer closer to the heart. This can be easily accomplished after numbing the back of the throat and administering mild sedation.

drink—especially hot foods or beverages—for about 2 hours, because your throat may be numb for a while. If you are given a sedative, do not drive for 24 hours.

EXERCISE ECHOCARDIOGRAPHY.

Echocardiography is also used in conjunction with exercise to obtain information about the heart under stress. Resting echocardiography is performed, and then you walk on a treadmill (see page 197) to your peak exercise level. At the end of the treadmill exercise, echocardiography is done immediately, while your heart rate is still high. The cardiologist evaluates the overall response of the heart to exercise and whether all parts of the heart muscle contribute equally to the contraction of the heart under stress. If some areas of the heart do not contribute as much, those areas are concluded to be supplied by coronary arteries that are at least partially blocked.

MEDICATION-INDUCED STRESS ECHOCARDIOGRAPHY. If you are unable to exercise on the treadmill for exercise echocardiography, a similar effect can be achieved by giving a medication (dobutamine or dipyridamole). The medication is given through a vein, and it increases the pumping capacity of your heart. The echocardiogram will show whether an area of your heart muscle does not respond to this stimulation. A lack of response indicates areas of the heart that are not getting enough blood flow.

OTHER ECHOCARDIOGRAPHIC TECHNIQUES. Other echocardiographic techniques are used in specific situations. *Contrast echocardiography* is a procedure in which echocardiographic images are obtained as fluid is injected into a vein. This may reveal abnormalities of blood flow within the heart or blood vessels. *Fetal echocardiography* can visualize the heart of an unborn baby and permit diagnosis of congenital heart disease before birth. *Intraoperative echocardiography* is useful for assessing heart function during surgical treatment—for example, during valve repair. *Echo-guided pericardiocentesis* is a procedure in which

excess fluid in the pericardial sac is drained by a needle inserted into the chest; the cardiologist precisely positions the needle by observing its location on an echocardiogram.

Additional techniques are being developed to analyze blood flow within the heart muscle, to equip catheters with ultrasound for accurately determining the structure of blood vessels, and to reconstruct three-dimensional images of the heart from echocardiographic information. These procedures are currently investigational and are not yet available for routine use in most medical institutions.

Are There Risks?

One of the assets of echocardiography is that it gives information about internal structures and blood flow without actually entering the circulatory system. There are virtually no risks to having this procedure. There is no known risk to the body of having ultrasound waves pass through it. Echocardiography involves no X-ray exposure.

During transesophageal echocardiography, there is a very small risk of an abnormal heart rhythm or minor injury to the throat. Exercise echocardiography and echocardiography performed with the use of medications to simulate exercise have a very slight risk of heart attack or rhythm problems, as do other exercise tests (see page 198).

CATHETERIZATION AND ANGIOGRAPHY

Cardiac catheterization can help determine the function of the heart muscle and the four heart valves and the condition of your coronary arteries. Although other tests provide valuable information about your heart, it is the only test that can provide an accurate "road map" of the coronary arteries.

What Are Catheterization and Angiography?

Catheterization refers to any procedure in which a catheter (a long, thin, flexible tube) is inserted into the body. For cardiovascular problems, catheters are inserted into the blood vessels or heart. Sometimes the term "angiography" (*angio* means "blood vessel," *graphy* means "record") is used synonymously with catheterization of the heart and blood vessels. Technically, angiography refers to the injection of contrast material (dye) through a catheter, and this dye can be visualized with X-rays. However, catheters are used to do more than angiography. Some catheters have miniature devices (sensors) at the tips that can measure oxygen in the blood and also pressures and blood flow within blood vessels and the heart. Some catheters are used to take a sample (biopsy) of the heart tissue. Catheters are also used to treat cardiovascular disease (see Angioplasty, page 270, and Valvuloplasty, page 261).

Even though other techniques, such as heart scanning and echocardiography, can provide a wealth of information noninvasively that could be revealed only through catheterization 10 years ago, some problems can still be detected only with catheterization techniques. In some situations, catheterization is used to confirm or add detail to problems identified by less invasive tests.

What Does Catheterization Show?

There are several types of catheterization; each type is used to obtain specific kinds of information. These

When is angiography needed?

It would seem that this invasive test, which allows your doctor to see the blood vessels, would be the final word for diagnosing problems in the coronary arteries or other blood vessels. This is often the case, but not always. Some people wonder why angiography is not recommended as a first-line test in the diagnosis of all heart disease, and others wonder why questions remain even after angiography is done.

Some of the reasons that it is not a first-line test have already been discussed: it is expensive, it requires special equipment and medical personnel, and it has some risks (although the likelihood of occurrence is small). Another important reason is that despite the extensive information it provides, angiography does not always provide the specific information that is needed. For example, abnormalities of the coronary arteries may be found on a coronary angiogram, but these abnormalities may not be the cause of your chest pain.

The coronary angiogram provides a road map. Simply looking at a road map of a city does not necessarily tell you what the traffic patterns are. To find out where the bulk of the traffic is in a city, perhaps a satellite view of the smog collections would be useful. To find out what the "traffic patterns" actually are for the oxygen and blood supply of the heart, the thallium scan may provide more valuable information. In many cases the two tests (or more) give information that is supplementary and adds to the whole picture.

include coronary angiography, left ventriculography, angiography in peripheral blood vessels, cardiac catheterization for congenital defects, pulmonary (lung) angiography, and biopsy.

CORONARY ANGIOGRAPHY. One of the main uses of catheterization techniques is coronary angiography. A liquid contrast agent is injected into the coronary arteries through a catheter. As the contrast agent fills the arteries, they are clearly visible on X-ray motion pictures and videotape (see Figure 25A, page A9).

Of course, it is not really the coronary artery that is being seen but the image of the contrast material in the hollow part (lumen) of the artery. If there are partial or total blockages of the coronary arteries by atherosclerotic plaque or blood clot, they show up as irregularities or places where the image of the contrast material cuts off. Thus, coronary angiography provides the doctor with a road map of the coronary arteries.

LEFT VENTRICULOGRAPHY. Often at the same time that a person undergoes coronary angiography, a contrast agent is also injected into the left ventricle. This procedure, called left ventriculography, shows how the left ventricle is pumping and reveals its shape and internal structures. It also shows whether there is any back leakage (regurgitation) through the mitral valve; if leakage is present, the contrast material can be seen flowing backward into the left atrium.

ANGIOGRAPHY IN PERIPHERAL BLOOD VESSELS. Similar techniques can be used to see blood vessels in other parts of the body. Angiography can be performed on the blood vessels to the brain (although this is not done by cardiologists but by neuroradiologists). Angiography can also be performed on the blood vessels to the legs or arms (arteriography), the aorta and its main branches (aortography), and selected blood vessels to specific organs, such as the kidney (renal arteriography). These procedures are done by vascular radiologists.

CARDIAC CATHETERIZATION FOR CONGENITAL DEFECTS. Other uses of cardiac catheterization include examining congenital malformations of the heart and assessing the degree of shunting of blood through a septal defect or through abnormal connections of the arteries (see page 52). Again, doctors can get much of this information from tests such as echocardiography, but catheterization may be used to confirm that information or to provide more information about areas, such as certain blood vessels, that cannot be seen on the echocardiogram.

The right atrium, right ventricle, and pulmonary artery can be studied by inserting a catheter into veins. The femoral vein in the groin or the internal jugular vein in the neck are the two most common sites of entry. The catheters can measure pressures and the amount of oxygen in the blood in the right side of the heart. Measuring oxygen is a useful way to assess whether blood is being shunted from the left side of the heart (where the blood has a high level of oxygen because it has just returned from the lungs) to the right side of the heart. If the amount of oxygen in the right ventricle is higher than the amount of oxygen in the right atrium, blood must have crossed from the left ventricle to the right ventricle through a hole in the septum separating the right and left ventricles (septal defect) (see bottom figure on page 55). Normally, blood going from the right atrium to the right ventricle has not gone through the lungs to pick up any oxygen.

PULMONARY (LUNG) ANGIOGRAPHY. Contrast material can also be injected through catheters into the pulmonary artery to visualize the arteries in the lungs. Pulmonary angiography is useful for determining whether there are any blood clots in or malformations of the pulmonary arteries. It can also be used to show the condition of the pulmonary arteries in certain congenital heart defects.

BIOPSY.   Catheters can be used to obtain small amounts of heart muscle for microscopic inspection (biopsy). A special catheter with small jaws on its tip which can be opened and closed by the cardiologist is usually inserted into the right ventricle through a vein. The open jaws are gently pushed up against the wall of the heart, and then a specimen is taken of the muscle and removed (see figure on page 220). More than one "bite" is needed to ensure that there is enough tissue to examine microscopically. The person undergoing this procedure does not feel the jaws of the catheter or the "bite."

Heart biopsy is useful for determining the presence of inflammation, abnormal protein deposits, or iron deposits that might explain cardiomy-

opathy (see page 38). It is also used to check for rejection of transplanted hearts (see page 257).

How Is Catheterization Done?

CATHETERIZATION IN THE CARDIAC CATHETERIZATION LABORATORY

Preparation.   The night before your catheterization, you will be asked to take a bath or shower and to scrub the inside of your right arm at the elbow joint or both sides of your groin. Do not eat or drink anything after midnight. Continue to take your medicines (with only a small sip of water) unless told otherwise by your doctor.

If the catheterization is not being done as an urgent procedure and you are otherwise healthy, you may be able to come to the hospital on the morning of your scheduled catheterization without spending the prior night in the hospital. Technicians and nurses may draw blood and obtain an

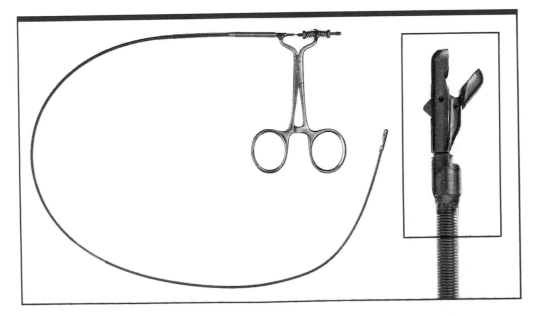

The biopsy catheter (or bioptome) is a thin tube with controls on one end and a small tip with "jaws" that can be opened and closed with the controls. The inset shows the "jaws" greatly magnified.

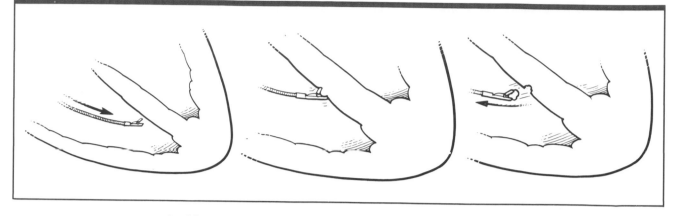

The biopsy catheter is inserted through a vein into the right ventricle. The jaws are opened, pushed against the inside of the heart wall and closed tightly, and then pulled back with a tiny "bite" of heart tissue that can be examined under the microscope.

ECG if it has not been done recently. They will discuss the procedure with you in detail.

Although the catheterization itself takes only about 30 minutes, preparations are extensive. Before the cathe-

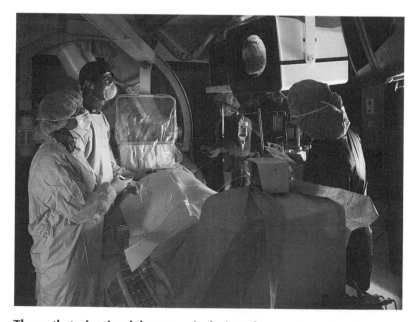

The catheterization laboratory is designed to perform invasive procedures efficiently, accurately, and safely. The catheterization team usually consists of one or two cardiologists, an anesthetist, an assisting nurse, and a camera operator. The procedure is done under sterile conditions.

terization, a technician will shave the hair off the small area where the catheter will be inserted through the skin. An intravenous (IV) line will be inserted into an arm vein. You will also be given a sedative to help you relax, but you will be awake. Your family should not expect you to return to your hospital room for 2 to 3 hours.

The Procedure. Catheterization is done in a specialized fluoroscopy (X-ray equipped) suite that is similar to an operating room. The room has a fluoroscopy camera, monitors, and much equipment, but not all of it will necessarily be used during your procedure. The staff will place sterile drapes around you so that the catheters and other instruments do not touch anything that is not sterile. Personnel in the catheterization suite include the cardiologist and assistant, one or more technicians, and an anesthetist.

The staff will be wearing lead aprons to protect them from repeated exposure to X-rays. However, the X-ray exposure to you from this single procedure is not harmful.

The X-ray table may be turned mechanically from side to side (so you may be secured to the table with straps around your waist, shoulders, and knees), or the camera may rotate about you. You will have ECG electrodes on your chest to monitor your heart and a blood pressure cuff on your arm to monitor your blood pressure throughout the study.

Adults undergoing catheterization usually are not given general anesthesia. You are awake during the catheterization because the cardiologist needs your cooperation for a good study. The cardiologist and members of the catheterization team will explain to you what is being done and any sensations you may expect to feel throughout the study.

To begin the catheterization, the cardiologist uses a local anesthetic to numb the site where the catheter will be inserted. You should have no pain or discomfort during the procedure. When the area is numb, the cardiologist inserts a needle into the blood vessel and then threads a very thin guide wire through the needle. After withdrawing the needle, the cardiologist usually pushes a short tube called a sheath over the guide wire and places it into the blood vessel. The sheath has a small one-way valve in it so that catheters can be inserted through it but no blood will leak out when there is no catheter in the sheath. Once the sheath is in the blood vessel, the cardiologist can insert and remove many different catheters without using a needle and with no discomfort to you. You may feel pressure or the movement of the catheters at the site of insertion, but there should be no pain. If pain develops, tell the doctor.

Sometimes rather than using the needle technique, the cardiologist may make a small incision to expose the blood vessel. This is done if the arm is used for access to the circulation. The catheter or sheath is inserted directly through a small nick that is made in the blood vessel. This is referred to as a "cutdown." If you have this procedure, it may take a little longer. You will have several stitches in your arm, and these will be removed in a few days.

A television screen shows an X-ray image of the catheter threading through the blood vessel; this helps the cardiologist position the catheter correctly. Once the catheter is in position, the cardiologist uses it to perform whatever tests are necessary, such as measuring pressures or oxygen or injecting contrast material. The cardiologist watches the screen to see where the contrast material goes. If contrast is injected into the left ventricle, you may feel a hot, flushing sensation all over your body for 15 to 30 seconds. This is normal, and this part of the procedure is usually done only once. You will be asked to hold your breath, which helps to get a clearer image. The cardiologist will tell you when it is okay to breathe normally. You may have to hold your arms above your head or to the side in a rather awkward position, again to help get a clearer picture of your heart.

The X-ray machine is very big and can be moved mechanically to many different positions to get different views. A series of X-ray pictures will be taken. The pictures are taken by the X-ray machine, not the catheter.

The cardiologist may insert several catheters into various areas of the heart to evaluate different aspects of your heart and coronary arteries. Different catheters may be used for various diagnostic tests, including drawing blood

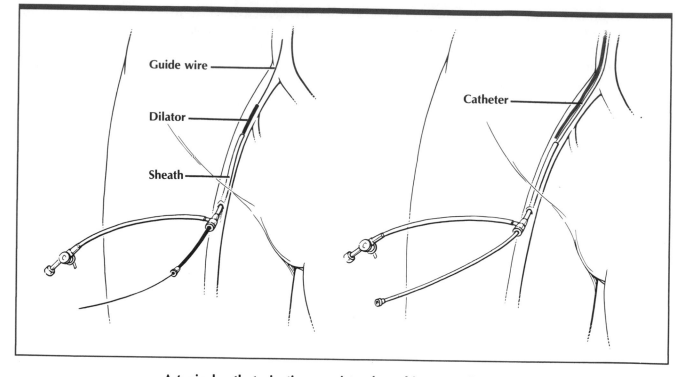

A typical catheterization consists of numbing a small area of your groin and inserting a needle into the artery. A very thin wire (guide wire) is inserted through the needle and the needle is pulled back and removed. The wire stays in place to keep the pathway into the artery.

Left, Then two short, narrow tubes, one (the dilator) inside the other (the sheath), are gently pushed over the wire into the artery. The dilator and guide wire are pulled out so that only the sheath remains in the artery. It has a one-way valve so that no blood flows out. The sheath maintains an open route into the artery.

Right, Now a catheter can be inserted into the sheath, through the artery, and up to the heart and coronary arteries. If necessary, the catheter can be removed and another inserted without any need for repeating the puncture with a needle.

samples, injecting dye, and taking pressure readings in the heart chambers and the arteries. Catheters with specific shapes and bends and sensors, and specially shaped or bendable guide wires that fit inside the catheter, are used to manipulate the tip of the catheter to the correct position.

You may feel your heart "skip" beats during the procedure, but this sensation is normal. You may also briefly feel flushed and warm all over, or you may become nauseated for a short time. These effects are common and should not worry you. Your heart rate and blood pressure are continuously being monitored by the doctor and technicians. Occasionally, the heart slows down briefly or temporarily pauses after an injection of contrast material into a coronary artery. If that occurs, you will immediately be asked by the doctor to cough vigorously. This helps the blood circulate during the temporary slowdown. You should report any chest pain to the doctor.

At the end of the procedure, the cardiologist removes the sheath and puts pressure over the site where it entered the blood vessel so that the puncture site can seal off naturally. You will be moved into a recovery room, where pressure is usually applied for about 15 minutes, and then a bandage and small sandbag are placed over the site to maintain pressure. You may spend more time in the recovery room to make sure there is no bleeding from the entry site or other complications. Do not move your affected arm or leg, raise your head, or strain the area for about 6 hours. You may be told to drink a lot of fluid to help flush the contrast material from your system. Most people can begin walking 6 to 8 hours after their catheterization.

CATHETERIZATION IN THE CARDIAC CARE UNIT. Some types of catheterization are not necessarily done in a catheterization suite or laboratory. Patients in the cardiac care unit (CCU) often receive a special type of catheter designed to measure pressures in the pulmonary arteries, which reflect the pressures in the left side of the heart and are very important for assessing your heart function. This catheter also is used to measure blood flow through the heart and therefore gives an index of how much blood the heart is capable of pumping. This information is very important for people who have had a heart attack or who are in heart failure (see page 36).

After a local anesthetic is injected, the catheter usually is inserted through an internal jugular vein in the neck or through the subclavian vein that runs under the collarbone. It is called a hemodynamic monitoring catheter, balloon flotation catheter, or Swan-Ganz

catheter (after the doctors who invented it). If necessary, it can be left in place for days at a time to monitor the function of the heart continuously.

Are There Risks?

A small bruise around the puncture site is not uncommon after a catheterization procedure. Elderly people with high blood pressure are especially susceptible to bruising. The bruise usually disappears in a few days or weeks. Infection at the site of a puncture is always a concern, but it is extremely rare because of careful sterile techniques.

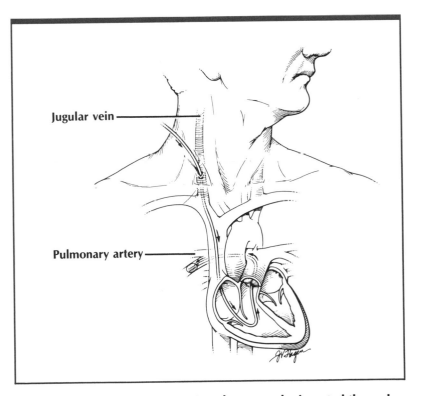

A balloon-flotation (Swan-Ganz) catheter can be inserted through a vein, such as the jugular vein. A small inflatable balloon on the tip "pulls" the catheter along as it floats in the bloodstream through the vein, heart, and pulmonary artery. This catheter is used for measuring pressures in the heart and pulmonary artery and for assessing blood flow (cardiac output). It can remain in place for days at a time.

Other uncommon problems at the site of the puncture include the formation of a bulge in the artery, blockage of the artery, irritation of nearby nerve fibers (which may cause localized numbness or tingling that is usually temporary), or bleeding in the first few hours after the procedure.

A rare problem is an allergic reaction to the contrast material, which may develop abruptly. This can be treated with drugs that counteract the symptoms.

Some complications may require urgent surgical correction. If these complications occur in a coronary artery, a heart attack is possible. Also, coronary angiography can result in irregular heart rhythms and cardiac arrest, which may require resuscitation. A blood clot or tear of the inner lining (dissection) extending from the aorta into a carotid artery may result in stroke. The risk of a severe complication, such as a heart attack or stroke, is very small—the likelihood of occurrence is between 1 in 100 and 1 in 1,000. If these complications occur, it is usually in a patient who is critically ill and in whom the catheterization was done under unstable emergency conditions. The catheterization personnel are highly trained to avoid and manage emergencies.

For some catheterization procedures, such as coronary or left ventricular angiography, the catheter is inserted into and threaded through arteries. In other procedures, such as measurement of right heart or pulmonary pressures or right ventricular biopsy, the catheter is placed into veins.

The risks for catheterization of the arterial circulation tend to be somewhat higher than those for the venous circulation because of the higher blood pressure in the arteries than in the veins. Higher blood pressure can make bleeding and bruising more likely. Also, there is the risk of a blood clot forming in the artery and blocking downstream flow. There is also a risk of perforating (poking through) the artery or causing dissection. Either the right or the left side of the heart may be perforated if a catheter is poked through the heart muscle. If this happens, blood can leak into the pericardial sac that surrounds the heart, which may require emergency drainage. Such events are rare.

Catheterization provides detailed information about your heart and blood vessels that cannot be obtained with other tests. Usually the benefits are worth the small but definite risk. However, complications have the potential to lead to a fatal outcome in very rare cases. It is important to recognize and consider the risks when deciding whether a procedure such as catheterization is warranted for a particular person.

ELECTROPHYSIOLOGY STUDIES

In certain situations, ECG and other related tests used to check the electrical function of the heart are inconclusive. They do not provide all of the necessary answers in some cases, or they may not be appropriate for certain problems. If someone collapses and requires resuscitation, doctors would not rely on a Holter monitor or a telephone transmitter (see page 199) to gather information about problems with the heart's rhythm. In these cases, electrophysiology studies are done in a controlled hospital setting to find out exactly where the problem is and what can be done to fix or control it.

People who undergo electrophysiology studies may have experienced dizziness, fainting spells or syncope (see page 29), palpitations (pounding or rapid heartbeat), or sudden cardiac death from which they were resuscitated.

What Do Electrophysiology Studies Show?

Electrophysiology studies are a type of catheterization in which electrode catheters (rather than hollow catheter tubes) are inserted through blood vessels (usually veins) and into the heart chambers, most commonly the right atrium and ventricle (see Figure 45, page A13). These catheters can sense electrical impulses in various regions of the heart and measure how the heart conducts the impulse from one area to another. By determining where and when impulses occur, your doctor can construct a "map" of the electrical wiring system of your heart.

The electrodes can also pace the heart with a small electrical current, just like a pacemaker electrode (see page 280). Pacing the heart can help in the mapping procedure and can also be used to try to induce or provoke certain abnormal heart rhythms so that they can be observed. "Spontaneous" abnormal heart rhythms that are causing symptoms usually can be reproduced in the electrophysiology laboratory. The doctor can then detect what may be causing the problem and test various medications during the study to see whether they prevent the problem.

A wide variety of heart rhythm medications are available (see page 279), but not every medication works equally well for a particular heart rhythm abnormality in a given person. The technique of inducing arrhythmias during electrophysiology testing allows medications to be evaluated during the rhythm abnormality, and their effectiveness can then be determined. If the abnormality is no longer inducible after you are given a medication, that medication has a good chance of preventing the "spontaneously" occurring rhythm abnormality in the future. Testing different medications in the electrophysiology laboratory enables the doctor to learn in a relatively short time which medications work best.

The response to pacemakers, which are used to prevent symptoms of some rhythm problems, also can be tested during electrophysiology studies.

Electrophysiology studies, like all tests, do not always give a perfectly accurate answer. To make an appropriate diagnosis and prescribe treatment, the doctor must consider the information from the electrophysiology study in combination with all the other available information.

How Is the Electrophysiology Study Done?

The procedure for an electrophysiology study is in some ways similar to that for catheterization. The procedure is done in a special catheterization suite or electrophysiology laboratory that has equipment for recording the heart's electrical signals and for electrically stimulating the heart. There is also fluoroscopic (X-ray) equipment for viewing the position of the catheter electrodes in the heart. Like catheterizations, electrophysiology studies are done under sterile conditions. Personnel in the room usually include the electrophysiology cardiologist, an assistant, a nurse, a technician, and an anesthetist.

The preparations for an electrophysiology study also are similar to those for a catheterization. You will have blood tests, X-rays, and ECG before the test. You may be told to stop taking some of your usual heart medications for 2 or 3 days before the test, but do not stop taking them unless told to do so by your doctor. You should not eat or drink for about 6 hours before the test.

A small intravenous (IV) catheter will be inserted into a vein in your arm. This will be used to give you any medications that may be needed during the test. General anesthesia is not routinely used for the procedure, but you may be mildly sedated.

A technician will scrub and shave the area (usually the groin) where the electrode wires will be inserted. After the area is injected with a local anesthetic, the catheters are usually inserted through the femoral vein in the groin using the techniques described for catheterization (see page 219). It is not uncommon in electrophysiology studies, however, to insert three or four catheter electrodes simultaneously for the purposes of "mapping." Several of these may be inserted through the same vein, such as the femoral vein, which has plenty of room to accommodate several at once. (A catheter is about the diameter of a strand of spaghetti, whereas your blood vessel is about the size of your little finger.) An-

other catheter may be inserted through the right jugular vein in the neck.

During the electrophysiology test, the doctor may stimulate your heart with tiny electrical impulses. You cannot feel these tiny impulses, but they may trigger the arrhythmia that has been causing your symptoms. In fact, you may feel the same symptoms that you had before (even passing out). You are in an extremely controlled environment with highly trained doctors and nurses available to relieve your symptoms promptly. In fact, this is the safest place for you to experience your symptoms, because the electrophysiology laboratory is equipped to handle them.

Because the electrode wires that sense your heart's electrical activity are in place, the doctor can see where the arrhythmia is occurring. This information is helpful for determining the appropriate treatment for your condition. The doctor can test medications or other pacing procedures during the study to determine what treatment best controls your particular arrhythmia.

Because the doctor is not only diagnosing the arrhythmia but also testing various treatments, electrophysiology studies can be quite lengthy. Depending on the problem and the findings during the study, a procedure may last less than an hour to more than 4 hours, during which you must lie flat on the procedure table.

The table itself may be tilted to bring you toward an upright position. This maneuver helps test your heart's response to changes in position by detecting any rhythm or blood pressure changes. You will be secured to the table with straps around your chest.

When the study is completed, the electrode wires will be removed, and pressure will be applied to the insertion sites, as with other catheterization procedures. Because the puncture sites are small, sutures are not necessary. Recovery time is usually short.

Are There Risks?

As with any catheterization procedure, there are some risks to electrophysiology studies. In general, the risk of a complication is less than 1 in 100. There may be bleeding, bruising, blockage (blood clot), or infection at the site where the wires were inserted. There is also a small risk of perforation of the heart, tearing or separation of the lining of a blood vessel, or stroke. All of these are rare.

In addition to the risks that any catheterization procedure poses, electrophysiology tests have risks that stem directly from the nature of the test. As mentioned, one of the goals of some electrophysiology procedures is to induce abnormal heart rhythms. In susceptible individuals, the procedure may result in severely abnormal heart rhythms, including ventricular fibrillation (see page 96), in which the ventricles twitch in an uncoordinated manner and are not able to pump enough blood to the body. If this occurs, prompt defibrillation is required. As drastic as this sounds, the possibility of fibrillation is precisely why the electrophysiology laboratory is equipped with all of the devices and trained personnel necessary for successful resuscitation. A defibrillator (a machine that is used to stop an abnormally fast heart rhythm with an electrical shock through paddles or adhesive patches that are attached to the chest) is always available during the test.

If ventricular fibrillation occurs, you become unconscious and do not feel the shock delivered by the defibrillator. If you experience markedly abnormal heart rhythms that do not result in unconsciousness but require treatment with cardioversion by a shock to the chest, you will be put to sleep briefly with a short-acting general anesthetic before the shock is done.

NONINVASIVE TESTS OF THE ARTERIES AND VEINS

Tests to determine the condition of the blood vessels and circulation do not necessarily require entering the arteries or veins with a catheter. Various noninvasive vascular tests assess blood flow to different regions of the body and also provide information about the condition of the blood vessels, such as whether there is a blockage or other problems. These noninvasive tests have the advantages of being virtually free of risk and are conveniently performed in either a clinic or a hospital.

In general, these tests do not provide the same degree of anatomic accuracy as angiography of the blood vessels. However, in some cases they provide more accurate detail about blood flow than angiography. Sometimes, the information that a noninvasive laboratory test provides is sufficient to make a specific diagnosis and determine treatment. Other times, it will show that further testing is required. Frequently, these tests are used for following the progression of vascular disease or checking on the effects of treatment.

Tests of Arteries

Many arterial diseases are caused by partial or complete blockage of an artery. A blockage in an artery has two basic effects on the circulation of blood through that vessel. Obviously, it decreases the flow of blood downstream from the blockage. It also decreases the blood pressure below the blockage. The same effect happens when a garden hose becomes kinked (or blocked). The jet of water slows to a trickle because the pressure downstream from the kink is too low to push the water out rapidly. Of course, the pressure upstream from the kink remains high. If you had another hose attached to a "Y connector" on your spigot, most of the water would flow through the unkinked hose.

Many noninvasive vascular tests of arteries are designed to measure and compare blood pressure and blood flow within various vessels. Comparing blood pressure above and below a blockage can help pinpoint the site and severity of blockages.

ARTERIAL BLOOD PRESSURE MEASUREMENT. A blood pressure measurement in your arm, part of the routine physical examination (see page 183), gives information about your *overall* blood pressure. For people suspected of having blockages in leg arteries, a blood pressure measurement in the legs is made and compared with that in the arm.

This test consists of putting blood pressure cuffs at various points along the length of your leg. Each cuff in turn is inflated to a point at which the blood flow downstream from the cuff is cut off. The cuff is then deflated slowly as a vascular technician determines the pressure at which blood flow resumes. Instead of using a stethoscope to hear the blood flow, as the doctor or nurse does when taking your blood pressure, the technician uses a small microphone-like device (Doppler ultrasound transducer) to "hear" blood flow. If the blood pressure is low when measured at your ankle but normal when measured at your thigh ("normal" is based on what the blood pressure is in your arm at the same time), the doctor concludes that there is a blockage between those two sites, perhaps near your knee. If the blood pressure is low at both the ankle and thigh, then the blockage lies still further upstream, perhaps near the region of the

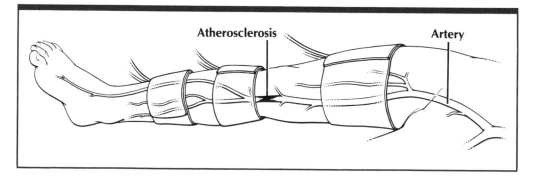

One way of determining whether there is a blockage in a leg artery is to determine the blood pressure at various sites in the leg. In this person, the blood pressure at the cuff closest to the waist would be about the same as the pressure in the arm. The blood pressure at the cuff near the foot would be lower than the arm blood pressure because of the partial blockage of the artery near the knee.

pulse in your groin or higher. If the blood pressure is reduced in both legs, the possibility of a blockage in the aorta (the main artery that branches to the leg arteries) must be considered.

Many other procedures performed in the noninvasive vascular laboratory to analyze blockages in the arteries are based on the same "theme," but with modifications to suit the specific problem being investigated. The same technique can be applied to determine whether and where a blockage is present in your arm, hand, or finger arteries.

Certain blockages in the arms may come and go, depending on the position of the arm. For example, some people are born with an extra rib that may actually crimp the artery under the collarbone. The effect of the compressed artery may be noticeable only when the arm is in certain positions. Doctors call this condition thoracic outlet syndrome. The technician or doctor may move your arms to various positions (called *thoracic outlet maneuvers*) while recording the pulse. Sometimes entirely normal arteries, however, show abnormalities during thoracic outlet maneuvers.

Pulse volume recording also uses a variant of the blood pressure-measuring technique. In this procedure, a blood pressure cuff is partially inflated around a limb and the form of the pulse on the cuff is measured. The shape of the pulse gives information about any blockage present upstream from the cuff. If the pulse is flattened, rather than showing the large difference between systole and diastole, then a blockage is present.

The use of noninvasive methods to check for blockages in the carotid arteries to the brain has required some

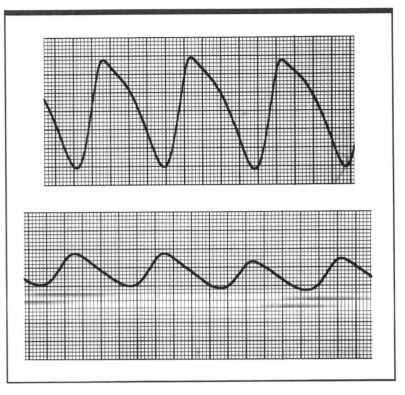

ingenuity. One cannot simply put a blood pressure cuff around the neck or head! However, blood pressure can be assessed in the eyeballs. Because branches of the carotid arteries supply the eyes, an indirect measurement of blood pressure in the carotid arteries can be obtained by measuring eye pressure. By painlessly touching small pressure-measuring devices (similar to contact lenses) to the front of the eye, doctors can determine whether the pressure is lower than normal or differs between the eyes. If the pressure in one eye is low, there may be a blockage in the carotid artery. This test is called *oculoplethysmography (OPG)*.

Another variation of making measurements with blood pressure cuffs is called *strain-gauge plethysmography*. For this, a blood pressure cuff is pumped up around your leg until it

The pulse volume recording in a limb with normal arteries shows normal full pulsations (*top*), but the recording of a limb with a blocked artery (*bottom*) shows flattened pulsations.

blocks blood flowing in the vein coming back from your leg below the cuff but does not impede blood flowing *to* your leg through the arteries. This is possible because the pressure pushing blood through the arteries is much higher than that in the veins, so it is easier to block blood flow through the veins. A special band (called a strain-gauge plethysmograph) placed around your leg below the pressure cuff detects tiny changes in the size (circumference) of your leg. With blood flowing into the leg, but not flowing out because the vein is being pressed shut by the cuff, the leg gradually "fills up" and the circumference increases. The rate at which it "fills up" tells the doctor how efficiently (or inefficiently) blood is flowing through the leg artery. The test is painless and free of risk; it takes about 10 minutes to perform.

It is often important to know the consequences of having a blocked artery. For example, the likelihood that an injury, skin ulcer, or surgical incision will heal is related to how much blood flow is reaching that region. Predicting whether healing can occur is often crucial for deciding on the best management. The staff of a noninvasive vascular laboratory can accomplish this by using *transcutaneous oximetry*. This is a procedure that measures the amount of oxygen in a region of skin with a special patch taped to the skin. If blood flow into the capillaries of the skin is reduced (because of an upstream blockage), then the amount of oxygen will be low. If the amount of oxygen is too low, then skin ulcers, injuries, or surgical incisions in that area may be slow or impossible to heal.

If you are suspected of having Raynaud's phenomenon (see page 105) and have no evidence of blocked arter-

ies in the fingers or arms, finger temperature may be measured before and after your hand is dipped into ice-cold water for 30 seconds. If the finger arteries develop spasm, it will take longer than normal for the finger to warm up again (because of slowed circulation to the finger).

Tests of Veins

Most noninvasive tests of veins are designed to examine whether there is blockage (usually due to a blood clot in the vein) or problems with the valves of the veins (see page 109). The pressure in the veins is very low compared with that in the arteries, so techniques to measure pressure are not as useful. Vein tests usually focus on the flow of blood through them.

VENOUS DOPPLER STUDY. This study takes advantage of ultrasound (sound that is too high-pitched to hear). As in the echocardiography laboratory (see page 209), ultrasound waves are directed through the skin and then are detected by a special "microphone" (transducer) after they "echo," or bounce back off the tissues of the body. When sound waves bounce off moving tissue (such as blood cells in the bloodstream), they change pitch in a characteristic way, called the Doppler shift. It is similar to a train whistle, which sounds different when the train is moving away from you (lower-pitched sound) than when it is coming toward you. This Doppler effect can be measured, and the speed of the bloodstream can be calculated. The machine that measures the Doppler effect of the bloodstream produces a whooshing sound that gives the technician or doctor information about the blood flow.

When used to study the vein circulation, Doppler techniques can indicate whether a vein is obstructed (suggesting the presence of a blood clot) and whether the pattern of blood flow is normal. If it is abnormal, it may reflect damaged valves in the veins which are causing venous incompetence (see page 109). To do a venous Doppler examination, the technician places a hand-held Doppler transducer at various places on your leg, applying pressure above and below the instrument and listening to the whooshing sounds. The test is painless and takes about 15 minutes.

IMPEDANCE PLETHYSMOGRAPHY.   This is a procedure very much like the strain-gauge plethysmography used to study the blood flow of arteries. For vein studies, however, the rate that the circumference of the leg *decreases* after the cuff is deflated is measured. This gives an idea about how efficiently the veins are able to let blood flow out of the limb. If they are inefficient, there may be an obstruction.

Variations of this test performed during exercise (deep knee bends) also provide information about the function of the venous valves and about obstruction of the veins.

Tests of Both Arteries and Veins

Some noninvasive tests are equally useful in the arteries or veins. *Duplex scanning* is used to detect blockages in the arteries or veins or to evaluate a wide variety of other circulatory problems such as arteriovenous fistula (abnormal direct connection between an artery and vein; see page 111), aneurysm (a bulge in a blood vessel), and venous obstruction or compression. For this test, the technician uses a combination of ultrasound imaging on a TV screen (like an echocardiogram, but of the blood vessel instead of the heart) and a Doppler microphone device to measure the speed of the blood flow. With this combination, specific blood vessels can be studied for abnormalities in flow and structure. The test is usually performed on the carotid arteries (see Figure 48A, page A15) or various peripheral vessels, such as the arteries to the legs.

SPECIAL TESTS TO VISUALIZE THE HEART

Although sophisticated diagnostic tests are available to study the structure and function of the heart, some newer procedures may provide even more information. Three recently developed diagnostic procedures are computed tomography (CT), magnetic resonance imaging (MRI), and positron emission tomography (PET).

Computed Tomography

Computed tomography (CT, or "CAT scanning") is an X-ray technique that has been extensively used to examine the brain and other organ structures. Although it is produced by an X-ray beam that passes through your body, it provides more information than an

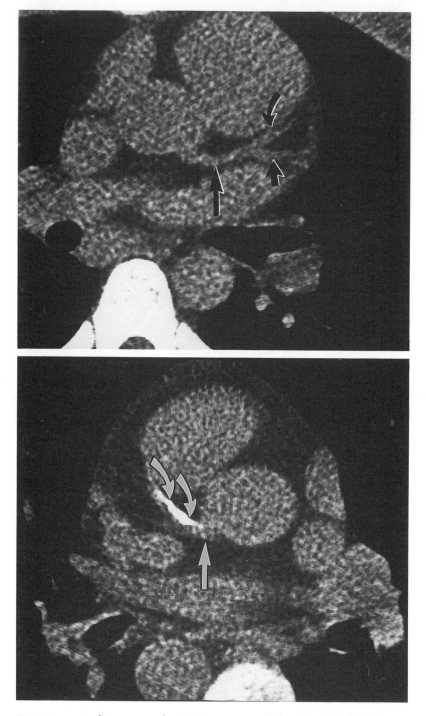

Fast computed tomography (CT) can reveal the fine detail in many structures of the heart. It can show portions of the coronary arteries and distinguish between those that appear normal (*top, black arrows*) and those with calcium deposits (*bottom, white arrows*), which indicate the presence of atherosclerosis and partial blockage of the artery.

ordinary X-ray. Part of the X-ray machine is rapidly rotated around your body so that images are obtained from all angles. A computer assimilates this vast amount of information and constructs a cross-section image of the body which can be viewed by the doctor on a computer screen or on X-ray film.

Because the heart is always in motion, special CT instruments were developed which allowed the heart to be seen clearly, rather than as a blur. These techniques are known as "cine CT" or "fast CT."

WHAT DOES COMPUTED TOMOGRAPHY (CT) SHOW?   The CT image can show body structures that cannot be identified on a normal X-ray. The CT scan shows "slices" of the body, as if it were divided into sections like a loaf of bread. Therefore, the CT scan allows your doctor to view the internal structures of your body, including the heart, pericardium, lungs, and blood vessels, in cross section.

HOW IS COMPUTED TOMOGRAPHY (CT) DONE?   The CT scanner looks like a giant doughnut. The ring of the doughnut contains the scanning equipment; it surrounds the part of your body being scanned. You lie flat on a movable table that slides into the doughnut's "hole." The machine directs X-rays in an arc through segments of your body. The procedure is painless; all you need to do is lie still. Sometimes a contrast material may be injected through a vein to enhance the image.

ARE THERE RISKS?   CT scans involve exposure to a small amount of radiation during the procedure. The benefits far outweigh the very low risk associated with this low level of radiation exposure.

Magnetic Resonance Imaging

Magnetic resonance imaging (MRI) is another technique that may be useful for investigating diseases of the heart. Rather than using X-rays to produce an image, magnetic resonance imaging uses magnetic fields and radio waves. The machine can detect small energy signals emitted by the atoms that compose the tissues of the body and can reconstruct images based on that information. The pictures produced with MRI are similar to those taken with X-rays, but they may show slightly different tissues.

WHAT DOES MAGNETIC RESONANCE IMAGING (MRI) SHOW? The procedure can be used to detect congenital defects and tumors and to evaluate ischemic heart disease and disease of the heart valves and pericardium.

ARE THERE RISKS? This procedure does not use ionizing radiation as do regular X-rays and CT. There are no known risks from MRI. Because the machine operates in a magnetic environment, certain patients cannot be scanned, including those with pacemakers or certain other internal metallic objects. Patients with artificial heart valves can be scanned safely.

Positron Emission Tomography

Positron emission tomography (PET) is an investigational imaging technique

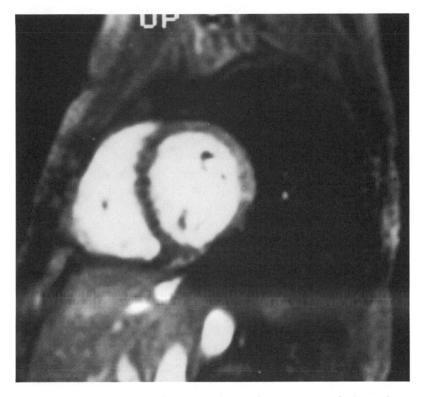

Magnetic resonance imaging (MRI) is another newer technique that can show details of the heart's anatomy.

that detects subatomic particles. Positron emission is detected by two different detectors placed on opposite sides of the body. This procedure requires very expensive equipment and materials. It is currently used primarily for scientific investigations.

WHAT DOES POSITRON EMISSION TOMOGRAPHY (PET) SHOW? This test is used mainly to measure blood flow and the metabolism of the tissues of the body, including heart muscle. This technique has a potential advantage of being able to characterize the way in which heart tissue actually uses energy, and this information may lead to new insights about heart cell metabolism and how oxygen is used to produce the required energy to make the heart contract.

SECOND OPINIONS AND HEART SPECIALISTS

Second Opinions

Despite the sophistication of testing procedures and the valuable information they can provide, it would be a mistake to think that tests provide the final answer in diagnosing heart disease. All tests have inherent differences in accuracy, and no test is 100 percent accurate, even under the best of circumstances. Tests do not make the diagnosis; they provide information that, when added with other information, leads to the diagnosis.

Physicians' most important contribution to evaluating a person is not their ability to arrange for tests or to do them, but to select and interpret diagnostic tests as they apply to a specific person's problem. To do this task, doctors must take into account all of the available data about the person. Doctors must know what each test can and cannot reveal and how the test results relate to the actual disease. The care and skill that are applied in doing a diagnostic test and then interpreting the results correctly in light of all the other information about the person determine how valuable a test is in leading the doctor to a diagnosis and to appropriate treatment.

Keeping all this in mind, it is not surprising that occasionally there is not complete agreement about the best treatment for an individual's problem. It may be advisable to get a second opinion before starting major therapeutic procedures.

There are several situations in which a second opinion might be a good idea: if a diagnosis is very serious; if the treatment advised by your doctor is risky, experimental, or controversial; or if it appears that you will need to have a major surgical procedure. Second opinions are sometimes useful when the diagnosis is clear but the choice of treatments is not so clear. Often, several significantly different treatments are available for a specific disease. You may also want to get a second opinion if your treatment is not providing you as much benefit as you had anticipated, or if you feel that your doctor has not given you enough information about the diagnosis and treatment methods. Insurance companies often require a second opinion before treatment is undertaken.

Ultimately, the most important "second opinion" about any health decision must come from you. Only you know your priorities and what impact the tests and treatments, each with its own risks and benefits, will have on your life. To render a meaningful second opinion, you must be fully informed about what the doctor found in the testing, just as you have fully informed the doctor about your symptoms and problems.

Specialists

Many of the tests that have been discussed are highly specialized. Medicine today offers more extensive care and more innovative treatments than ever before. Knowledge about diseases and treatments is growing so rapidly that specialties and subspecialties have developed in an effort to manage this proliferation of knowledge.

Gone are the days when one person could know everything about all of the possible ailments that can affect you. The medical profession has evolved

How to choose
a cardiologist if you need one

To choose a cardiologist, you have several options:

- The most useful and reliable option is a referral by a trusted family physician, general practitioner, or internist or a referral by a subspecialist who has been treating you for a different problem.

- Another way to find a cardiologist is through a friend who has been satisfied with a particular doctor. Another is to choose a specialist with a good general reputation in your community.

- If you cannot find a cardiologist through your primary care doctor or referral by a friend, you can look to several directories for help. The 370,000 physicians recognized as specialists by the American Board of Medical Specialties (ABMS) are listed in many telephone directories throughout the country, noting their specialty or subspecialty. In addition, you may call the ABMS toll-free at 1-800-776-CERT (1-800-776-2378) to verify a doctor's certification.

- The following references can also provide information about a doctor's professional background. Look for them at your public library, medical society, or libraries at a hospital or university medical school:

  American Medical Directory. This is a directory of physicians in the United States, Puerto Rico, the Virgin Islands, and certain Pacific Islands and U.S. physicians temporarily located in foreign countries. This is published by the American Medical Association. It lists only physicians who belong to the AMA, whether board certified or not. It provides such information as name, address, type of practice, and medical school attended.

  ABMS Compendium of Certified Medical Specialists. This is published by the American Board of Medical Specialties (ABMS). It lists physicians who are certified by the examining boards of recognized specialty organizations. It provides information such as a doctor's medical school and internship training, type of practice and hospital affiliation, and address and telephone number.

  Directory of Medical Specialties. This is published by Marquis Who's Who. It provides, in a short curriculum vitae, information similar to that in the ABMS Compendium.

- Some hospitals have set up informational telephone lines staffed by people who can direct you to a doctor in your area. These lines are usually advertised in newspapers or on radio or television. In addition, university hospitals, medical schools, and medical societies can supply you with a list of affiliated cardiologists.

from the traditional "hometown doctor" to a complex network of medical specialists. It should be obvious after reading this chapter that specialists are needed to perform many of the different diagnostic tests and to interpret the data. It is reassuring to know that your family doctor has numerous sources for specialized assistance with the complex problems of some patients. For some people, however, this expansion has made it harder to know where to turn for help.

If you want a second opinion, let your doctor know that you would like to talk to another doctor or specialist just to confirm the diagnosis or the appropriateness of the procedure. Indeed, your primary care doctor (family practice physician or general internist) is the best source of advice about whom to consult.

PART 5

What Can Be Done to Treat Heart Disease?

Once you find out that you have some form of heart disease, the most pressing question is "What can be done about it?" Tremendous strides have been made in the fields of cardiology and cardiac surgery, so that treatment options are now available which have a great impact on the course of most cardiac illnesses.

Open-heart surgery was first performed only about 35 years ago, signaling the beginning of an era in which effective therapy became available for previously untreatable disorders of the heart. Options for treating heart disease now include a broad array of medications; complex surgical techniques; methods of using catheters to treat coronary artery disease, valvular disorders, and rhythm abnormalities; sophisticated implantable electronic devices to monitor and to treat automatically both fast and slow heart rhythms; and procedures to replace a defective heart. In many situations, more than one form of treatment is available. Appropriate management entails selecting the treatment that provides the best outcome for the particular medical problem while keeping risks, inconvenience, and expense to a minimum.

EMERGENCY TREATMENT

Not all medical treatment requires a doctor. Numerous cardiac problems develop rapidly without warning and are immediately life-threatening if intervention is not undertaken at the instant they occur. Consequently, survival depends on the response of individuals who are in the vicinity of the cardiac victim, *before medical attention is available*. No one can predict when the need for a rapid life-sustaining response may be required. Thus, everyone is well advised to obtain and to maintain the fundamental skills for dealing with emergencies in which the bystander, not the doctor, can make the difference between life and death.

Emergencies Requiring Expert Medical Assistance

Recognition is the first step toward successful treatment of most cardiac emergencies. As a rule, if you think there is a possibility that a situation

Information to give the operator in an emergency call

1. The location of the emergency. Provide as much useful information as possible, including the address, nearby intersections, or other landmarks. This information is vital—even "enhanced 911," which can display to the operator the location of the telephone you are calling from, is ineffective if the telephone is not at the precise site of the emergency.
2. Give the telephone number you are calling from. There may be a need to call back.
3. Summarize the problem briefly by describing what happened.
4. Tell how many victims need help and what their conditions are.
5. State what is being done for the victim. You should not hang up first. Let the operator hang up first so you are sure that the operator has obtained all the necessary information.

Urgency vs. emergency

Symptom	Suspected diagnoses	Possible associated features	Action
Chest pain, pressure, tightness, heaviness	Myocardial infarction (heart attack) Unstable angina	Duration more than 15 minutes Shortness of breath Sweating Pallor Nausea, vomiting Palpitations Faintness	Any unexplained chest pain warrants immediate attention even if none of the other features are present. The presence of associated features increases concern. *Transport to emergency room, preferably by ambulance. Give nitroglycerin if available*
Loss of consciousness (syncope)	Serious arrhythmia Stroke Seizure Extremely low blood pressure Sudden cardiac death	Palpitations Fast or slow pulse Convulsions Sweating Pallor Chest pain Loss of bladder or bowel control	Any unexplained loss of consciousness requires *immediate transportation to an emergency room, preferably by ambulance.* The person should be positioned on the back with the legs and feet elevated. Evaluate for possible need to perform CPR The other features are important to note and discuss with the doctor
Shortness of breath	Myocardial infarction (heart attack) Sudden congestive heart failure Sudden aortic or mitral regurgitation Pulmonary embolism	Chest pain Wheezing Ankle and leg edema Palpitations Fever	Any unexplained new or worsened shortness of breath warrants immediate attention, preferably by *ambulance transportation to emergency room.* If the onset of symptoms has been more gradual, early evaluation is advisable but the level of urgency may be less

(continued on page 240)

Urgency vs. emergency (continued)

Symptom	Suspected diagnoses	Possible associated features	Action
Sustained rapid palpitations, regular or irregular rhythm	Arrhythmia	Light-headedness Passing out Chest pain Shortness of breath	Without associated symptoms, urgent transportation (by car) to doctor's office or acute care facility is warranted If associated symptoms are present, transport to emergency room, preferably by ambulance
Skipped beats or irregular nonrapid rhythm	Arrhythmia	Light-headedness Passing out Chest pain Shortness of breath	Usually does not require emergency evaluation. Make appointment with doctor. However, associated symptoms, if present, may require more urgent evaluation
Edema, leg swelling	Congestive heart failure Deep vein thrombosis (and possible associated pulmonary embolism)	Inflammation Redness Pain, tenderness Hot Shortness of breath Chest pain	Signs of inflammation may indicate thrombosis (clot) in leg vein. Rapid transport to doctor or hospital is recommended. Shortness of breath or chest pain requires emergency evaluation. Edema from heart failure usually is not sudden or an emergency but requires early evaluation and treatment

may require emergency medical help, do not hesitate: *get help immediately*. If it turns out not to be an emergency, there is no harm done. However, if you do not call for an ambulance, contact a doctor, or get to an emergency room during a real emergency, the consequences can be tragic.

All circumstances that warrant immediate attention cannot be exhaustively listed. Judgment and common sense are the final determinants of action. Many emergencies are simple to recognize as such. Others may be less clear. In these, the key to decision making is recognizing the significance of symptoms that were discussed in Part 2, "What Is Heart Disease?" (page 19). Ultimately, "If in doubt, check it out" is a reliable rule of thumb.

Sudden Cardiac Death

In sudden cardiac death (or cardiac arrest), the heart stops beating and breathing ceases abruptly. The victim is unconscious. Sudden cardiac death is distinct from actual death, which is defined as the irreversible loss of brain function. The importance of recognizing and responding to sudden cardiac death is that brain death may be avoided. Sudden cardiac death is potentially reversible.

Many instances of sudden cardiac death occur in people with other forms of heart disease who are recognized to be at high risk. However, up to 50 percent of sudden cardiac deaths occur in individuals with no previously suspected heart disease. In any case, if sudden cardiac death is witnessed and responded to appropriately, the victim may be given a second chance at life.

Sudden cardiac death is *not* the same as a heart attack or stroke. The usual cause of sudden cardiac death is ventricular fibrillation (see page 96). The heart ceases to beat effectively, and consequently the brain is deprived of oxygenated blood. Ventricular fibrillation almost never returns to a normal rhythm on its own, so if the victim does not receive immediate help, the brain will die. Respiration is one of the brain-controlled functions that come to a halt during sudden cardiac death, and this event compounds the problem even further. These fundamental abnormalities dictate what the immediate course of action must be. Unless oxygenated blood flow to the brain is restored in less than 4 to 6 minutes,

potentially reversible cardiac death becomes permanent brain death. The technique for maintaining breathing and circulation is appropriately termed *cardiopulmonary resuscitation (CPR)*.

A person who experiences sudden cardiac death as a result of ventricular fibrillation has the best chance of surviving if a bystander starts CPR within 4 minutes and if advanced life support is begun within 8 minutes of collapse. Of the persons who are resuscitated, about 40 percent will have another episode within 2 years. Special interventions may need to be undertaken to minimize their future risk of death; but to have the opportunity for prevention, they must survive the initial episode. That is where CPR is vital.

Cardiopulmonary Resuscitation (CPR)

If CPR is performed properly and early enough, an estimated 100,000 to 200,000 lives could be saved every year in our country. A bystander who can perform CPR until advanced cardiac life support can be started is the most important lifesaving link in the emergency medical system.

CPR can be performed by "anyone, anywhere, using only our hands, our lungs, and our brains," according to the American Heart Association. It involves a sequence of actions that will get oxygen into a person's lungs and help blood circulate through the body until more advanced medical care can be given.

You cannot learn CPR by reading a book! It is important to practice the skills until they become automatic. Ideally, everyone should take a course in CPR. CPR can be easily learned in a setting where trained instructors demonstrate how it is done and then supervise practice drills on mannequins designed to mimic a victim of sudden cardiac death. The course is offered by many organizations, including the American Heart Association, the American Red Cross, local fire departments, community health services, and local hospitals. Your skills in CPR may never be required. However, if they are, it may be the most important thing you can do for another person, whether it is a loved one or a stranger. If you live with or near a person who has heart disease and a possible predisposition to rhythm disorders, you especially should learn CPR.

Two important goals in maintaining the brain's oxygen supply can be accomplished by CPR: ensuring that sufficient oxygen reaches the blood in the circulation of the lungs, and that the oxygenated blood reaches the brain. The first goal is achieved by mouth-to-mouth breathing, the second by chest compressions.

How can the breath we breathe out keep someone else alive? Fortunately, the air we breathe in contains 21 percent oxygen, which is more than enters the bloodstream. Consequently, three-fourths of the oxygen is breathed *out* again when we exhale. That exhaled oxygen can be breathed into a victim's lungs. It is sufficient to keep the brain alive when the blood is squeezed out of the lungs and heart, through blood vessels to the brain.

Emergency Signs of Sudden Cardiac Death
- Sudden loss of consciousness
- No breathing
- No pulse

What to Do
- Assess situation

- Call out for help. If someone responds, he or she should immediately call the local emergency telephone number (usually 911). If no other bystander is available, make the phone call yourself.
- Begin CPR

OVERVIEW OF CPR TECHNIQUES.
CPR involves a combination of mouth-to-mouth rescue breathing and chest compressions. It keeps some oxygenated blood flowing to the brain and other vital organs until appropriate medical treatment can restore a normal heart rhythm.

The American Heart Association, which sets guidelines for CPR, has an easy-to-remember way of describing the three basic rescue skills. They call it the ABC's of CPR:

- **A**irway
- **B**reathing
- **C**irculation

Airway. For successful resuscitation, the first action is immediate opening of the airway, which may be obstructed by the back of the tongue or by the epiglottis (the flap of cartilage that covers the windpipe). When someone is unconscious, muscle control diminishes and the tongue is likely to drop back against the back of the throat and impede the passage of air to the lungs. When the head is tilted back and the lower jaw (chin) is moved forward, the tongue and the epiglottis are lifted. This technique usually opens the airway.

Breathing. Mouth-to-mouth rescue breathing is the quickest way to get oxygen into a person's lungs. It must be performed until the person can breathe alone or until advanced medical assistance takes over.

If the victim has a heartbeat but is not breathing, you must maintain an open airway and provide breaths (for an adult, once every 5 seconds, or 12 times a minute). If the person's heart has stopped, you must perform chest compressions along with the rescue breathing.

Circulation.   Chest compressions replace the heartbeat when it has stopped. Compressions help maintain some blood flow to the lungs, brain, and coronary arteries. You must also perform mouth-to-mouth breathing anytime you perform chest compressions.

Performing CPR in Adults and Children Older Than 8 Years.   The following description of CPR reflects the procedures recommended by the American Heart Association. It should be considered a refresher for those who have taken a CPR course, because periodic review may be useful.

Assess Situation and Get Help
1. **What to do:** Tap or gently shake the victim's shoulder. Shout "Are you okay?"
   Reason: Avoid resuscitative efforts on someone who may be merely soundly sleeping or intoxicated or who has only fainted.
2. **What to do:** Shout for help. If someone responds, have him or her call 911 (or other emergency number) for help. If you are alone, make the call yourself.
   Reason: CPR alone cannot save a victim of cardiac arrest. More than 80 percent of nonhospitalized

people who have cardiac arrest have ventricular fibrillation, and defibrillation is their chance for survival. So, first, summon advanced cardiac life support, then start CPR. Basic CPR buys some time until medical rescue efforts are started.

Airway
3. **What to do:** Position the victim on his or her back. The victim should be placed on a firm, flat surface—a bed or couch is not firm enough—with the head at the same level as the heart. Kneel to the side of the victim so that you are at a right angle to him or her. This positioning should take no more than 10 seconds.

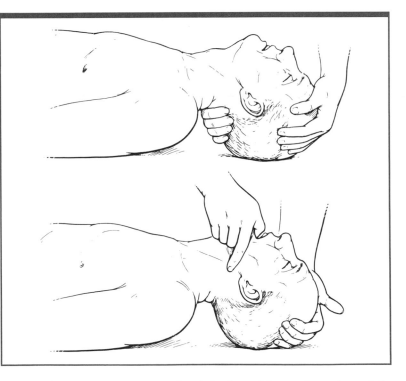

Position the victim so you can check for breathing and a pulse—followed by cardiopulmonary resuscitation (CPR) if necessary—by laying him or her flat on a firm surface, extending the neck, and opening the mouth and airway by lifting the chin forward.

Reason: To produce effective blood flow to the brain, CPR must include compression of the chest between the rescuer's hands and a firm surface. On a soft surface, adequate compressions cannot be given because of bouncing. Oxygenated blood will not reach the brain if the head is higher than the heart.

4. **What to do:** Lift the chin gently with one hand while pushing down on the forehead with the other to tilt the head back. Avoid completely closing the mouth.
Reason: This maneuver opens the airway.

Breathing

5. **What to do:** While maintaining the open airway, determine whether the victim is breathing.
   - Position your ear directly near the victim's mouth.
   - Look at the chest for movement.
   - Listen for the sounds of breathing.
   - Feel for breath on your cheek.

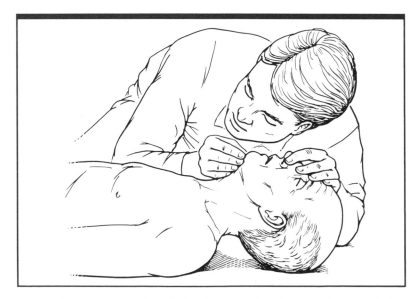

Determine whether the victim is breathing by simultaneously listening for breath sounds, feeling for air motion on your cheek and ear, and looking for chest motion.

Reason: Hearing and feeling are the only true ways of determining the presence of breathing. If there is chest movement but you cannot feel or hear the breath, the airway is still obstructed. Accurate diagnosis is important—rescue breathing should not be performed on someone who is breathing.

6. **What to do:** Pinch the person's nostrils while maintaining pressure on the forehead to keep the head tilted. Open your mouth wide, take a deep breath, and make a tight seal around the person's mouth. Breathe into the person's mouth two times initially. Give one breath every 5 seconds and completely refill your lungs after each breath. Always watch for the person's chest to rise with each breath.

   Each breath into the victim's mouth should take 1½ to 2 seconds. Then allow the lungs to deflate.
   - Feel air going in as you blow.
   - Feel the resistance of the person's lungs.
   - Feel your own lungs emptying.
   - See the rise and fall of the person's chest and abdomen. (If the rescue breaths do not inflate the lungs, start the obstructed airway sequence [see page 246]).
   Reason: This step in CPR provides the lungs with oxygen.

Circulation

7. **What to do:** Place two or three fingers on the Adam's apple (voice box) just below the chin. Slide your fingers into the groove between the Adam's apple and muscle, on the side nearest you. Maintain head tilt with the other

hand. Feel for the carotid pulse in the neck for 8 to 10 seconds.

Reason: This maneuver establishes that there is *no* pulse. A pulse is a sign of an effective heartbeat; if one is present, do not do CPR.

8. **What to do:** Prepare to begin chest compressions by positioning your hands and body appropriately. First, locate the bottom of the sternum (breastbone) at the point where the lower ribs on each side converge. Second, place the heel of your hand approximately 2 inches up from the bottom of the sternum. Third, place the other hand on top of the first. Your shoulders should be directly over your hands, and your elbows should be straight and locked.

Reason: Precise hand placement and proper distribution of weight are essential to produce effective compressions without injury to the victim. Proper positioning also reduces your own fatigue.

9. **What to do:** Compress the chest smoothly and evenly, using the heel of your hand and keeping your fingers off the person's ribs. You must apply enough force to depress the sternum 1½ to 2 inches at a rate of 80 to 100 compressions per minute. Use your weight to compress the chest vertically downward 1½ to 2 inches.

Between compressions, release the pressure and allow the chest to return to its normal position. To ensure that your hands remain in the proper location, do not lift them off the chest.

Count aloud to establish proper rhythm: "one-and-two-and-three-and-four-and" . . . up to 15.

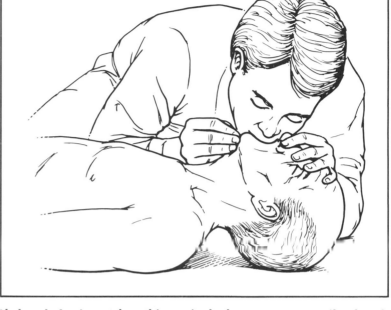

If the victim is not breathing, pinch the person's nostrils closed, make a seal around the mouth, and breathe into his or her mouth twice.

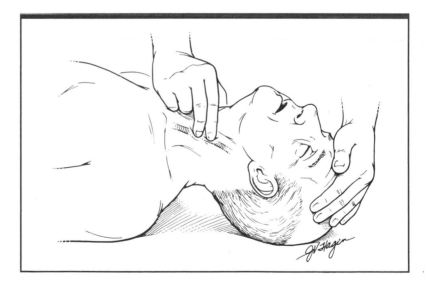

Feel for the carotid artery to see whether the victim has a pulse.

Reason: This technique promotes the most effective blood flow. Half of the compression/relaxation phase is downward to squeeze the blood out of the

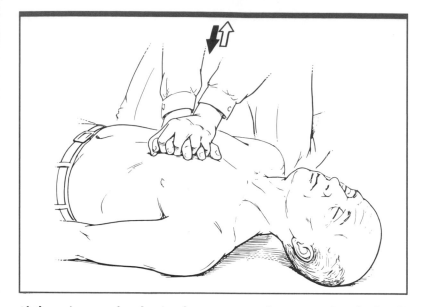

If there is no pulse, begin chest compressions. Your hands should be located over the lower part of the breastbone, your elbows kept straight, and your shoulders positioned directly above your hands to make best use of your weight. Push down about 1½ to 2 inches at a rate of 80 to 100 times a minute. The "pushing down" and "letting up" phase of each cycle should be equal in duration. Don't "jab" down and relax. After 15 compressions, breathe into the victim's mouth twice. After every 4 cycles of 15 compressions and 2 breaths, recheck for a pulse and breathing. Continue the rescue maneuvers as long as there is no pulse or breathing.

If the victim's chest does not rise when you breathe into his or her mouth, the airway is probably blocked. Try to dislodge the obstruction, such as a piece of food, by performing a Heimlich maneuver. Because the victim will be lying down, place your hands slightly above the navel and press upward, firmly and rapidly.

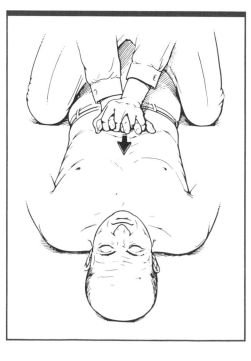

heart, and the other half is upward to allow the heart to fill. It is tempting to "jab" downward and to relax slowly; that is *incorrect* technique. With each compression you want to squeeze the heart or increase the pressure within the chest so that blood is pushed to the vital organs.

10. **What to do:** Continue to ventilate properly: after every 15 compressions, deliver two rescue breaths.
 Reason: Adequate oxygenation must be maintained. Remember, you are maintaining the circulation in order to deliver oxygen to the body.

11. **What to do:** At the end of four cycles, each consisting of 15 compressions and two rescue breaths (which should take a little more than a minute), check for return of the pulse for 5 seconds. If there is no pulse, resume CPR. If there is a pulse but no breathing, give a rescue breath every 5 seconds (12 per minute).
 Reason: These actions establish whether there is a spontaneous return of pulse or breathing.

If the Airway Is Obstructed

1. **What to do:** If you find that your rescue breaths do not inflate the lungs, first reposition the head and try again to give rescue breaths.
 Reason: The most common cause of airway obstruction is improper head tilt.

2. **What to do:** If the rescue breaths still do not inflate the lungs, give 6 to 10 abdominal thrusts below the diaphragm (the Heimlich maneuver). With the victim still lying down, straddle his or her thighs and place the heel of one of your hands on the midline of the abdomen

slightly above the navel and well below the tip of the breastbone. Place your other hand directly on top of the first hand. Press into the abdomen with quick upward thrusts.

Reason: Such thrusts can force air upward into the airway from the lungs with enough pressure to expel whatever is blocking the airway.

3. **What to do:** Remove the foreign body from the victim's mouth or throat. Open the mouth, pull the lower jaw forward, and sweep deeply into the mouth along the cheek with a hooked finger. Dentures should be removed.

Reason: You may now be able to remove the obstruction even if it has not been fully expelled from the mouth or throat. The hooked-finger sweeping technique avoids accidentally pushing the foreign body further back into the throat.

4. **What to do:** Open the airway and attempt to give five rescue breaths. Reposition the head using the head-tilt/chin-lift technique.

Reason: By this time, another attempt must be made to get some air into the lungs.

5. **What to do:** Repeat the entire sequence until you successfully inflate the lungs. If the airway remains obstructed, alternate the maneuvers in rapid sequence: abdominal thrusts, finger sweep, attempt to ventilate.

Reason: You must be persistent in trying to relieve the obstruction rapidly. As the person becomes more deprived of oxygen, the muscles will relax and maneuvers that were ineffective before may become effective.

Remember, chest compressions without ventilation are useless, be-

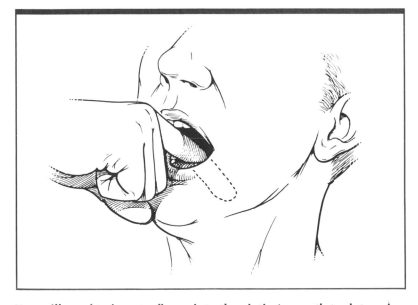

You will need to insert a finger into the victim's mouth to determine whether the obstruction has been expelled and to remove it from the mouth or throat.

cause there will be no oxygen to circulate. The first thing you need to do is to open the airway.

Performing CPR in Infants and Children. There are special considerations for administering CPR in infants younger than 1 year and in children aged 1 to 8 years. For infants and children, administer CPR for 1 minute before calling the local emergency telephone number (911).

1. **Infants (Younger Than 1 Year).** To perform chest compressions on an infant, imagine a line drawn between the nipples. Measure one finger's width below that line. (These instructions are only guidelines because of the variations in sizes of infants' chests and rescuers' fingers.) Make sure your fingers are not below the breastbone. Compress the chest ½ to 1 inch at least 100 times a minute, using only two fingers, not the heel of your hand.

To perform cardiopulmonary resuscitation (CPR) on an infant, cover the mouth *and nose* with your mouth and give one rescue breath for every five chest compressions. Compress the chest ½ to 1 inch at least 100 times a minute, *using only two fingers.*

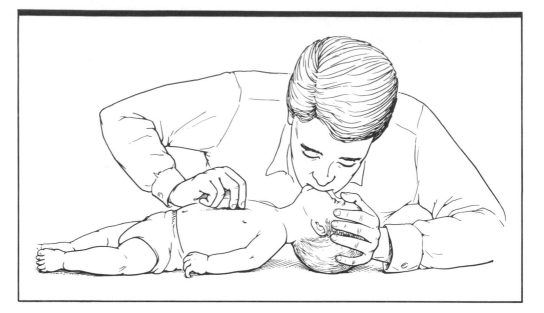

Give one rescue breath for every five compressions.

Do 10 cycles of compressions and rescue breaths, then check the pulse in the inner part of the upper arm. If there is no pulse, give one rescue breath and continue compressions with rescue breaths. Check the pulse every few minutes.

2. **Children (1 to 8 Years Old).** In children aged 1 through 8, the hand position for chest compressions is the same as that for adults, but use the heel of only one hand, not both hands. Compress the chest 1 to 1½ inches 80 to 100 times per minute. Give one rescue breath for every five compressions.

Do 10 cycles of compressions and rescue breaths, and then check for the pulse in the neck. If there is no pulse, give one rescue breath and continue compressions with rescue breaths, checking the pulse every few minutes.

When to Stop CPR.   Once you start CPR, you are obligated to continue un-til the person recovers (regains pulse and breathing), another trained individual takes over, or you are too exhausted to continue.

Many states have "Good Samaritan" laws that protect professionals and laypersons performing CPR "in good faith." Under most Good Samaritan laws, laypersons are protected from lawsuits if they perform CPR, even if they have had no formal training.

Advanced Cardiac Life Support

The emergency medical system is a team approach to handling emergency medical situations. It begins outside the hospital with persons trained in CPR (basic life support), after which trained rescue personnel take over and use more advanced procedures and equipment for sustaining life (advanced cardiac life support).

INTRAVENOUS (IV) CATHETER. Rapid administration of medications and fluids is essential. Advanced cardiac life support personnel place an intravenous (IV) catheter to provide access to the circulation.

ENDOTRACHEAL INTUBATION.
Mouth-to-mouth ventilation is an indispensable stopgap measure, but far higher concentrations of oxygen can be administered directly into the lungs by means of a tube inserted through the nostril or mouth into the windpipe (trachea).

Oxygen can be pushed through the tube by repeatedly squeezing an inflated rubber balloon, which functions as a pump. The tube can also be attached to a mechanical ventilator if extended assistance with breathing is required. The tube ensures that all the air goes to the lungs (not to the stomach) and makes it easier to clear secretions from the lungs.

DEFIBRILLATION.
Defibrillation is the most effective way to stop ventricular fibrillation. Emergency medical personnel apply "paddles" or electrode patches to the chest in order to deliver a shock to the person's heart. This shock "jolts" the heart into a more normal rhythm by briefly inactivating all the cardiac cells simultaneously, so that the normal rhythm mechanism has a chance to regain control. Defibrillation is more likely to be successful the sooner it is applied. Effective CPR may provide the necessary time for a defibrillator to arrive on the scene. Some defibrillator machines are capable of "interpreting" a person's heart rhythm and delivering a shock when and if it is necessary. If ventricular fibrillation is the cause of sudden cardiac death and paramedics with a defibrillator reach the victim in time, ultimately about 25 percent of victims

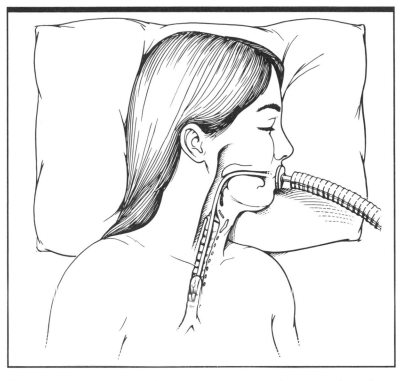

Oxygen can be delivered best to a person who is not breathing through a tube inserted directly into the trachea (windpipe). The oxygen can be delivered by a ventilator machine or by a "bag" pump controlled by a caregiver. A small inflatable cuff at the end of the tube keeps the air from leaking backward, and it also prevents stomach fluids from getting into the lungs.

are able to leave the hospital without evidence of brain damage.

AUTOMATIC CHEST COMPRESSION.
A repetitive action such as chest compression can be done as well by a machine as by a person. Mechanical devices have been developed which can take the place of volunteers or paramedical personnel. Not only does the device not fatigue during a rescue effort, and thus the compression remains strong and effective throughout, but also it enables the advanced rescue team to perform other vital tasks such as endotracheal intubation or insertion of intravenous (IV) catheters. Automatic chest compres-

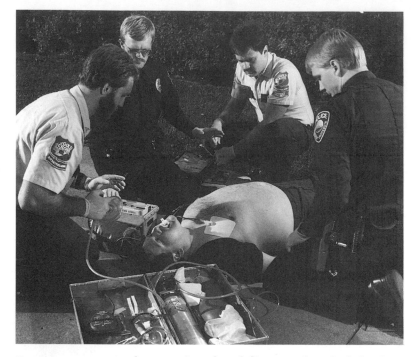

Emergency personnel are equipped to deliver an electrical shock to defibrillate the heart of a victim with ventricular fibrillation or other catastrophic fast heart rhythms.

sion devices are especially useful during transportation of the victim in an emergency vehicle.

EXTERNAL PACEMAKER. In contrast to ventricular fibrillation, in which a large electrical impulse is required to reset a disorganized heartbeat, sometimes a heart does not beat at all or beats too slowly to circulate blood effectively. A cardiac pacemaker is a device designed to deliver an electrical stimulus to the heart repeatedly, which causes it to contract. The energy required to make the heart contract repeatedly is less than that used to defibrillate the heart. Pacemakers are useful when the heart rhythm is drastically slow or the heart has no rhythm. Most cardiac pacing uses wires inserted through veins and into the heart so that the stimulus is delivered directly to the heart muscle. External cardiac pacemakers, however, use patches on the chest to transmit electrical stimuli through the chest wall to the heart. This external system is useful in emergencies, when inserting a wire through a vein may be extremely difficult or takes too much time.

TREATING PROBLEMS OF HEART MUSCLE (CONGESTIVE HEART FAILURE)

Treatment of congestive heart failure is aimed at correcting the cause, if possible. If correction is not possible, treatment is aimed at optimizing the heart's performance. Many types of medical therapy are available to help relieve symptoms and potentially prolong life.

Correcting the Cause

When the cause of heart failure can be corrected, the problem may resolve. For example, if a faulty valve is decreasing the heart's pumping effi-

ciency, repairing or replacing the valve may resolve the heart failure (see page 261). Likewise, if a section of the heart muscle is not getting enough oxygen because the coronary artery supplying it is blocked, restoring blood flow to that region may improve the function of the heart muscle enough to reverse the heart failure. If the cause of the heart failure is a persistent fast heartbeat that causes inefficient pumping, correcting the rhythm problem may reduce the heart failure. Because heart failure is a condition that can stem from various causes, there are various treatments, depending on the specific problem.

Medications for Heart Failure

The basic principles of treating heart failure without a correctable cause focus on augmenting the pumping function of the myocardium, reducing the work load of the heart, reducing the sodium and fluid retention that causes swelling (edema), and preventing thromboembolism (blood clots).

STRENGTHENING THE HEART'S CONTRACTIONS: INOTROPIC MEDICATIONS. In most cases of heart failure, the heart does not pump enough blood to meet the body's needs. The contractions are too weak. Thus, it seems logical that strengthening the contractions would improve your condition. Medications that increase the strength of contraction of the heart muscle are called inotropic medications (*ino* means "fiber," *tropic* means "to influence"). Digitalis, dopamine, dobutamine, and amrinone are examples of inotropic agents (see Table 7, page 306).

Digitalis is one of the oldest medications available for heart failure; it was first used more than 200 years ago (its source was the foxglove plant). Digitalis increases the strength of heart muscle contractions. This medication seems to work best in people who have severe heart failure. It is also beneficial in people who have atrial fibrillation because it slows the commonly associated rapid heart rate.

Despite the long history of digitalis use, its exact role and which people benefit from its use still remain impre-

Causes of heart failure: can they be reversed?

Causes of heart failure that *can usually be* reversed

- Heart valve defects
- Chronic fast heart rates
- Metabolic abnormalities

Causes of heart failure that *may be* reversed

- Severe high blood pressure
- Infections
- Alcohol poisoning of the heart muscle
- Hemochromatosis (abnormal iron deposits in heart muscle)
- Coronary circulatory abnormalities ("hibernating myocardium")

Causes of heart failure that are *usually not* reversible

- Idiopathic dilated cardiomyopathy (see page 41)
- Amyloidosis (abnormal protein deposits in heart muscle)
- Extensive injury of the heart muscle from heart attacks
- Restrictive cardiomyopathy

cise. Studies are currently under way for systematically testing the risks and benefits of digitalis in people with reduced pumping function of the heart.

Other medications have been developed to increase the strength of contraction, but they are given only intravenously. They are very useful for people in advanced stages of heart failure who require hospitalization in the intensive care unit.

Unfortunately, there may be drawbacks to the use of certain inotropic agents. Like all medications, each inotropic agent has side effects (see Table 7, page 306). During drug-testing trials, the use of some experimental inotropic medications led to an even higher rate of complications and death than did the use of a placebo (inactive) medication. Although these specific inotropic medications never came to be prescribed routinely, some doctors have speculated that the use of standard inotropic agents to force a weakened heart to beat harder puts an excessive work load on an already laboring muscle. This may actually accelerate its weakening process. Thus, in the past decade, many doctors have expressed reservations about long-term use of inotropic agents. Nevertheless, these agents are useful in appropriately selected individuals.

REDUCING THE WORK LOAD OF THE HEART: VASODILATORS.

With the recognition that there may be disadvantages to forcing increased work from a weakened heart with inotropic agents, other medical strategies for treating heart failure have been developed. Rather than making the heart work harder, another strategy is to reduce the work load and increase the efficiency of the heart.

A pump must work harder to squeeze fluid (or blood) through narrow tubes (or arteries) than to squeeze the same amount of fluid through wider tubes. Thus, the main way to reduce the work load of the heart in congestive heart failure is to widen or dilate the arteries with medications called vasodilators (see Table 6, page 304). Vasodilators were initially developed with the intention of treating high blood pressure, and they are also used for that condition.

Several types of vasodilators have been used to treat heart failure (see Table 7, page 305). The most widely used are the angiotensin converting enzyme (ACE) inhibitors. These medications act by decreasing the hormones in the circulation which constrict or narrow arteries and raise blood pressure. Studies and experience have shown that the ACE inhibitors and other vasodilators are effective for improving the pumping efficiency of the heart, reducing symptoms, and increasing survival of people with heart failure. In fact, of all the medications used for heart failure, only vasodilator therapy has been shown to prolong life and also to reduce symptoms.

REDUCING FLUID ACCUMULATION: DIURETICS.

One of the hallmarks of congestive heart failure is the accumulation of fluid (edema) in the legs, abdomen, liver, and lungs (see page 38). Fluid accumulation may occur despite treatment with vasodilators and inotropic agents, especially in severe or rapidly developing cases of congestive heart failure. Thus, one aspect of the treatment strategy is to reduce fluid accumulation by using diuretic agents.

Diuretic agents promote urine production by the kidneys. As increasing amounts of water and sodium are removed from the blood by the kidneys, the edema fluid is absorbed from the tissues back into the bloodstream and is eliminated, and swelling is thus reduced. Therefore, diuretics do not really treat the heart failure itself, but they try to reverse some of the effects, and relieve some of the symptoms, of heart failure.

Diuretics can relieve shortness of breath and swelling within hours or days, whereas other agents such as digitalis or vasodilators may take weeks or months. There are several types of diuretics (see Table 7, page 305), and they vary in potency and speed of action. Sometimes a combination of diuretic agents is used.

PREVENTING BLOOD CLOTS: ANTI-COAGULANTS. People with heart failure are at risk of forming blood clots within the heart chambers or in the veins of the legs. Because the weakened heart pumps blood less vigorously, blood flow may be sluggish, and this condition increases the chance of clot formation along the inner surface of the heart muscle. If a fragment of clot were to dislodge, stroke or other complications might result. Thus, many people with heart failure receive long-term oral therapy with anticoagulants (blood thinners) to prevent this. A common anticoagulant is warfarin (see Table 9, page 311)

Warfarin acts by preventing the liver from using vitamin K to produce clotting proteins. A blood test called the prothrombin time ("protime") measures the level of certain blood clotting factors necessary for clotting. Your doctor uses the results of this test to determine the amount of medication you need.

Various medications can affect your prothrombin time, so check with your doctor before taking any new medications. Aspirin can increase the effect of anticoagulants (by inhibiting the natural clotting action of platelets). It can also cause irritation of the stomach lining, which may lead to internal bleeding. Thus, aspirin should usually be avoided while you are taking anticoagulants. Rarely, large amounts of vitamin K from foods (such as green leafy vegetables) or vitamin supplements that include vitamin K may decrease the action of warfarin.

Complications of Therapy

All medications for heart failure have limitations despite their potential for improving the condition. The problems with some inotropic agents occasionally increasing complications and death rates have already been mentioned. Vasodilators should not be given if a person's blood pressure is already low, because the vasodilators will lower it further. ACE inhibitors may lead to worse kidney failure in people with kidney disease.

Diuretics should not be given if blood pressure is too low, because they will lower it further by decreasing the volume of blood in the blood vessels. Furthermore, as diuretics eliminate the excess fluid from the body,

Basic principles for treating congestive heart failure

1. Reduce the work load on the heart
   - Maintain a comfortable activity level to help the body and circulatory system adapt and stay fit.
   - Decrease physical activity during periods of worsened heart failure.
   - Avoid isometric work (such as heavy lifting), which increases blood pressure (and decreases cardiac output).
   - Decrease emotional stress.
   - Lose weight if weight is above ideal.
   - Control high blood pressure.
2. Control sodium and water retention
   - Rest in bed during periods of worsened heart failure to enhance removal of water and sodium in the urine, then gradually increase activity.
   - Restrict sodium in your diet (see page 150).
   - Restrict intake of fluids.
3. Medications
   - Decrease work load of heart with vasodilators.
   - Control sodium and water retention with diuretics.
   - Improve pump function with inotropic medications.
   - Prevent thromboembolism with anticoagulants.
4. Heart transplantation

other substances are eliminated along with it. The most common chemical abnormality caused by some kinds of diuretics is a lowering of the body's supply of potassium. Potassium maintains the electrical stability of your heart and nervous system. Low levels of potassium can lead to heart rhythm abnormalities. Digitalis is more likely to cause side effects (including some heartbeat irregularities) when potassium levels are low.

Because of the loss of potassium, many people taking certain types of diuretics must take supplemental potassium. If you are taking a diuretic, it may be advisable to eat potassium-rich foods, such as bananas, cantaloupe, grapefruit juice, honeydew melon, orange juice, baked or boiled potatoes, avocado, flounder, halibut, prunes and prune juice, cooked soybeans, dates, and figs. Your doctor can measure the level of potassium in your blood and advise you if you need extra potassium.

Magnesium is another mineral that can be depleted by diuretics. Low magnesium levels can lead to muscle weakness and irregular heart rhythms. Foods rich in magnesium include beans, nuts, poultry, fish, green vegetables, grains, and citrus fruits.

What Can You Do?

In the past, people with heart failure were told to rest and lead a sedentary life. This advice is still true for people having an episode of severe heart failure. Increased bed rest during these episodes reduces the work load on the heart and also redistributes fluids in the body, thus helping the kidneys get rid of excess sodium and fluid.

However, all but the most severely debilitated people with chronic heart failure are now encouraged to continue with regular activities that are within their comfort zone. If you are too sedentary you can get out of shape, which will make activities seem even harder. However, you should not engage in activities that make you short of breath.

Dietary considerations are important. Limiting salt (sodium) intake is essential (see page 150). Unless sodium is restricted, medications will be relatively ineffective. Often, periods of worsening heart failure can be traced back to eating sodium-containing foods. Overeating and being overweight add to the work of your heart.

If you have trouble getting a good night's rest because of difficulty breathing, use pillows to prop up your head and avoid eating a big meal just before bedtime. If frequent nighttime urination is a problem, your doctor can change the time you take your medication.

Heart Transplantation

In some situations, the heart becomes so weak that conventional medical treatment has little impact. The possibility of heart transplantation may need to be explored. This procedure can significantly reduce the symptoms and increase the rate of survival in some people with severe heart failure. Individuals receiving transplants at experienced medical centers have 1-year survival rates of approximately 85 to 90 percent, and heart transplantation is now considered a standard form of care in end-stage heart failure. Nearly 2,000 heart transplantations are performed yearly in the United States.

SELECTING TRANSPLANT CANDIDATES. To use the limited supply of donor hearts optimally and to help ensure successful heart transplantations, great effort is made to identify not only the individuals who have the greatest need but also those with the greatest likelihood of gaining from transplantation. People who are most likely to benefit are usually younger than 65 years and have irreversible heart disease causing a life expectancy of less than 2 or 3 years. One difficult part of deciding whether a person should be a candidate for a heart transplant involves estimating how long the person can live without a transplant and how the disease will progress over the waiting period. The transplant candidate must be able to comply with medical recommendations, must be motivated for transplantation, and must not have major contraindications for transplantation.

Contraindications to heart transplantation include pulmonary hypertension (high pressure in the arteries to the lungs), infection, noncardiac disease that significantly limits life expectancy or will be worsened by using immunosuppressive medications after transplantation, unresolved drug (including tobacco) or alcohol abuse, extreme obesity, and inability to adhere to a schedule of medications and medical evaluations. These characteristics make it less likely that a heart transplantation will be successful.

Potential candidates for a heart transplant must undergo rigorous testing to determine whether a heart transplantation is advisable. Tests include a careful assessment for evidence of infection, other diseases that would compromise the transplantation, and the likelihood that the immune system would reject a transplanted heart. Other organ systems must be healthy.

When doctors recommend a heart

Heart donation

There is a shortage of donor hearts for transplantation. Many members of the general public are not yet aware of the vital need for organ donation. Up to 30 percent of people waiting for a heart transplant die before a donor heart becomes available. Therefore, educational efforts to inform more people of the need for healthy donor hearts is a high priority. Although no one would wish for another person to die so that a heart would be available for transplantation, when deaths occur the families often find comfort in helping another person or persons through organ donation. A single donor may provide lifesaving organs (heart, lungs, kidneys, liver, and pancreas) for six or more recipients.

Families should talk about this issue before the situation arises. The decision to donate a loved one's organs is much easier if families know beforehand what the person would want. Many states now have laws and regulations that promote the process of seeking permission for acquiring donor organs.

transplant, you are put on a waiting list. Once you are on the waiting list, you may have to relocate to be within 2 to 3 hours of the hospital. People on the waiting list are given beepers so the hospital can reach them anytime, wherever they are. Have your suitcase packed and your travel plans ready so you can get to the hospital promptly.

By law, heart transplantations are done on a "first come, first served" basis. The only exception is if you become so ill that you must be hospitalized in an intensive care unit, requiring intravenous medications, a ventilator, or other devices to support life. In these cases, you move to a higher position on the waiting list.

THE TRANSPLANTATION PROCEDURE AND HOSPITALIZATION.
When a donor heart becomes avail-

able, tests will be done to determine the donor's blood type and whether there is evidence of infection, including human immunodeficiency virus (HIV), which causes acquired immunodeficiency syndrome (AIDS). Matching the blood type helps prevent the body from rejecting the donor heart. Determining whether there may be hidden infections allows doctors to determine whether a heart is appropriate to use and to plan preventive treatment against activation of any infection that may be carried in the heart. If the blood type matches and the donor heart is healthy, the transplantation proceeds. The size of the donor heart should be relatively proportional to the size of the recipient's body frame, but a precise match is unnecessary. There is no problem transplanting between people of different sexes or races as long as the size difference is not extreme.

If you are next on the waiting list and have the same blood type as the donor, you will be notified to come to the hospital promptly for the heart transplantation. Once the donor heart is removed from the donor, it can remain outside the body for only 4 to 6 hours before the transplantation must be completed.

Before the operation, you will have blood tests, and urine samples and a chest X-ray will be taken to ensure that your condition is satisfactory. You will also take a shower with special cleansing soap to help prevent infection. An intravenous (IV) catheter will be inserted.

The heart transplantation itself is a relatively uncomplicated procedure for skilled heart surgeons to perform. After you are connected to a heart-lung machine (see page 273), the surgeon removes the failing heart by making incisions in the atria, aorta, and pulmonary arteries, and the donor heart is then connected at these sites (see Figures 14 and 15, page A5).

After the operation, you will be monitored closely in the intensive care unit for several days. As with most heart operations (see What to Expect Before, During, and After a Heart Operation, page 275), you will temporarily require supportive measures to speed recovery. Drainage tubes inserted through the skin of the chest and upper abdomen during the operation will remain in place for a day or two to remove excess fluid or blood from the chest cavity. A breathing tube may be left in place for a day or so until you are able to take adequate breaths and clear secretions by coughing on your own. A catheter in the bladder will simplify urination and allow accurate measurement of the fluid balance in your body. A nasogastric tube in your stomach will remove stomach juices because the intestines will require time to begin working. Because you will be temporarily unable to take water, food, or medications by mouth, they will be given through intravenous tubes. As a precaution, the surgeon will insert pacemaker wires that can be connected to a pacemaker; if they are never needed, they can simply be removed without a further operation.

During your recovery period in the hospital (which will last from 1 to 3 weeks), numerous specialists may participate in your care: the heart surgeon, cardiologists, and lung and infectious disease specialists may all contribute. Specialized nurses, respiratory and physical therapists, pharmacists, and dietitians are essential for the success of the transplantation.

AFTER THE TRANSPLANTATION.

Treatment after a transplantation includes medications to help prevent rejection of the donor heart. Your body's immune system recognizes and defends itself against foreign substances such as disease-causing organisms (bacteria or viruses). It also recognizes an organ from another person as a foreign substance and attempts to destroy it. The medications suppress your immune system to minimize the chances that it will attack the new heart.

Suppressing the immune system, however, reduces your body's ability to fight infection. Infection is one of the complications of transplantation, sometimes with types of infections that usually do not occur in an otherwise normal person. The transplant team takes great care to prevent infections and to detect them immediately if they do occur so that they can be treated quickly. For a time after the transplantation, visitors to your room may be required to wear a hospital gown and a mask to minimize the chance of exposing you to germs. After you leave the hospital, you may be advised to wear a mask when in public places until your doctors think that you are no longer at high risk of acquiring an infection. Medications used to suppress the immune system have other potential side effects, too, including high blood pressure, diabetes, kidney function problems, weight gain, and certain types of cancer. Medications and doses are tailored to meet your own needs, and they are monitored closely.

REJECTION.

When the body's immune system attacks the donor heart, it is said to be "rejecting" the organ. Rejection episodes may occur anytime after the operation, but most often they occur within the first few months. Rejection is controlled by adjusting the immunosuppressive medications. Immunosuppressive agents help prevent your immune system from rejecting your transplanted heart. The level of medication in your blood, white blood cell counts, and other values must be monitored to check your response to the medications. Any doctor or dentist caring for you must be informed of the heart transplant and the immunosuppressive medications.

To detect rejection, endomyocardial biopsies are done at regular intervals after the transplant operation (see page 219). The doctor takes a tiny piece of tissue from your heart and checks it under a microscope for signs of rejection. Biopsy specimens are taken every week for the first 6 weeks after opera-

Possible complications of heart operation

- Bleeding (hemorrhage)
- Heart attack (myocardial infarction)
- Stroke
- Infection
- Reaction to anesthetic medications
- Heart rhythm abnormality
- Prolonged dependence on a ventilator for breathing
- Death

The chance of any complication is low, but it varies depending on the specific type of operation, the overall condition of the patient, and the skill of the surgical team. The chances of a complication should always be discussed thoroughly before any operation, and they should be weighed against the anticipated benefits of the operation (or complications of *not* having an operation). Keep in mind that no matter how low the risk of any operation or treatment, it is never zero.

tion, once every 2 weeks from 6 weeks to 3 months after operation, once a month from 3 to 6 months after operation, and once every 3 to 6 months thereafter.

LONG-TERM DEVELOPMENTS.
Now that people who have received transplants are living longer, doctors are finding that some problems develop years after the transplantation. Coronary arteries of the transplanted heart may develop widespread narrowing. Because the nerves have been cut in the transplanted heart, transplant recipients do not usually feel angina if their coronary arteries are not

supplying enough oxygen to the heart muscle. Therefore, doctors perform coronary angiography (see page 217) yearly to look for possible narrowing of the coronary arteries.

Your doctors will also continue to examine you for any evidence of tumor formation, especially of the lymph glands, because immunosuppressive medications may increase the chances of this occurrence.

ARTIFICIAL DEVICES.
Because of the shortage of donor hearts, researchers are studying the possibility of using artificial pumping devices or total artificial hearts to help people with severe heart failure who would otherwise be incapacitated or die soon. Some people have received artificial hearts as a "bridge" to transplantation when their own hearts were unable to keep them alive until a donor heart was available. Other devices have been developed that do not replace the human heart but rather help it to pump more effectively.

All of these devices are experimental and need outside power sources entering through the skin to help them work. This requirement means that the person is limited to activities within the range of connections to the power source. However, progress is being made toward totally implantable devices that do not require wires or tubes passing through the skin.

Operations for Other Diseases of Heart Muscle

Hypertrophic cardiomyopathy (overgrowth of heart muscle, see page 43) causes symptoms because the muscle blocks the blood flow from the left ventricle to the aorta. Medical treatment is directed toward reducing the

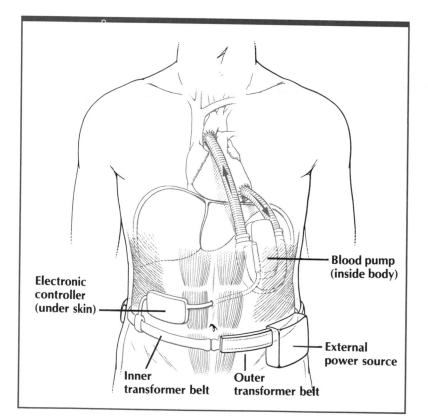

Electronic controller (under skin)

Blood pump (inside body)

External power source

Inner transformer belt

Outer transformer belt

This is one design of a totally implantable artificial heart. A power source transfers energy through the skin from an outer transformer belt to an inner one under the skin. The energy then powers an artificial pump that draws blood from a person's damaged left ventricle and pumps it into the aorta, which distributes it throughout the body.

effect of the obstruction, promoting efficient relaxation of the heart, and avoiding rhythm disorders that may be associated with this problem.

Because the obstruction increases when the heart contracts, medications are used to reduce the contraction strength of the heart. These medications, which include beta-adrenergic blockers (see page 264) and certain calcium blockers (see page 264), have the opposite effect of the inotropic agents. If rhythm problems are present, antiarrhythmic medications may be needed (see Table 8, page 307).

If medications do not relieve the symptoms adequately, an operation may be advisable in which the portion of overgrown heart muscle that is blocking the flow of blood is removed (excised). This procedure is called a myotomy/myectomy (*myotomy* means "cutting into muscle tissue," *myectomy* means "removing muscle tissue"). This procedure can be very effective for reducing symptoms, but its use must be balanced because, like all surgical procedures, it carries certain risks. Pacemaker treatment of some patients, even if they do not have a slow heartbeat, seems to help reduce the effect of the blockage.

TREATING CONGENITAL HEART DISEASE

The general issues in deciding how to treat congenital heart disease were discussed on pages 48–57. Some congenital heart defects such as bicuspid aortic valve or a small ventricular septal defect may be so minor that operation is not needed. Some defects such as an atrial septal defect, a patent ductus arteriosus, or a ventricular septal defect are straightforward abnormalities for which well-established surgical procedures are indicated. Other defects such as transposition of the great arteries or truncus arteriosus may be extremely complex, and the decision whether to operate and what type of operation to perform is a difficult process that may require evaluation and treatment in a highly specialized surgical facility.

Operation for congenital heart disease follows one of the following three strategies.

1. **Palliation:** The goal is to make the person have as few symptoms as possible and live as long as possible without actually correcting the defect, because the defect cannot be totally corrected. An example of a palliative procedure is the Blalock-Taussig anastomosis for tetralogy of Fallot (see figure on page 50).

2. **Staged operations:** An operation is done to correct the problem partially and to allow the person's heart and blood vessels to adapt or to grow so that a second, more completely corrective, operation can be done in the future. An example of a two-stage procedure is one in which the pulmonary arteries enlarge in response to the Blalock-Taussig shunt in the palliative procedure so that a conduit (tube) can be placed between the right ventricle and the pulmonary arteries.

3. **Total correction:** Either the defect is repaired or a procedure is done that reverses the effect of the congenital heart problem. An example of a complete repair is interruption of a patent ductus arteriosus.

TREATING VALVE DISEASE: OBSERVATION, MEDICATION, CATHETERIZATION, OR OPERATION?

Disease can affect any of the four valves in the heart, but it is more common in the mitral and aortic valves on the left side of the heart than in the tricuspid and pulmonary valves on the right side. Valves may open incompletely (stenosis) or allow blood to leak backward (regurgitation). Because it is sometimes difficult to predict how valve disease and its effect on the heart muscle will progress, it is difficult to always select the best treatment.

Observation

If the valve disease is not causing symptoms or causing damage to the heart muscle's contracting function, your doctor may take a "wait-and-see" approach. Continue with regular examinations to make sure that the valve disease is not worsening or causing a deterioration in the overall function of the heart muscle.

Medication

It is important to prevent or manage problems that can result from the disturbance in blood flow through damaged valves. One potential problem is infective endocarditis (see page 58). You should let your doctor or dentist know that you have a valve problem and that you need preventive antibiotics before any dental or surgical procedure that could introduce germs into your system.

Because valve disease can cause reduced pumping efficiency of the heart,

leading to symptoms of heart failure, you may need medications such as digitalis, diuretics, or vasodilators to augment contraction of the ventricles, to prevent or control fluid retention, or to reduce the work load on your heart (see page 252). Sometimes valve disease can also lead to heart rhythm problems, and you may need medication to help control your heart rhythm. Valve problems cause abnormal blood flow through your heart, which may lead to the development of blood clots. Anticoagulant medications (blood thinners) are used to help control this problem when valve disease is complicated by atrial fibrillation, heart failure, or blood clots.

The development of symptoms in people with some types of valvular heart disease is a signal that the valve problem must be corrected. Further observation or medications alone will be insufficient, and the inadequate function of the valve and heart muscle will only continue to deteriorate. In other types of valvular heart disease, your doctor may recommend that the valve problem be corrected even in the absence of symptoms in order to prevent deterioration of the heart muscle and to prolong life.

In these situations, treatment consists of two basic strategies, depending on the nature of the valve problem: 1) altering the valve, or 2) replacing the valve. Altering the defective valve to improve its function can sometimes be done with catheterization procedures, but most of the time it requires operation. Replacing the valve always requires an operation.

Catheterization Techniques (Balloon Valvuloplasty)

Catheterization techniques can be used to widen heart valves that are stenotic (narrowed) and limit blood flow. Percutaneous balloon valvuloplasty (*percutaneous* means "through the skin" [with a catheter], *valvulo* means "related to the valve," *plasty* means [re]"shaping") is a procedure in which one or two balloons mounted on catheters are guided into the heart through blood vessels, positioned through the stenotic valve, and then inflated (see Figure 24, page A8). This procedure enlarges the opening through the valve and improves the blood flow.

As with any heart catheterization procedure, there are potential risks, in addition to the increased chance of causing further damage to the valve structure with manipulation of the balloon. However, in the right people, the risks are small compared with the probability of relieving symptoms promptly. In addition, the hospital stay is usually much shorter with valvuloplasty than with open-heart valve operations.

Balloon valvuloplasty has become the preferred method of treating properly selected people with symptomatic *pulmonary valve stenosis* or *mitral stenosis*. For mitral stenosis, one or two catheters are inserted through the femoral vein (in the groin) and threaded up to the right atrium of the heart. The doctor punctures a sharp-tipped catheter through the atrial septum and passes the balloon catheters through the small hole. The balloon catheters (with the balloons deflated) are positioned midway through the mitral valve and inflated. The stiff leaflets that have become "stuck" to one another split open to allow more blood to flow through. When the catheter is removed, the tiny hole in the atrial septum seals on its own.

Mitral balloon valvuloplasty may not be appropriate if there is too much calcium buildup on the valve or if it is already allowing blood to leak backward. It is also not performed if there is a blood clot in one of the heart chambers, because of the risk of dislodging it. Under these circumstances, the valve must be replaced.

Balloon valvuloplasty is also used for *aortic stenosis*, but it is not the preferred approach to this problem because of only relatively small improvements that frequently last less than 1 year. Nevertheless, it may be useful in people with other illnesses who could not withstand open-heart operation.

Operation

Balloon catheter procedures are *not* appropriate for some symptomatic individuals with mitral stenosis, for most persons with aortic stenosis, or for any person with mitral or aortic regurgitation. For these valve problems, operation on the valve is indicated (see What to Expect Before, During, and After a Heart Operation, page 275).

VALVE REPAIR.   Many cases of *mitral regurgitation* can be repaired: the surgeon can modify the original valve (valvuloplasty) to eliminate back leakage of blood. This procedure is most effective when the cause of mitral regurgitation is breakage of chordae tendineae (which tether the valve leaflets), misshapen billowy valve leaflets that do not close properly, or enlargement of the ring of tissue around the base of the valve leaflets. The valve is repaired by reconnecting the valve leaflets to their tethers or by cutting out sections of excess valve leaflet tissue so that the valve leaflets close snugly. Sometimes repairing the valve includes "cinching" the surrounding ring of heart tissue tighter to ensure that the leaflets close adequately. This is called annuloplasty (*annulo* means "ring," *plasty* means [re]"shaping").

If your natural valve can be repaired, the result is usually better and longer lasting, and you may not require additional medications such as the anticoagulants that may be necessary with artificial valves. Surgeons cannot repair valves that are very heavily calcified or that have been significantly destroyed by disease.

Some people with *mitral stenosis* undergo surgical revision called mitral commissurotomy, in which the surgeon cuts between the valve leaflets that have become "stuck" together. The natural separations between leaflets are called commissures, hence the name meaning "to cut the commissure." Because percutaneous mitral balloon valvuloplasty is usually as effective as mitral commissurotomy, operations are being used less frequently.

VALVE REPLACEMENT. To replace a damaged heart valve, the surgeon removes (excises) it and sutures an artificial (prosthetic) valve at the site. This is the treatment of first choice for aortic valve disease that needs treatment beyond medications. Replacement of the mitral valve is necessary if either repair or balloon valvuloplasty is judged to be unlikely to provide a satisfactory result.

Mechanical prosthetic valves are constructed from metal and synthetic materials. Bioprostheses are made from animal or human tissue. An animal tissue bioprosthesis is usually made from a pig's heart valve, or it is fashioned from the pericardium of a cow. Animal tissue valves are often called heterografts (*hetero* means "different," and in this usage it means different from humans). A human tissue bioprosthesis consists of a heart valve donated from someone who has died. These are called homografts (*homo* means [hu]"man"). Unlike heart transplants, the valves can be preserved and are no longer living tissue. They also do not cause rejection.

The surgeon and cardiologist will discuss with you what type of prosthetic valve would be best for you. Each type has particular advantages and disadvantages. Mechanical prostheses (see Figures 20, 21, and 22, page A8) include ball valves, tilting disk valves, and double-tilting half-disk (bileaflet) valves. The advantage of all of these is that they are extremely durable. The disadvantage of mechan-

Which prosthetic valve is right?

Situation	Recommended valve
Advanced age with expected limited life span Bleeding tendency Anticipated difficulty with anticoagulation (such as future pregnancy)	Bioprosthesis (tissue valve from human or animal)
Young age with expected long life span No reason to avoid anticoagulation	Mechanical prosthesis

ical valves is that you will need to take an anticoagulant (warfarin) for the rest of your life, because blood has a natural tendency to clot on the valve. This clotting could either plug the valve or result in an embolism.

The advantage of bioprostheses is that they usually do not require anticoagulation. However, heterografts are not as durable as mechanical valves. About 30 to 50 percent of people who get heterograft valves need a second new valve by 10 years after the first

implantation. Homografts may be more durable than heterografts, but they are in more limited supply and are used only to replace a defective aortic valve.

All prosthetic valves are prone to infection, which is difficult to treat with antibiotics once it develops. Therefore, it is extremely important to take appropriate precautions (endocarditis precautions; see page 59) before any dental or surgical procedure if you have a prosthetic valve.

SURVIVING HEART ATTACK AND CORONARY ARTERY DISEASE

Coronary artery disease restricts the flow of oxygen-containing blood to the heart muscle. It can result in stable and unstable angina, heart attack, and sudden death. Because coronary artery disease is so common in our population and because its consequences can be so serious, doctors are continuously searching for better ways to diagnose and to treat it. In recent years, there have been many innovations in diagnosing and treating coronary artery disease. New medications, procedures, and operations that improve blood flow to the heart muscle can help minimize symptoms and lengthen life in people with coronary artery disease.

The initial and overriding goal of treatment for all these problems is to balance the supply of blood flow to the jeopardized portions of the heart muscle with the demand for oxygen by the muscle. The strategies and methods used depend on the specific underlying problem causing the inadequate blood flow, the severity of symptoms, and the future risk posed by the

coronary artery problems. There are different strategies for stable angina, unstable angina, coronary spasm, and heart attack (see below). Strategies include medications, interventional procedures with catheters, and coronary artery bypass operation.

Medications

The medications used to treat *stable angina* (see page 73) act either by promoting blood flow through the coronary arteries or by reducing the demand of the heart muscle for oxygen, or both. This effect allows the myocardium to function better even with a reduced supply of oxygen. Unfortunately, no medication reliably removes or dissolves the cholesterol plaques that clog arteries. Some studies, however, suggest that some medications may lessen the severity of blockages.

Medications that *increase the flow of oxygenated blood supply* to the heart do so mainly by relaxing the smooth muscle in the walls of the coronary arteries, allowing them to dilate as much as possible. This relaxation permits an increased flow of blood through the artery, but it does not eliminate the blockages from atherosclerotic deposits.

Medications that *reduce the heart's demand for oxygen* act in one of the following ways:

1. They slow the heart rate; the fewer times the heart beats per minute, the less oxygen it requires.
2. They decrease the vigor of heart muscle contraction; more vigorous contractions require more oxygen. Unless the heart is already severely weakened, most people can tolerate some reduction in the intensity of their heart muscle contraction.
3. They reduce the size of and pressure inside the ventricles. The less pressure and stretch on the heart muscle of the ventricles, the less oxygen the muscle uses.

People who have only mild or infrequent spells of angina may need only a medication to eliminate the symptoms at the time of their infrequent episodes. This strategy is called "p.r.n.," from the Latin *pro re nata*, which means "according to circumstances." Nitroglycerin pills (see Table 1, page 296) that are dissolved under the tongue or nitroglycerin spray that is sprayed into the mouth at the onset of symptoms eliminates the chest discomfort in most people with stable angina. The discomfort usually ends within several minutes after taking the nitroglycerin. This treatment may be all that is needed.

People who have symptoms that occur under predictable circumstances, such as during climbing a flight of stairs, may be advised to use their nitroglycerin *before* the activity. Other people with more prominent or frequent symptoms may benefit from taking medications regularly to try to prevent or reduce the number and intensity of episodes of chest discomfort or breathlessness. This is a *prophylactic* (preventive) medical strategy.

Other medications that are used to treat angina include nitrates, calcium channel blockers, and beta-adrenergic blockers. Nitrates (which include nitroglycerin and medications with a more prolonged effect) decrease the demand of the heart for oxygen by reducing heart muscle stretch, and they increase blood supply to the heart muscle by relaxing the coronary arteries. Calcium channel blockers interrupt the normal flow of calcium through cell membranes in heart muscle and blood vessels. This effect produces dilation of the coronary and other arteries, and blood flow to the heart increases. It also diminishes the heart's demand for oxygen by decreasing blood pressure, heart rate, and the vigor of heart muscle contraction. Not every calcium channel blocker produces these effects to the same extent. Beta-adrenergic blockers decrease the heart rate and blood pressure, and the heart's work load thus decreases.

More than one medication is often needed to get the best effect. If the symptoms progress, the doctor may recommend increasing the dosage of some or all of the medications. If symptoms are not adequately controlled by medications, further treatment may be required.

The medical treatment for *unstable angina*, which is angina that is becoming more frequent, more easily provoked, or more intense or prolonged, is more urgent than that for stable angina. Unstable angina usually results from blood clot formation in a coronary artery that is partially blocked with atherosclerosis.

Many people with unstable angina belong in the hospital so their condition can be evaluated and treatment can be started as soon as possible to try to prevent a heart attack. Almost everyone with unstable angina requires coronary angiography (see page 217) to determine whether they are good candidates for coronary angioplasty or coronary artery bypass operation (see page 377). Frequently medical treatment first is used to stabilize the situation before angiography is done. Exercise testing (such as a treadmill electrocardiography test) usually is not recommended in people with unstable angina, because it poses an additional unnecessary risk.

Even when angioplasty or a bypass operation is anticipated, people with unstable angina usually receive medications to reduce their immediate risk and to stabilize their condition. Any of the medications used for stable angina may also be used to treat unstable angina.

In addition, oxygen is usually given to people in the hospital with unstable angina. Breathing oxygen gives the blood more oxygen to release to the heart tissues even when the amount of blood reaching the heart muscle is reduced.

In people with unstable angina, a thrombotic occlusion (total blockage due to blood clot) may develop in the coronary arteries at the sites of an atherosclerotic blockage, which could lead to a heart attack. Anticoagulants and aspirin are used to reduce the tendency for blood clotting until the blockage is treated by angioplasty or bypass operation. Heparin is the anti-coagulant that is used in hospitalized patients. It is administered intravenously, and the dose can be adjusted rapidly to provide just the right amount of blood-thinning effect. Aspirin reduces the tendency for platelets in the blood to clump together and cause blood clotting.

With *coronary spasm*, the main problem is an abnormal tendency for the coronary arteries to constrict and narrow intermittently, causing reduced oxygenated blood supply to the heart muscle. This may occur even when atherosclerosis is not present, although the two conditions may coexist.

The primary goal of therapy for coronary spasm is to relax the arterial smooth muscle spasm that is causing the narrowing. Medications used for this are agents that relax the blood vessels, such as nitroglycerin, other nitrates, and calcium channel blockers (see Table 1, page 296, and Table 3, page 299).

A *heart attack (myocardial infarction)* occurs when a region of heart muscle is damaged because of complete interruption of its blood supply. The usual cause of the blockage is a blood clot forming inside a coronary artery at a site of atherosclerosis.

The goals of treating or managing a heart attack are threefold:

1. Reverse the blockage to allow blood flow to resume into the jeopardized area of the heart muscle. The resumption of blood flow is called reperfusion, and it is done to "salvage" the heart muscle (myocardial salvage).

2. Eliminate symptoms (supportive care).

3. Monitor, prevent, and treat the complications of heart attack (intensive care).

Methods to reperfuse heart muscle

1. Administering medications that dissolve blood clots (thrombolytic agents)
2. Opening the blocked area of the coronary artery with a catheter that has a balloon tip (see page 270)
3. Performing emergency coronary artery bypass graft operation (see page 272)

Medical Treatment for Reperfusion

Heart muscle can survive longer than the brain without blood flow, but the duration is limited. Unless the blood flow is restored within 30 minutes to several hours, the heart muscle will be irreversibly damaged. The jeopardized portion of the heart muscle will die, form a scar, and no longer contribute to the overall pumping function of the heart.

If salvage of heart muscle is to be successful, blood flow must be restored (reperfusion) before the heart muscle cells have been irreversibly destroyed. Reperfusion is more successful the quicker it is achieved after the onset of the heart attack and its symptoms. That is why it is so important to get to the hospital at the first sign of heart attack. Prompt therapy can make the difference between heart muscle death and heart muscle salvage.

CLOT-DISSOLVING MEDICATIONS (THROMBOLYTIC THERAPY). The most common method of reperfusing heart muscle during a myocardial infarction is the use of medications that dissolve blood clots (thrombolytic agents). Thrombolytic agents, including streptokinase, urokinase, anistreplase, and tissue plasminogen activator (tPA) (see Table 4, page 301), are a monumental step forward in preventing disability and death among people having heart attacks. In the past, only pain medications and supportive measures were available for the treatment of myocardial infarction. Now, with the availability of thrombolytic agents, the damage can be prevented or minimized if you get to a hospital soon enough.

Thrombolytic agents are administered through an intravenous catheter. They can be given as soon as a heart attack is diagnosed on the basis of symptoms and abnormalities on the electrocardiogram. In addition, there must be no condition that might cause a serious bleeding problem, such as recent injury or operation, recent stroke, very high blood pressure, or ulcer disease. Usually, the thrombolytic agent can be given promptly on arrival in the emergency room.

About 80 percent of people having a heart attack who receive a thrombolytic agent within 2 hours of the onset of symptoms have reperfusion. Successful reperfusion reduces the size of the heart attack and helps preserve the overall pumping function of the heart.

If the thrombolytic agent is given later than 2 hours after the onset of symptoms, the benefits diminish. Much of the damage has already occurred, so there is less improvement even if the coronary artery is opened. Thus, early recognition of the symptoms of heart attack and prompt transportation to the emergency room are needed.

SUPPORTIVE CARE. Whether or not thrombolytic treatment is undertaken or successful, additional treatment is usually required. Other medications for the emergency treatment of heart attack include the use of oxygen, just as in cases of unstable angina. Nitroglycerin is also given either under the tongue or by vein to reduce symptoms by decreasing the heart's demand for oxygen and by improving the blood flow through the coronary arteries as much as possible.

Heart attacks can be very painful, so narcotics such as morphine are given when necessary. Medications such as beta-adrenergic blocking agents may be helpful for reducing pain and enhancing survival, especially in people with high blood pressure or a fast heart rate. Beta-adrenergic blockers make the heart beat more slowly and less forcefully, so it requires less oxygen. Inotropic agents and diuretics (see Table 7, page 305) may be used if there is evidence of congestive heart failure, and occasionally calcium channel blockers are used to decrease the heart's demand for oxygen. If blood pressure is too low, or if shock develops (see page 34), medications that elevate blood pressure (vasopressors) and inotropic medications may be needed.

Because people with heart attacks are at a higher risk for the development of blood clots inside their hearts near the dead heart muscle, they receive heparin, an anticoagulant (blood thinner), to inhibit this tendency. Blood clots can re-form in the coronary artery at the sites where thrombolysis has already dissolved the original blood clot. Thrombolytic medications dissolve blood clots that have *already* formed; anticoagulants prevent *new* blood clots from developing. Even when thrombolysis is unsuccessful or is not done, anticoagulation may be advisable to prevent further coronary thrombus (blood clot) from forming.

People who have had heart attacks are also at risk for the development of blood clots inside the left ventricle at the site where the heart damage occurred. If fragments of blood clot break off from this site, they may travel to other parts of the arterial circulation and cause complications such as stroke.

Like anyone having prolonged bed rest, people with heart attacks are at risk for the development of blood clots in the veins of their legs. For all of these reasons, anticoagulants are administered to people who are hospitalized with a heart attack.

INTENSIVE CARE: THE CARDIAC CARE UNIT.   Even though thrombolytic agents may successfully dissolve the blood clot, they do not remove the underlying partial blockage by atherosclerotic plaque. Thus, you may have continuing risk of angina or even the recurrence of a blood clot and another heart attack. Although all of the medications (thrombolytic agents, nitroglycerin, narcotics, oxygen, and anticoagulants) can be started in the hospital emergency room, an integral part of managing people with heart attacks is hospitalization in the cardiac care unit (CCU). There are more than 1,200 coronary intensive care units in hospitals throughout the country.

In the CCU, you are evaluated to see whether further treatment is needed after the clot-dissolving thrombolytic agent is given in the emergency room. You may undergo coronary angiography, which will help the doctor determine whether balloon dilation or a bypass operation is needed. In most cases, coronary angiography and further treatment can be deferred for a few days or weeks until your condition has stabilized.

Since the development of CCUs in the past 30 years, the survival of people with heart attacks has improved, even before the days of thrombolytic agents. Some experts credit CCUs with reducing in-hospital deaths by about 30 percent for people who have had a heart attack. CCUs allow medical personnel to monitor patients carefully and to respond quickly to any of the complications that might occur after a heart attack. These complications include congestive heart failure, rhythm abnormalities, development of a ventricular septal defect, mitral valve regurgitation, development of a ventricular aneurysm, rupture of the ventricular wall, clot formation, recurrence of angina or extension of the heart attack, pericarditis, and shock (see pages 75–82).

The CCU is best equipped to manage these problems because it is staffed with a highly trained medical team whose members are constantly moni-

Electrocardiographic monitoring of all patients in an intensive care unit is centralized. Both automatic computerized detection and human observation are used to alert caregivers quickly of any abnormality needing immediate treatment.

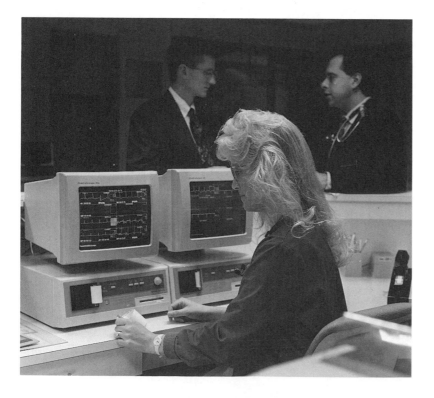

toring the electrocardiogram, the hemodynamics (pressures in the heart, circulation, and blood flow), and the oxygen level in the bloodstream. Specialized nursing personnel and medical technicians are available around the clock. Emergency resuscitation equipment such as defibrillators (see page 283) and facilities for inserting emergency catheters and pacemakers are available.

Other equipment used in the CCU is designed to help the staff watch closely for early signs and symptoms of complications and to administer prompt treatment when necessary. *Continuous electrocardiographic monitoring* allows around-the-clock observation of the person's heart rhythm. The electrocardiogram is recorded continuously and can usually be observed in the person's room and at a central panel of monitors that are watched continuously. The monitors are often equipped with automatic computers that can recognize problems and sound an alarm if ominous changes occur.

People who have had heart attacks are prone to heart rhythm abnormalities, including ventricular fibrillation (sudden cardiac death; see page 241), ventricular tachycardia (see page 95), or slow heartbeats (see page 86). Often during the very early phases of a heart attack, rhythm-controlling medications are given by vein to reduce the likelihood of a rapid dangerous heart rhythm or ventricular fibrillation. If dangerous rhythms develop, nursing personnel and doctors use *medications and defibrillators* as necessary.

Many, but not all, persons who have had heart attacks, as well as other people requiring hospitalization in CCUs (such as those with very severe congestive heart failure), have a special *moni-*

toring catheter inserted through a vein and threaded into the right-sided chambers of the heart and the pulmonary artery (see page 223). It is called a hemodynamic catheter, or a Swan-Ganz catheter (named after the inventors). The catheter measures pressures inside the heart and pulmonary artery and is used to determine the amount of blood pumped by the heart per minute (cardiac output). This information gives medical personnel a very early and sensitive means of determining the efficiency with which the heart is functioning. The catheter continuously tells doctors whether there is any change in the pumping function of the heart so that they can start appropriate treatment.

The catheter is usually inserted through a needle puncture into a neck (jugular) vein, subclavian (under either collarbone) vein, or an arm vein. A small balloon at the tip of the catheter can be inflated to help it move through the vein circulation into the heart and out into the pulmonary artery.

After a heart attack, a slow heart rhythm may develop or your electrocardiogram may show clues that you may be at risk for development of a slow heart rhythm. This potentially dangerous situation can be corrected by inserting a *temporary pacemaker* wire through the same vein used for the monitoring catheter. The electrode tip touches the inner wall of the right ventricle. The end of the electrode wire that is outside the body is attached to a small pacemaker unit that can deliver stimulation to the heart muscle to make it beat at an acceptable rate.

Often the problem with the slow heart rate corrects as the heart muscle begins to heal, and the temporary pacemaker can be removed. Sometimes the slow heart rate is permanent, or the risk of development of a slow heart rate in the future is high enough that you need a permanent pacemaker.

Besides emergency treatment, one important aspect of the CCU is to start the process of rehabilitation from the heart attack (see page 312). In the hospital, you gradually increase your level of physical activity and start regaining your strength. Most CCUs also have a "step-down" area where close monitoring can be continued at a somewhat less intense level for people who have recovered from the immediate effects of their heart attack.

Surgical and Catheter Treatment

The underlying problem in most cases of angina or heart attack is one or more atherosclerotic blockages of the coronary arteries. It stands to reason that removing or reducing the blockage would solve the problem. If medications and changing life-style factors (such as diet, exercise, and smoking) are not adequate treatment, your doctor may recommend coronary angioplasty or a coronary artery bypass operation to remove or bypass the blockage in your coronary artery.

The use of angioplasty or bypass operation is reserved for people who do not get enough relief from medications alone or who have had an exercise (or other type of stress) test or coronary angiography that shows they are at higher risk for future heart attack or death. People have a higher risk if they have decreased pumping function of the heart and blockages in all three coronary arteries or the left main coronary artery. (The left main coronary artery supplies most of the left ventricle, the main pumping chamber.)

CORONARY ANGIOPLASTY. Coronary angioplasty is a procedure in which a specially constructed catheter with a small balloon on the tip is inserted in an artery in the groin or arm. It is threaded into the coronary arteries and used to open up the blockage. The complete name for this procedure is percutaneous (through the skin) transluminal (inside an artery) coronary angioplasty (blood vessel reshaping), or PTCA.

Not every blockage of a coronary artery is amenable to treatment with a balloon catheter. Some blockages may be too long or in places that are difficult to reach with a catheter. In these cases, bypass operation may be advised. However, as doctors have gained experience with this technique, increasingly complicated and severe disease has become accessible to this form of treatment.

The PTCA Procedure. Before the PTCA, you will have had a chest X-ray, electrocardiography, and blood tests. A member of the medical team who will perform the PTCA will make sure you understand the rationale, procedural aspects, and risks associated with PTCA. Do not eat or drink anything after midnight the night before your PTCA. You may take the medications ordered by your doctor with a small amount of water. You might also receive medications to decrease clotting of your blood or to relax the muscles in your coronary arteries.

On the day of the procedure, an intravenous (IV) catheter is inserted, and a sedative is given. Small electrode pads are placed on your chest to moni-

tor your heart rate and rhythm. Your groin is washed with an antiseptic solution and a sterile drape is placed over your body. After injection of a local anesthetic, a short tube called a sheath is inserted into the leg artery. A guide catheter, which is a hollow, flexible tube, is then inserted through the sheath and moved to the narrowed coronary artery while the doctor watches it on a televised X-ray image. You may feel pressure, but you should not feel sharp pain in the groin area during the procedure.

The doctor injects a small amount of contrast agent (which appears on the X-ray image like a dye) through the catheter to see the exact location of the blockage. A smaller catheter with a tiny deflated balloon at the tip is inserted through the guide catheter until the balloon crosses the blocked area of the artery. The balloon is inflated for 30 to 120 seconds and then deflated. This inflation stretches open the artery wall and increases the diameter of the artery (see Figures 37 and 38, page A11). It is common to experience chest pain while the balloon is inflated, because it blocks the blood flow to an area of your heart for a short time. Tell the staff if this occurs. The pain usually disappears after the balloon is deflated. The doctor usually inflates and deflates the balloon several times.

The balloon catheter is removed, and more pictures (angiograms) are taken to see how the blood flow through the artery has improved. The guide catheter is then removed. The average procedure takes about 30 to 90 minutes.

During the recovery period, your electrocardiogram continues to be monitored for 12 to 24 hours. A nurse checks your vital signs, foot pulses, and PTCA site frequently. Tell your nurse of any discomfort, pain, or anything that bothers you after the PTCA.

After the procedure, the sheath usually is left in your leg artery for 4 to 24 hours. A salt (saline) solution with blood thinner (heparin) mixed in it flows through the sheath to keep blood from clotting inside the sheath. You must not bend your leg at the hip or the knee from the time the PTCA is completed until 6 hours after the sheath has been removed, so you will be on complete bed rest for that time.

After the sheath is removed, pressure may be applied to the groin area for up to 6 hours to prevent bleeding and promote healing at the puncture site. After the pressure is removed you may sit up and walk around your room with the help of your nurse.

Your doctor may prescribe medications such as nitroglycerin to relax the coronary arteries, calcium antagonists to protect against coronary artery spasm, or a combination of aspirin and dipyridamole to help prevent blood clots in the previously blocked coronary artery.

You will probably be released from the hospital 1 or 2 days after the PTCA. Many people return to work the next week. You will be given follow-up instructions when you are released. You may be asked to return 6 months after the PTCA for a follow-up evaluation, which may include angiography or an exercise test.

Results of PTCA. More than 90 percent of PTCA procedures are initially successful. Successful PTCA reduces the blockage, improves symptoms, and is not associated with complications such as heart attack or emergency coronary bypass operation.

Risks of PTCA. As with all procedures that involve inserting catheters into the coronary system, there are risks with PTCA. The insertion of a catheter can injure or puncture the artery, and operation is then necessary to correct the complications. Also, after the inside surface of the artery has been touched by the balloon, the risk of blood clots forming on the site is increased slightly.

Despite these possibilities, the overall risks are very low, especially in relation to the benefits that might be achieved. The risk of death from PTCA is less than 1 percent, and the risk of precipitating a heart attack is less than 4 percent. Occasionally the blockage is made worse, and coronary artery bypass grafting is required to correct the problem. This happens less than 5 percent of the time.

Although PTCA is successful in reducing the amount of blockage in 90 percent of people, the procedure does have an Achilles' heel: about one-third or more of the blockages return to their original severity in less than a year. The blockage causes a return of angina, but only rarely (less than 5 percent of the time) does it cause a heart attack. A second PTCA is often successful and resolves the problem, but coronary artery bypass grafting may be necessary.

NEW CATHETER TECHNIQUES.
Much research on catheter methods of opening coronary arteries is directed at lowering the rate of recurrence of the blockage. Medications have been investigated that might reduce the chance of further atherosclerosis or blood clot developing at the site of dilation. Other types of dilating catheters have been studied, including a cutting

or shaving type (atherectomy catheter), which actually shaves off and removes plaque from the inside of the artery, and laser-tipped catheters that "vaporize" the blockages with a tiny laser beam. In addition, stents, which are like tiny scaffolds used to hold the artery open, are being studied.

The *atherectomy* catheter has a metal cylinder about 1 inch from the tip that contains a rotating disk that spins at 2,500 revolutions per minute (see Figure 39, page A11). Plaque is exposed to the rotating cutting blade and shaved off. The plaque fragments are stored in a collection chamber in the tip of the catheter until it is withdrawn. When the collection chamber is full, the cardiologist withdraws the catheter, which can be cleaned and reinserted. The procedure is repeated four to six times to open the artery adequately.

Using a catheter with a *laser* at the tip, doctors can focus rapidly pulsating beams of light that vaporize the tissue into gases that are dissolved in the bloodstream and eliminated in the body's natural waste system (see Figure 40, page A11). Lasers may be useful in areas where balloons are suboptimal, such as long areas of narrowing.

Even though these newer techniques are initially successful, so far none of them have made a significant impact on the recurrence of blockage. Thus, it is important for people who have had PTCA to reduce their risk factors for recurrence by quitting smoking, lowering cholesterol levels, maintaining a healthy weight, controlling diabetes and high blood pressure, and getting regular exercise.

CORONARY ARTERY BYPASS GRAFTING.

Another way to manage a coronary blockage is to create a detour for the blood to go around it. This is the principle of coronary artery bypass grafting (CABG). This type of operation was first performed in 1969, and now about 300,000 bypass operations are performed every year in the United States.

Bypass operation is usually appropriate in people who have a blocked left main coronary artery, people with disease in many vessels and poor function of the left ventricle (the main pump of the heart), and people with debilitating angina. In these people, a bypass operation can enhance and prolong life.

For a bypass operation, the surgeon reroutes blood flow around the site of your coronary blockage in one of two ways.

1. A saphenous vein is taken from your leg and is used as a bypass tube or conduit. The saphenous vein is not crucial for blood flow in the leg. (It is the vein that is often involved with varicose veins and is "stripped" if necessary.) One end of the vein is connected to the aorta near where the coronary arteries normally originate, and the other end is connected to the coronary artery downstream from the blockage. This allows blood to flow around the blockage from the aorta to the coronary artery (see Figure 41, page A11).

   Saphenous veins are long and easy to remove from the legs. Removing them does not impair the circulation in the legs.

2. A second technique for bypass operation is to use one or both of two arteries that normally arise from branches of the aorta. These arteries are called the internal mam-

The heart-lung machine

During a coronary artery bypass grafting or open-heart operation, a heart-lung bypass machine performs the functions of the heart and lungs and keeps you alive while the operation is taking place.

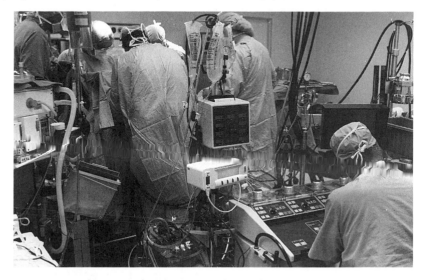

A heart-lung machine in the foreground is taking the blood returning to the patient's heart from all parts of the body, providing it with fresh oxygen, and then pumping it into the aorta, which distributes it throughout the body. The heart and lungs are "bypassed" by this procedure, allowing the surgeon to operate on a motionless heart without blood blocking his or her vision.

The heart-lung machine takes blood returning from the body through your veins to the right atrium and diverts it into an apparatus that oxygenates the blood as your lungs would. After the blood is oxygenated, it is pumped into your aorta downstream from the heart. From there it can flow to all of your organs (except the heart and lungs). No blood flows through the heart, so it can be stopped.

In coronary artery bypass grafting, this stopping of the heart allows the surgeon to make the delicate maneuvers that are necessary without having to deal with a "moving target." In operations for congenital heart disease and valve disease, it allows the heart to be opened and the blood to be drained out so the surgeon can see what he or she is doing.

During the operation, the heart does not receive a continuous blood supply through the coronary arteries, although the surgeon may intermittently allow blood to flow through them. To prevent the heart from suffering damage, it is cooled down and chemicals are used to slow its metabolism and reduce its need for oxygen.

When the operation is completed, the heart is restarted with an electrical shock.

mary arteries (also called the internal thoracic arteries). With this technique, the surgeon does not entirely remove the artery as in the procedure in which the saphenous vein is used. Rather, the surgeon disconnects the downstream end of the artery from the inner part of the chest wall and reconnects that end of the artery to the coronary artery downstream from the blockage (see Figure 41, page A11). This procedure allows blood to flow through the aorta and through the artery as it normally would, but it ends up in the coronary artery instead of along the inner surface of the chest wall. There are enough other arteries in the chest wall to supply an adequate amount of blood when the internal mammary artery is diverted.

Multiple saphenous vein segments or both the right and the left internal mammary arteries can be used to bypass different blockages. Furthermore, one bypass graft can be used to bypass more than one blocked artery (sequential grafts).

The Coronary Artery Bypass Procedure. The events preceding and following coronary artery bypass grafting are very similar to those with most cardiac surgical procedures (see What to Expect Before, During, and After a Heart Operation, page 275). For the operation itself, an incision is made along the midline of your chest, through your breastbone. For a part of the operation, the functions of your heart and lungs will be assumed by a heart-lung machine (see The heart-lung machine, page 273). Incisions are also made along the inside of your leg if the surgeons intend to use a saphenous vein for a bypass graft. More than one bypass is usually needed, so you may have more than one incision in the legs.

Coronary artery bypass grafting usually takes 3 to 6 hours, depending on the complexity of your operation. The more bypasses that must be attached, the longer it will take. As many as eight or nine segments of arteries may be bypassed, but the average number is four or five.

Results of Coronary Artery Bypass Grafting. The goal of coronary artery bypass grafting is to restore adequate blood flow through the coronary arteries so that you can enjoy a more productive and active life. Coronary

Preoperative autologous blood collection

If you are anticipating an operation, you can use your own blood for transfusions. Autologous blood is your own blood that has been collected and made available for you during operation. It is the safest blood product available for transfusion, because it eliminates the risk of transfusion-related diseases and reduces the risk of blood transfusion reactions.

When a surgical procedure is planned, your doctor will discuss your blood needs with you. Eligibility for preoperative autologous blood collection is based on your medical condition.

The blood donation procedure is safe and simple and requires about 1 hour of your time. You may make autologous donations at a frequency of 1 unit of blood per week. You should donate the last unit of blood at least 72 hours before your scheduled surgical date.

Blood can be stored as a liquid for 5 weeks. Frozen storage techniques may be used to extend the period of storage significantly for some blood components such as red blood cells and plasma.

artery bypass grafting substantially improves symptoms in 90 percent of the people who have it done, and it prolongs life in people with either left main coronary artery disease or blockages in two or three of the major coronary artery trunks, especially if the pumping function of the heart is also reduced.

In general, about 40 percent of people who have bypass operations have evidence of new blockage within 10 years after operation. Angina can recur in people with coronary artery bypass grafts for several reasons: blockages can develop in the bypass grafts, new blockages can develop in the coronary

arteries that were not originally bypassed, and there may be blockages in coronary artery branches that are too small to bypass. Internal mammary arteries seem to stay open longer than saphenous vein grafts, so there is an increasing trend to use that approach.

Risks of Coronary Artery Bypass Grafting. The risk of dying from the operation is about 2 percent in people undergoing scheduled operation for angina. The risk is about 8 percent if the procedure is done in an emergency situation such as a heart attack, when the person's condition is unstable.

WHAT TO EXPECT BEFORE, DURING, AND AFTER A HEART OPERATION

Anyone anticipating a heart operation looks forward to relief of the problem. However, there are some natural fears and doubts that accompany a major operation. For most people, knowing more about what to expect can ease some of the feelings of uncertainty. Do not hesitate to ask your doctor, surgeon, and others involved in your care any questions you may have.

Almost all types of "open heart operation" involve some of the same steps before, during, and after the procedure. Outlined below are procedures that coronary artery bypass grafting, a valve replacement operation, repair of a congenital defect, and some operations for cardiomyopathy and pericarditis have in common. Procedures that are exclusive to heart transplant operations are discussed on page 254.

Timing of Operation

Most operations can be scheduled days or weeks in advance, depending on the medical urgency of the problem and on your and the surgeon's schedule. If the severity of the symptoms warrants emergency operation, it is done right away.

The Week or Two Before Heart Operation

Once your heart operation is scheduled, your doctor will discuss with you some of the following standard instructions to prepare for the operation:

- Do not take aspirin or ibuprofen (such as Advil, Motrin-IB, or Nuprin) for at least 10 days before the procedure. These medications reduce the function of platelets, so excessive bleeding during or after operation is more likely to occur. Acetaminophen (such as Tylenol, Datril, Anacin 3, or Panadol) does not promote bleeding, so it can be taken if needed.

- If you need to take an anticoagulant (warfarin; see Table 9, page 310), you may be admitted to the hospital several days before your scheduled operation. During this time, your medication can be changed to a shorter-acting intravenous anticoagulant (heparin, see Table 9, page 310) whose use can be discontinued temporarily for the operation.

- Continue to take all other medications until reporting to the hospital, unless your doctor tells you otherwise.

- Report any signs of infection, such as fever, chills, and respiratory symptoms (including coughing or a runny nose), that occur within a week before operation.

Preparations at the Hospital

You will probably be admitted to the hospital the afternoon or evening before the next day's operation. Sometimes, patients are asked to report to the hospital in the early morning the day of the operation.

In preparation for the operation, you will have blood tests, a chest X-ray, and electrocardiography unless these were recently done.

Each hospital has its own procedure for giving you the details about any final instructions or preparations. Usually, representatives of the surgical team (surgeon, cardiologist, anesthesiologist) will visit with you and your family the evening before or the morning of the operation to discuss what time your procedure is scheduled, perform a brief physical examination, and gather a medical history. You may have an opportunity to attend a class or watch a video about heart operation and what can be expected after it. Family members should make sure they understand the instructions about where they are to wait during the operation and when they can expect information about the progress of the operation. You and your family will also learn about the facilities and special monitoring in the intensive care unit where you will spend the first few days after operation.

Your doctor will tell you which medications to continue taking up until the time of the operation. Generally, medications for angina are allowed. Do not eat or drink anything after midnight the day of operation because anesthesia is safer if it is given when your stomach is empty.

The final preparations include shaving or removing most body hair (which can harbor bacteria) from your neck to your ankles and showering with a special cleansing soap.

You may receive medication to help you relax before going to the surgical suite. In a surgical preparation area, an intravenous (IV) catheter may be inserted. This procedure involves inserting a needle into a vein. A small, flexible catheter slides over the needle and remains in the vein; the needle is withdrawn. Anesthetic medications and other medications can be administered through the IV catheter.

During the Operation

You will be given a general anesthetic to put you to sleep during the operation. The surgeon makes an incision and opens the chest. Depending on the type of operation, the opening is made lengthwise through the breastbone or crosswise between ribs. A heart-lung bypass machine (see The heart-lung machine, page 273) performs the functions of your heart and lungs during operation, allowing the surgeon to make the necessary repairs while your heart remains motionless.

A breathing tube, called an endotracheal tube, is inserted through the nose or mouth. It serves three purposes: 1) helps you breathe during anesthesia, 2) assists in clearing secretions from the lungs, and 3) decreases the work load on the heart by assisting breathing. The tube may remain in place after operation for a few hours or days, according to your need for breathing assistance.

Your family will be informed when the major part of the operation is over, which is when you are taken off the heart-lung bypass machine and your heart resumes functioning on its own. You will probably remain in the surgical suite for observation for another 1½ to 2 hours before being moved to the intensive care unit (ICU). When you arrive in the ICU, a surgical team member will describe the operation and your condition to your family.

What to Expect in the ICU

While you are in the ICU, many monitoring devices are used by the health care team. A catheter device inserted through a neck vein during operation will measure blood pressure and pressures in the chambers of the heart (Swan-Ganz catheter; see page 269). It is threaded through a vein into the right atrium and ventricle and into the pulmonary artery. The catheter monitors the pressure in the right side of the heart and the amount of blood flowing through the heart, both of which are very useful means of determining how efficiently the heart is performing.

Tubes inserted through the chest wall during the operation drain excess fluid or blood from around the heart into a container on the bedside cart. A catheter removes urine from the bladder to assist the nurse in recording urine output. A tube may be passed through the nose and throat into the stomach (nasogastric tube) to remove stomach juices to allow the intestines time to begin working again. Fluids, nutrition, and medications are given through the intravenous (IV) catheter in an arm vein. Throughout your stay in the ICU, all fluid intake and output will be closely monitored.

Your heart rhythm will be monitored continuously with electrocardiography. Many people experience minor changes in heart rhythm after an operation. Many factors may contribute to these changes in rhythm, including handling of the heart during operation, catheters used to monitor pressures within the heart, changes in potassium and sodium levels, and stress (the body's normal response to fear and anxiety). Some changes in heart rhythm may require temporary treatment with medications.

The endotracheal tube (or breathing tube) is left in place until you are able to breathe deeply and cough to clear lung secretions. Although the tube is not painful, it is uncomfortable. While the tube is in place, you will not be able to speak because the tube passes through the voice box. Nurses will help with communication. The endotracheal tube is removed when blood tests show that there is enough oxygen in your blood and when you are able to cough up secretions. When the tube is removed, you will wear an oxygen mask and you may have a raspy voice or a sore throat for a few days.

To assist with recovery, you must breathe deeply and cough. Some types of movement will cause discomfort. You will receive medication to decrease the discomfort.

A stay in the ICU is not restful. Because of all the activity associated with monitoring your condition around the clock, you (and your family) may be distracted by the frequent visits by members of the health care team and the sounds of the equipment. Despite the commotion, it is reassuring to realize that the activity is directed at ensuring your rapid recovery so that you can safely leave the intensive care setting.

The length of stay in the ICU varies, depending on the complexity of the surgical procedure. When the surgeon decides that the special facilities of the ICU are no longer required, you will be moved to a step-down area where close monitoring is continued, but at a somewhat less intense level.

What to Expect in the Step-Down Area

Your heart rhythm will continue to be monitored with electrocardiography. Monitoring allows the doctor to evaluate whether any change in rhythm requires treatment. Results of blood tests also help the doctor manage your care.

Generally, you will wear an oxygen mask for the first day in the step-down area, and then as needed. The moisture from the oxygen mask helps loosen and clear secretions from your lungs.

Coughing is crucial to keep the airways clear. Coughing has several beneficial effects. It clears secretions that can block airways and prevent oxygen from reaching the air sacs, where it passes into the blood. If secretions block airways, pneumonia can develop more easily. Coughing also requires taking a deeper breath first, and this promotes reexpanding zones of lung that were compressed during the operation. Nurses will help you with turning in bed, coughing, and deep-breathing exercises. The nurses may continue to do chest physiotherapy—gentle thumping on the chest in different positions—to assist in clearing secretions.

You will be encouraged to increase activity levels gradually, even while monitoring continues. As your strength increases, extend the time you spend out of bed and walking. Short rest periods help as you increase the amount of activity. Support stockings help blood circulation in your legs.

Your fluid intake and output will be closely monitored. Tell your nurse of any fluid you drink between meals. Urine output will be measured throughout your hospital stay to calculate the fluid balance in your body. Being neither too "wet" nor too "dry" is important for your recovery. You will be weighed each day as another indicator of the balance between your fluid intake and output. It is common to weigh more the first few days after operation because of the fluids given during the operation, but you will gradually lose the weight.

Your appetite may be poor for a few days. However, it is important to take in enough liquid and food for nourishment and to promote healing. A dietitian can help you make food selections based on your doctor's prescription. Talking with a dietitian gives you and your family a chance to learn more about heart-healthy eating that you can continue at home.

It is natural to feel emotional "ups and downs" during recovery. You will probably have both "good" and "bad" days after the operation. The entire health care team—cardiologists, surgeons, nurses, dietitians, and therapists—is available for support.

There is no standard length of stay in the cardiac surgical step-down area. Your surgeon determines when special monitoring is no longer necessary. Even though monitoring is discontinued, you may need to recover further in the step-down area or general hospital unit until dismissal.

RESTORING RHYTHM CONTROL

The rhythm of the heart can malfunction in various ways (see page 82). Depending on the nature of the problem, management may require the use of medications, pacemakers, shocking the chest wall (defibrillation or cardioversion), placement of an internal cardioverter-defibrillator, operation, or catheter techniques to eliminate abnormal rhythms. This section discusses the different categories of treatment of abnormal heart rhythms.

Medications

Drugs that treat rhythm disorders are called antiarrhythmics (see Table 8, page 307). Virtually all antiarrhythmic drugs are used in treating fast or irregular rhythms, except for atropine and isoproterenol, which are given intravenously in emergency situations to speed up slow heart rates. Antiarrhythmic drugs act by various mechanisms. Certain antiarrhythmic medications may be useful for one type of rhythm disorder, whereas others are appropriate for another rhythm disorder. Conversely, two people with the same rhythm disorder may respond differently to the same medication. Choosing the correct medication requires an accurate diagnosis of the rhythm disorder (see page 83) and an understanding of its mechanism.

Most antiarrhythmic medications work by changing the electrical behavior of the heart. Modifying electrical conduction alters the setting in which rhythm disorders can start or continue, thus minimizing their occurrence or severity.

Several principles of treatment with antiarrhythmic drugs are very important for both patients and doctors to understand.

All antiarrhythmic medications can cause side effects. Indeed, one of the most worrisome side effects of some antiarrhythmic medications is their tendency to *provoke* rhythm disorders. Ironically, although an antiarrhythmic medication may benefit 9 out of 10 people, it may make 1 out of 10 worse. Cardiologists have become much more aware in the past several years that medications given to help people may actually hurt them or increase their chances of dying. This fact was revealed in a recent study of antiarrhythmic medications in heart attack victims with rhythm disorders; people receiving certain antiarrhythmic medications had a higher rate of dying than those who were given inactive pills (placebos).

A medication must be thoroughly justified and its benefit documented before it is prescribed by doctors. There must be a clear-cut reason for you to use an antiarrhythmic medication, and you must be carefully observed for your response once it is started.

Not all rhythm disorders require treatment. Some rhythm disorders that may cause symptoms such as palpitations pose less risk to the person than the medication that might be used to treat them. Your doctor may encourage you to tolerate and not worry about certain rhythm disorders such as ventricular premature contractions that may cause palpitations. You may try avoiding factors that affect your heart rhythm and rate, such as tobacco, alcohol, and caffeine.

An important part of rhythm management is determining the efficacy (success) of the medication in accomplishing what it is supposed to do. Depending on the circumstances, efficacy can be measured by 1) the effect of the medication on your symptoms, 2) the effect on your heart rhythm as observed on the electrocardiogram or monitor, or 3) the ability of the medication to prevent your heart from being artificially stimulated into a rhythm disorder during electrophysiology testing (see page 224). In some cases, this process of assessing efficacy can be lengthy and tedious. However, it is important and should not be compromised.

A drug that is effective for one person with a rhythm disorder may not be as effective for another person with the same rhythm problem.

No antiarrhythmic medication can work unless it is present in the bloodstream at adequate levels. It is some-times useful to measure the level of the drug in the bloodstream. If the rhythm disorder is not well controlled and testing shows that the drug level in the bloodstream is low, increasing the dose may help. The need for maintaining effective levels in the bloodstream means that it is important to take the medication as prescribed—avoid skipping doses unless instructed to do so.

Pacemakers

An abnormally slow heart rate requires treatment 1) if it causes symptoms such as fatigue, shortness of breath, or faintness or passing out, or 2) if the heart rhythm poses a significant risk of symptoms developing suddenly in the future. The only effective treatment for a slow heart rate is a pacemaker.

Pacemakers were originally designed to be used for one purpose: to maintain an adequate heartbeat when the heart beats too slowly or pauses. Now, more sophisticated devices not only keep the heart beating at an acceptable rate but also mimic a normal heartbeat and speed or slow the heart rate according to the person's needs.

WHAT IS A PACEMAKER?   A pacemaker has two main parts: a pulse generator that contains the batteries and electronic circuitry, and the wires (electrodes or leads) that carry an electrical impulse from the pulse generator to the myocardium (heart muscle). The batteries and electronics of the pulse generator are contained in a watertight casing about the size of a pocket watch which is usually made of the metal titanium. The electronics can receive signals from a programmer (somewhat like the remote control of a television), so that the settings can be altered by your doctor even after the pacemaker is implanted. The flexible electrode wires, which conduct electricity, are covered by an insulating material (much like a household electric cord) such as silicone rubber or polyurethane.

HOW DOES A PACEMAKER WORK?

At its simplest, a pacemaker can sense your heartbeat and respond accordingly. If it senses that the heart rate is too slow or if there is no heartbeat, the pacemaker emits tiny electrical impulses (too small to feel), which stimulate the heart to contract. If the pacemaker senses that the person's heart is beating fast enough, the pacemaker will go "on demand" and stand by until it is needed. The instant the heart goes too slow or pauses, the pacemaker begins pacing.

The pacemaker is told (programmed) to know what heart rate it should accept as satisfactory or below which it should start pacing. Various other functions can also be programmed, such as the strength of each impulse that is emitted and the sensitivity of the pacemaker's ability to detect your natural heartbeat.

More sophisticated pacemakers are capable of additional functions that may help certain people.

Dual-Chamber Pacemakers. Two-wire, or dual-chamber, pacemakers consist of a pulse generator and wires to both the right atrium and the right ventricle. This type of pacemaker (see Figure 46, page A14) can sense when the heart's own pacemaker (the sinus node) is firing.

In people with complete heart block (see page 89), the message from the sinus node is blocked at the atrioventricular node and does not reach the ventricles. With a dual-chamber pacemaker, however, the message from the sinus node is sensed by the pulse generator, which then causes the heart to contract by sending an impulse to the ventricle. This maintains the normal sequence of the heartbeat (the atrium beats first, followed by the ventricle), and the pacemaker can adjust its rate according to how fast the sinus node tells it to "fire." Your sinus node speeds up when you exert yourself. Thus, if you have a dual-chamber pacemaker, it will be "told" by the sinus node to stimulate the ventricles to beat faster, too. Acceleration of the heartbeat is important for ensuring that you can achieve a normal activity level.

Some people with a one-wire system (in which only the ventricle is stimulated) experience an uncomfortable feeling of neck throbbing, chest fullness, or faintness when the pacemaker paces (this is called pacemaker syndrome). Dual-chamber pacemaker systems avoid these symptoms.

Rate-Responsive Pacemakers.

Some people do not have a normal sinus node that can be tracked by a dual-chamber pacemaker. People with atrial fibrillation or an irregular or slow sinus node do not benefit from the dual-chamber pacemaker. These people can be treated with other pacemakers with advanced features that make them more closely mimic normal heart function.

These pacemaker models can sense indicators of physical activity that they then use to alter the heart rate. Just as a normal heart speeds up its rate during more activity and slows down during rest, the pacemaker changes its rate according to the activity it senses.

For example, one type of pacemaker senses motion of the body. When the body begins to move rapidly, the pacemaker concludes that the person is walking, running, climbing stairs, or doing some other type of exercise. The pacemaker raises the heart rate proportionately to the amount of activity it senses.

Another pacemaker senses the depth and rate of breathing. When breathing becomes heavy and fast, this pacemaker concludes that exertion is occurring and increases the heart rate.

Another pacemaker senses the temperature of the blood inside the ventricle. When you exercise, your blood temperature increases slightly because exercising muscle cells give off heat. This pacemaker increases heart rate as temperature increases.

PACEMAKER IMPLANTATION.
Implantation of a pacemaker is a relatively minor surgical procedure that is performed using local anesthesia. It takes about 1 hour. If you are not in the hospital already, you will be admitted the morning of or evening before your pacemaker implantation. You should not eat or drink anything after midnight. Your heart is monitored before, during, and after implantation. An intravenous (IV) catheter is inserted for administration of fluids and medications.

Your chest is cleaned with a special antibacterial soap and shaved if necessary. A special X-ray machine is positioned over you to help your doctor correctly place the pacemaker lead wires. The area of your incision, just below the collarbone, is numbed with a local anesthetic, and additional medication may be given through the IV catheter to help you relax.

The doctor inserts the lead wires into a vein under the collarbone and threads them into the right side of your heart. Tests are done to make sure that the wires are in the best possible location for pacing your heart. When the wires are positioned correctly, the doctor attaches them to the pulse generator, which is then positioned in a "pocket" beneath the skin and fat of your chest wall. The pacemaker is programmed so that the stimulus is strong enough to pace your heart, but not so strong as to waste battery energy.

You are taken back to your hospital room after the procedure. You can eat regular meals as tolerated. The pacemaker nurse or doctor will talk to you and your family about your pacemaker, including information about checking your pulse, your activity level, your incision, and telephone monitoring for follow-up care.

LIVING WITH YOUR PACEMAKER.
Your incision may be mildly tender for several weeks. After the initial swelling goes down, you may feel or see the outline of your pacemaker under the skin. You may shower or bathe 48 hours after your pacemaker implantation. Most people can be dismissed from the hospital 1 to 2 days after implantation of the pacemaker system. Occasionally, dismissal on the same day is possible.

For several weeks after implantation, you are advised not to drive (to make sure the pacemaker is working as it should and to avoid having the discomfort from the healing incision hamper your driving skills). You should temporarily avoid vigorous above-the-shoulder activities, golf, tennis, swimming, bicycling, bowling, and lifting anything that weighs more than 15 pounds. These activities may compromise the stability of the pacemaker lead as it becomes securely attached to the inner wall of the heart.

Contact your doctor if you experience increased swelling, redness, or drainage from the incision or a fever above 100° Fahrenheit.

Fortunately, there is very little that you must do to ensure that the pacemaker works properly. Activities that emit strong electromagnetic fields that may interfere with the function of the pacemaker, such as arc welding, should be avoided. In addition, you should avoid contact sports or shooting a shotgun or rifle from the shoulder where the pacemaker is positioned. Pacemakers are not harmed by airport monitoring devices, but they may cause the metal detector to signal. Airport security personnel are aware of this and can be of assistance. Modern pacemakers are not affected by microwave ovens.

Because pacemakers are battery-driven, they eventually wear down. It is not always possible to predict when this will happen, because it depends in part on how often the pacemaker is actually pacing versus being on standby. If your pacemaker has to stimulate your heart only occasionally, the batteries will last longer. However, if it has to stimulate your heart most of the time, the batteries will wear out sooner.

The batteries generally last between 5 and 15 years. The battery status, as well as the pacemaker function, can be monitored by telephone, so you usually do not have to make frequent office visits. A special telephone monitoring system is provided to you so you

Pacemaker precautions

- Do not arc-weld. Electromagnetic fields may interfere with your pacemaker function.
- Do not do mechanical work on a running car engine. Small electromagnetic fields are present.
- If you are to undergo magnetic resonance imaging (MRI), inform the doctor or medical staff that you have a pacemaker, because this procedure can pose problems for your pacemaker.
- If you have any type of operation in which electrocautery is used to control bleeding, precautions should be taken by your doctors to ensure normal pacemaker function throughout the operation.

can send an electrocardiogram and special signals over the telephone to a central monitoring office. These transmissions are recommended every 2 to 3 months.

When the pacemaker begins to send signals that the battery is weakening, you will be told to schedule an appointment for replacing the pulse generator. There is plenty of lag time to do so, and although there is generally no reason to delay, it usually need not be done urgently. The batteries are replaced by replacing the entire pulse generator; the original leads are checked, and they are generally satisfactory for continued use.

Defibrillation and Cardioversion

Some fast or chaotic heart rhythms are not effectively treated by medications. Rhythms such as ventricular fibrillation cause such catastrophic consequences (sudden cardiac death) that there is no time to begin a medication. Others, such as atrial fibrillation, may not respond to medications. Fortunately, an alternative form of treatment is available for these conditions.

EXTERNAL DEFIBRILLATION AND CARDIOVERSION.

Administering an electrical shock to the heart through the chest wall can convert the heart to a normal rhythm. When this procedure is used in people with ventricular fibrillation, it is called defibrillation. When it is used in people with less severe rhythm disorders, it is called cardioversion (conversion of cardiac rhythm to normal).

Defibrillation and cardioversion are thought to work by momentarily stopping the heart and the chaotic rhythm. This often allows the normal heart rhythm to take over again.

The size of the electrical shock ranges from 20 joules to 400 joules, which is thousands of times stronger than a pacemaker stimulus. A shock of this size can cause a person's entire body to twitch vigorously. When it is used for defibrillation of ventricular fibrillation, the person is unconscious and unaware of the shock. When cardioversion is done electively, you are put to sleep first for 2 or 3 minutes with a short-acting general anesthetic agent.

Elective cardioversion refers to cardioversion that is not done in an emergency; it is scheduled ahead of time. It is most commonly performed in people who have atrial fibrillation that has not responded to medications. Although you can survive and function well with atrial fibrillation, it is usually worth trying to restore normal sinus rhythm.

For at least 3 weeks before attempted cardioversion of atrial fibrillation, warfarin (see page 253) usually is given to prevent any formation of clot inside the fibrillating atria which might be dislodged by the shock and cause complications such as a stroke.

Before the cardioversion, you should not eat for 8 hours. An intravenous (IV) catheter is placed in your arm and you breathe oxygen through a face mask. A short-acting anesthetic is given through the vein, which puts you to sleep for 2 to 3 minutes. During that time the electrical shock is administered by a doctor. If necessary, two or three shocks may be given.

After the cardioversion, you wake up and are monitored for several hours, after which you may leave. You may be somewhat drowsy, so you should arrange transportation home ahead of time. If warfarin was used, it should be continued for another 2 to 4 weeks. The decision of whether to continue taking antiarrhythmic medications after cardioversion should be made by you and your doctor according to the likelihood that the rhythm will recur.

Most defibrillations and cardioversions are done in a hospital or by ambulance teams. In addition, a special type of defibrillator is now available which enables individuals untrained in interpreting electrocardiograms to administer lifesaving defibrillation in an emergency (see figure on page 250). Adhesive patches are applied to the chest wall, and they can sense the type of heart rhythm. The defibrillator then delivers a shock in an appropriate fashion. Although machines and computer chips are not infallible, this device improves the odds for people who require emergency defibrillation.

INTERNAL CARDIOVERTER-DEFIBRILLATOR. People who experience ventricular fibrillation are at risk of recurrence. People with ventricular tachycardia (see page 95) also may have serious symptoms such as loss of consciousness, and they may progress from ventricular tachycardia to ventricular fibrillation. Because no medication is 100 percent effective, special measures to manage any recurrence are often warranted.

Medications may be used to try to reduce the risk of recurring ventricular fibrillation or ventricular tachycardia, but a "safety net" may be desirable in case these rhythms occur despite the medications. Internal cardioverter-defibrillators provide this safety net and are being used increasingly.

Like pacemakers, internal cardioverter-defibrillators are battery-driven devices that are implanted in the body. However, they are larger than pacemaker generators (about the size of a package of index cards), and currently they cannot be fitted conveniently beneath the skin under the collarbone. Instead, they are implanted beneath the skin and muscle of the abdomen. Technologic advances will result in reduced size of future devices (see Figure 47, page A14).

Also, like pacemakers, wire electrodes are used to attach the pulse generator to the heart. The site of attachment and type of electrodes vary. Usually a combination of wires is used. Some wires are used for sensing the heartbeat and are inserted through veins into the inside of the heart. They can also be used for pacing, just like a regular pacemaker, should the need arise. Other wires may be attached to the outside of the heart, including "patches" that are sewn

onto the surface of the heart. These are used for delivering the shock to the heart when it is required. Some models do not require attaching electrode patches to the outside of the heart, but instead they use electrodes that go under the skin of the chest near the heart. Sometimes, the electrodes that deliver the shock are positioned inside the heart. Careful testing determines which specific design of internal cardioverter-defibrillator and which lead placement are used to give the most reliable response.

Because the implantation procedure is more involved than that with a pacemaker, and because people receiving internal cardioverter-defibrillators may have more dangerous problems, the average hospital stay after implantation is 3 to 7 days. You will stay in the intensive care unit after the operation, and the recovery is longer than with pacemaker implantation.

Internal cardioverter-defibrillators can sense the heart's rhythm and respond in a fashion that is designed to convert the heart to a normal rhythm. Some of these devices can tell when ventricular tachycardia occurs; they may then attempt to convert the rhythm by pacing the heart in special patterns that the cardiologist has programmed. If several of these attempts are unsuccessful, or if the chaotic rhythm of ventricular fibrillation develops, then the internal cardioverter-defibrillator directly shocks the heart. This is similar to the conventional external defibrillator, but the advantage of the internal device is that it is always with the person and ready to deliver a shock when needed.

The shock may feel different for each person and each event. It may feel like a kick or thump in the chest.

You will not feel the shock if you first pass out from the abnormal heart rhythm.

The devices are capable of functions besides defibrillation and cardioversion. Some include a pacemaker so that pacing therapy may be used if a slow heartbeat develops. They also can record on microchips information about any shocks that have been used. This helps your doctor determine whether the shocks were appropriate and optimally effective. You will return to the doctor for follow-up on a regular basis to have the device checked for proper function and to determine whether any shocks were needed since your last visit.

Although the use of this device may be lifesaving (and the evidence is clear that it frequently is), it does not prevent the loss of consciousness that may come when ventricular fibrillation starts. It takes about 10 to 30 seconds for the device to sense the abnormal rhythm and then give the shock. You may become dizzy or pass out during this time. Consequently, people with an internal defibrillator must still avoid activities such as driving a car that would put them and others at risk if ventricular fibrillation were to occur. However, the cardioverter-defibrillator significantly reduces the chance of dying from ventricular fibrillation.

Surgical and Catheter Treatment

Some fast rhythm disorders do not respond adequately to medications and are not appropriately treated with internal defibrillators. For example, some people have atrial fibrillation that causes the ventricles to beat exceedingly fast despite the use of medications (see page 92). This fast rate can be extremely uncomfortable or even potentially dangerous. Other people have fast rhythms that emanate directly from the atrioventricular node.

Some people have an abnormal "bridge" (in addition to the normal atrioventricular node) that electrically connects the atrium with the ventricles. This allows electrical impulses to travel from the atrium to the ventricle without going through the atrioventricular node. This condition, called Wolff-Parkinson-White syndrome (WPW; see page 95), can predispose a person to exceedingly rapid and potentially dangerous heart rhythms.

If medications are ineffective in any of these situations, other approaches are available.

SURGICAL TREATMENT. The "bridge," or accessory pathway, in WPW can be disconnected by a surgeon's scalpel. Operation has been a solution for this condition for several years, but now it has been largely replaced by catheter techniques.

Under some circumstances, rhythms such as ventricular tachycardia are found to emanate from a specific site in the heart muscle. If other means fail, removing that site surgically may prevent the rhythm from happening over and over again.

CATHETER ABLATION. Nonsurgical techniques with a special "ablation" (*ablation* means "elimination" or "removal") catheter have been perfected to the point that they are often used to treat WPW, rapid atrial fibrillation, or fast heart rates originating from the atrioventricular node.

Using special electrophysiologic studies (see page 224), specialists can determine where the accessory pathway is located in people with WPW (this technique is called mapping). The doctor inserts a special catheter so that it lies close to the pathway and then passes radiofrequency energy through it. The tip of the catheter heats up and destroys the precise area of the heart that contains the abnormal bridge of tissue (the accessory pathway).

If the atrioventricular node behaves abnormally by transmitting electrical impulses to the ventricle too fast (such as during rapid atrial fibrillation) or by initiating fast heartbeats, it can also be selectively damaged by radiofrequency ablation to slow the heart rate.

Catheter ablation procedures are proving to be effective in the management of these selected problems. Depending on the cause of the fast heart rate, radiofrequency ablation procedures may result in complete heart block, requiring a pacemaker. For example, to control the heart rate in people with rapid atrial fibrillation, radiofrequency ablation causes complete heart block in more than 90 percent of cases. The regular paced rhythm is a vast improvement over the symptomatic fast heart rates that were previously occurring. Ablation of the bridge in WPW very rarely causes complete heart block.

TREATING CIRCULATORY PROBLEMS

The many types of vascular problems that can jeopardize the circulatory function of the heart and blood vessels were discussed in Diseases of the Arteries and Veins, page 97. A wide range of therapeutic options are available. This section discusses the typical treatments for each of the general categories of vascular disease.

Atherosclerosis

Atherosclerotic disease in the arteries of the body impedes the blood flow to organs and tissues.

If you have intermittent claudication of the legs, your doctor will encourage you to walk (see page 99). Walking at least several times a day to the point of your limitation will improve your claudication over time.

Atherosclerotic arterial disease of the legs may improve with walking because of the development of collateral blood vessels, which are like the body's own bypass response. Although collateral vessels will not return the circulation to normal, they may reduce symptoms enough to eliminate or delay the need for more aggressive treatment. Walking also produces a "training effect" by improving muscle efficiency; the leg muscles can perform more work with the blood supply they receive.

MEDICATIONS. Your doctor may recommend aspirin to reduce the likelihood that platelets will clump at sites of atherosclerosis, form a blood clot, and cause further blockage. A medication called pentoxifylline tends to make red blood cells "softer." It makes the blood "slippery" and better able to flow through narrowed areas. For some people with claudication, this medication allows them to walk greater distances.

SURGICAL TREATMENT. If symptoms are severe and the blockage is bad enough to threaten the survival of muscle or skin tissue or to hamper the function of the organ the blood vessel supplies, then a bypass operation or a surgical "coring out" (endarterectomy) may be required. In suitable candidates, opening the blockage with a balloon catheter is possible, just as with the coronary arteries. Other types of catheters that use laser energy or mechanical devices to open the artery may be used in certain circumstances.

Arterial Thrombosis and Embolism

Just as in the coronary arteries, blood clots can develop at other sites of atherosclerosis and rapidly block a vessel (thrombosis) or break into fragments and block branches of vessels farther downstream (embolism). The result is a sudden cessation of blood flow to the areas supplied by the artery and branches. With the sudden blockage, there is no time for collateral arteries to develop. The body cannot compensate for this reduction in blood flow, and emergency medical attention is required.

Treatment may involve dissolving the blood clot with a thrombolytic agent (similar to the use of thrombolytic medications in myocardial infarction; see page 266) or removing the blood clot surgically. The clot must be removed within a few hours or the tissue supplied by the blocked artery may die, and amputation may be required.

MEDICATIONS. Thrombolytic medication that dissolves the clot may be given through a catheter directly to the affected area. People who have had arterial thrombosis or embolism or who are at risk of their development are treated with anticoagulants (blood thinners) to reduce the likelihood of blood clotting and future problems.

SURGICAL TREATMENT. The surgeon can remove a clot in an artery by making a small opening in the artery upstream from the blockage and passing a balloon-tipped catheter down past the blood clot (the clot is soft). Once the balloon is downstream from the blood clot, the doctor inflates it and pulls the catheter back to the opening in the artery. The balloon pulls the blood clot upstream where

A blood clot that has lodged in an artery can often be removed by passing a catheter beyond the clot and inflating a small balloon at the tip of the catheter. When the catheter is pulled back, the clot is dragged back to where it can be readily removed.

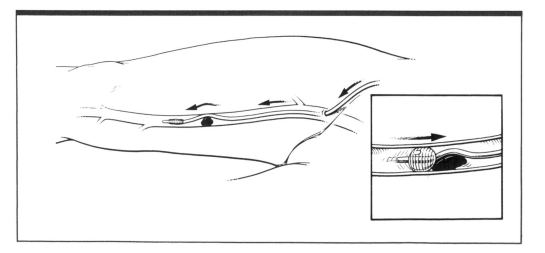

the doctor can remove it. Occasionally, it is necessary to replace or bypass the blocked vessel.

Aortic Aneurysm

Bulging in the aorta (aortic aneurysm) usually occurs in the abdominal portion of the aorta but may also be present in the chest (see Figure 49, page A15). Aneurysm carries a risk that the aorta may rupture (spring a leak).

If the aneurysm is small and you have no symptoms when it is discovered, your doctor may recommend careful monitoring at regular checkups to determine whether it is enlarging. Treatment is usually unnecessary until the aneurysm reaches a size at which the possibility of rupture is significant. For an abdominal aortic aneurysm, operation should be seriously considered when the diameter is 5 or 6 centimeters (about 2½ to 3 inches) or when a smaller aneurysm is enlarging rapidly.

MEDICATIONS.   Drugs have no specific value in aortic aneurysm, except that treating high blood pressure is prudent. The only way to reduce the risk of rupture is to repair the bulge surgically before a rupture occurs. Once the aneurysm ruptures, it may be too late to do anything, because rupture is often fatal within minutes to hours. Emergency operation is the only hope for survival when that occurs.

SURGICAL TREATMENT.   The operation for an aortic aneurysm is safe and relatively uncomplicated. It consists of replacing the area of the bulge, where the arterial wall is weak, with a tube made of synthetic material. With time, the normal lining cells of the blood vessel grow into the inner surface of the tube, producing a durable conduit for blood to flow through.

Aortic Dissection

Dissection of the aorta, in which the layers of the aortic wall separate from one another (see page 102), is a medical emergency. Not only does it cause pain but also the risk of impending death is very high if the tear should go completely through the wall.

Once the presence of dissection is established by tests such as computed tomography, echocardiography, magnetic resonance imaging, or aortography, an emergency surgical procedure is usually advisable. Occasionally, some specific variations of aortic dissection may be treated with medication alone.

MEDICATIONS.   As you might imagine, if the blood pressure is high in the aorta, the likelihood of extending the tear increases. Therefore, the first treatment action is to keep the blood pressure low by using intravenous medications. Narcotics may be required for control of pain.

SURGICAL TREATMENT. Operation for aortic dissection consists of either replacing a portion of the aorta where the tear originated with a synthetic material, or "tacking down" the tear with a suture (a "stitch") so that blood can no longer force its way through the opening. If repairing the dissection involves replacing parts of the aorta where vessels branch off to the brain, arms, kidneys, or other organs, the surgeon must disconnect the branch vessels and reconnect them to the synthetic tube.

Arteritis (Inflammation of the Arteries)

The inflammation of arteritis (*itis* refers to "inflammation") can result in obstruction of the arteries, which reduces the supply of blood reaching the affected areas.

MEDICATIONS. Inflammatory conditions of the arteries are usually treated with medications that reduce inflammation. The most potent anti-inflammatory medications are corticosteroid drugs. These medications are all related to cortisone. The side effects from these agents are minimized by giving them in the smallest dose needed to control symptoms adequately, and they are decreased or discontinued as the condition resolves.

SURGICAL TREATMENT. Some types of arteritis may cause blockage of the vessels, even after the active inflammation has been treated or has gone away. Occasionally, an operation may be needed to bypass or open the blockage.

Arterial Spasm

The first step in treating arterial spasm is to determine whether there are any provoking factors and to avoid them. Some medications, such as ergotamines used for treating migraine headaches, may provoke arterial spasm. Cold temperatures can provoke Raynaud's phenomenon (see page 105).

MEDICATIONS. As with coronary spasm, treatment may include the use of medications that prevent the smooth muscle in the artery wall from over-contracting. Thus, vasodilators (see page 252) are the preferred medications.

Venous Thrombosis

As with most problems, the best way to treat venous thrombosis is to prevent it. Preventive measures are aimed primarily at people who have had thrombosis before or who are at greater risk of it developing because of prolonged bed rest, immobility resulting from operation or other diseases, or injury to the legs and leg veins.

PREVENTION. People in these situations, such as those in the hospital recovering from operation or a heart attack, are often given anticoagulants until they are able to get up and move around. Anticoagulants are given temporarily in relatively low doses. The usual method is to give small injections of heparin under the skin twice a day. This dosage is enough to minimize the risk of a blood clot forming inside a vein, yet it is low enough to avoid most of the complications of blood thinning such as a tendency to bleed or bruise.

Support stockings are recommended for individuals confined to bed or who have had damage to the veins of the legs. The stockings help prevent pooling of blood in the veins and thus decrease the chance that it will clot.

MEDICATIONS. If venous thrombosis does develop (see page 105), you will require full doses of anticoagulants. The treatment of deep vein thrombosis of the legs requires hospitalization so that heparin can be given in full doses, usually by vein. After about 5 days of effective heparin therapy (the effectiveness is measured by blood tests that monitor the ability of the blood to clot), your treatment will be switched to warfarin. Treatment for deep vein thrombosis with warfarin, which is taken by mouth, is usually continued for 3 to 6 months.

People on anticoagulation therapy must have periodic blood tests to measure the prothrombin time ("protime") to make sure that the blood's tendency to clot has been reduced enough but not too much (see page 192). The prothrombin time is compared with a normal prothrombin time. For anticoagulation to be effective, the prothrombin time should be about 1.3 to 1.5 times more than the duration of the normal prothrombin time, but this varies among different laboratories.

Because deep vein thrombosis may lead to venous insufficiency, in which the veins are unable to return the blood to the heart adequately (see page 109), measures to reduce this consequence include the use of support hose and periodic leg elevation.

Pulmonary Embolism

If a thrombus (clot) in the deep veins of the leg breaks loose, it is carried by the blood through the veins into the heart and out into the pulmonary arteries, where it lodges and obstructs blood flow to a portion of the lungs. Depending on the size of the pulmonary embolism, the results may range from no symptoms, to chest pain and shortness of breath, to shock and death.

MEDICATIONS. For pulmonary emboli that do not immediately threaten survival, blood thinners are used to prevent the embolism from getting worse. You must be hospitalized and given heparin, after which you are treated with warfarin for 6 months to a year.

For more extensive pulmonary embolism, the use of thrombolytic agents to dissolve the blood clot has been shown to improve the blood flow and promote survival.

SURGICAL TREATMENT. For particularly life-threatening pulmonary emboli, an emergency operation may be required to remove the blood clot from the lung arteries.

Pulmonary Hypertension

Pulmonary hypertension, regardless of the cause, is seldom completely reversible if it is bad enough to cause symptoms of breathlessness, chest pressure, or blacking out.

MEDICATIONS. Vasodilators have been shown to improve pulmonary hypertension in some people, but they rarely normalize the elevated blood pressure in the lungs completely and must often be used in high doses. The use of vasodilators should be started in the hospital during careful monitoring with a pressure-measuring (Swan-Ganz) catheter in the pulmonary artery (see page 223). Some people with pulmonary hypertension treated with vasodilators may become worse if the vasodilators lower their "regular" blood pressure more than their pulmonary blood pressure.

A blood thinner (warfarin) has been shown to increase lifespan in people with pulmonary hypertension. Your doctor may also recommend the use of oxygen on a regular continuous basis, because one of the consequences of pulmonary hypertension is a low level of oxygen in the bloodstream.

SURGICAL TREATMENT.   On rare occasions, people with pulmonary hypertension may have a large thrombus (clot) in the pulmonary artery (presum-ably from an old pulmonary embolism), even though they do not have a specific history of having a pulmonary embolism. In these cases, the pulmonary hypertension may be improved or reversed by surgical removal of the blood clot. Lung transplantation or heart-lung transplantation may be a consideration for people with severe pulmonary hypertension.

TREATING PERICARDIAL PROBLEMS

Pericardial Effusion and Tamponade

The accumulation of excessive fluid in the pericardial sac surrounding the heart (pericardial effusion) can make the heart's pumping task more difficult and lead to tamponade, a condition in which the heart is compressed in the sac too tightly to expand properly. It may lead to low blood pressure, shock, or symptoms of rapidly developing heart failure. This situation requires urgent treatment by draining the fluid from the pericardial sac surrounding the heart.

PERICARDIOCENTESIS.   Pericar-diocentesis (*centesis* means "puncture") is the technique for removing excess fluid from the pericardial sac. To drain the fluid, the doctor anesthe-tizes an area of skin over the chest wall or upper abdomen next to the heart and inserts a needle directly into the fluid-filled pericardial sac. Echocardi-ographic images (see page 209) may be useful to guide the path of the needle into the pericardial space. The fluid can be drained off either through the needle or through a soft catheter that can replace the needle. If there is concern that the fluid may reaccumulate, a catheter can be left in place for several days if necessary to continue draining the fluid.

Even in cases of pericardial effusion in which there is no tamponade, it may be advisable to remove at least some

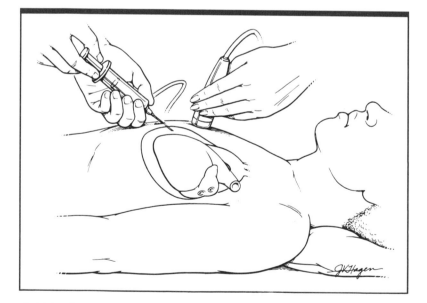

Fluid in the pericardial sac can accumulate enough to press on the heart and impair its pumping function. The fluid can often be removed by inserting a needle through the skin and into the distended pericardial sac, using guidance by an echocardiogram. The fluid can then be drained through the needle.

of the fluid so that it can be inspected to help determine the underlying cause (see page 113).

Pericarditis

Pericarditis (see page 112) is inflammation of the pericardium. It may cause pain and irritation. Inflammation is one of the causes of excess fluid in the pericardial sac.

MEDICATIONS. Pain may be substantially alleviated during the natural healing process, by anti-inflammatory medications. Aspirin, the most common anti-inflammatory agent, is often effective. Sometimes other anti-inflammatory agents such as indomethacin may be used. These medications have anti-inflammatory actions similar to those of corticosteroids, although they are not corticosteroids. Thus, they are sometimes called nonsteroidal anti-inflammatory drugs (NSAIDs). The reduction of inflammation produced by any of these medications also reduces the resulting pain.

Rarely, corticosteroids may be required to alleviate the pain of pericar-

ditis. However, a recurring pattern may develop in which the symptoms of pericarditis are reduced by the corticosteroid, so use of the corticosteroid is stopped. Without the drug the pain recurs. Treatment with corticosteroids should be avoided because of the significant number of side effects associated with their use, and because of the increased risk of recurrent pericarditis.

SURGICAL TREATMENT. If recurrent pericarditis is a problem, as it sometimes is, your doctor may advise a surgical procedure to remove the pericardium from the surface of the heart. This usually ends your symptoms.

In conditions in which the pericardium becomes thickened and stiff, the resulting pericardial constriction (see page 113) may significantly impede the pumping function of the heart. Surgical "stripping" of the pericardium (pericardiectomy: removing the pericardium from the surface of the heart) may be required to reverse this problem. Fortunately, there are rarely any noticeable disadvantages to being without the pericardium.

MEDICATIONS FOR THE TREATMENT OF HEART DISEASES

The tables on the following pages contain information about various medications that are used to treat many aspects of heart disease. For each medication there are specific reasons why it may be especially right (or wrong) for your health problem. The tables in this book cannot tell you which, if any, medication is best for you—this can be determined only by your doctor after

appropriate evaluation. The information in the tables is intended to provide you with background information about medications you may be taking, as well as similar medications.

Names of Medications

Each medication has several names. The *generic name* is the name that refers to all medications with the same chemical structure, regardless of which manufacturer makes them. Some medications are made by more than one manufacturer; each pharmaceutical company uses a different *proprietary* (or *brand*) *name*. In general, medications with the same generic name are equal. However, they usually are combined with other substances to make a dosage form such as a tablet, capsule, or liquid (1 milligram of a medicine, for example, is too small to handle conveniently so it is combined with an inactive substance). Differences in the inactive substances may affect the way the same generic medication acts. As a result, the dosage form must be the same to be considered equivalent. Your doctor may permit use of a generically equivalent medication. If so, you can discuss your options with your pharmacist. Not all medications are available generically, because they may still be under patent protection.

Doses of Medications

For a medication to be useful, an adequate amount must get into the bloodstream and go to the organs and tissues where it produces its effect. Once the medication is in the body, the body (usually the kidneys or liver) begins to eliminate it. If no more medication were taken, eventually there would no longer be any left in the body. If a sustained effect is desired, an appropriate amount must be taken periodically to maintain an effective level in the body. The size and timing of the dose depend on how much is needed to produce the beneficial effect, how well it gets into the bloodstream (for example,

how much is absorbed from the intestines), and how rapidly the body eliminates it.

Some medications also come in a form that provides them with a longer duration of action, so that doses do not need to be taken as frequently. The names of these "long-acting" or "sustained-release" medications usually have an abbreviation after the brand name, such as LA, SR, XL, or CD.

The specific dose of a medication that is best for you must be determined by your doctor. This information is not included in the tables, because there is no "right" dose for everyone.

Indications for Medications

The reason a medication is given is the "indication" for its use. Nearly every medication that is prescribed has been approved for one or more indications by the Food and Drug Administration (FDA) after tests showed it was effective and safe. Some medications are useful for indications that have not been formally approved by the FDA. A medication approved for treatment of high blood pressure may be very effective for the treatment of angina also and can be used for that purpose, even if it is not officially listed as approved for that indication.

Thus, not all medications in the tables have been FDA-approved for the use listed in the table in which they appear. Rather than listing each medication in numerous tables, a medication's multiple uses are shown in the "Uses" column of a single table. For example, if you take metoprolol (a beta-adrenergic blocker) for blood pressure control, you will not find it in

Table 6, "Medications for High Blood Pressure." Rather, you will be referred to Table 2, "Medications for Angina: Beta Blockers" (page 298), which provides information about the entire "family" of beta-adrenergic blockers. However, not every beta-adrenergic blocker is necessarily used commonly for the treatment of angina. The "Heart Drug Directory" (page 343) is a useful index of commonly used heart medications which will help you find your medication in the tables.

Combinations of Medications

Sometimes more than one medication is needed for treatment of a problem. Some combinations of medications are used frequently enough that pharmaceutical companies have combined them into a single tablet or capsule and have given the combination its own brand name. A few combinations are shown in the tables, but many are not, so you may need to look up the separate components if you want to learn about a combination medication you are taking.

Side Effects

Medications may have undesirable effects in some people. Sometimes it is because of an allergy to the medication. Some medications produce unpleasant or even dangerous effects in one person but not in another. If given in high enough doses (overdose), every medication will produce toxic effects. What may be an effective dose in one person may be too high for another individual.

In the tables, some of the more commonly encountered or serious side effects are listed for each medication. Not every side effect is necessarily included. The fact that a side effect is listed also does not mean it will occur in you.

Precautions and Contraindications

Some individuals are at higher risk of having an adverse effect from a medication. For them, certain precautions should be kept in mind; the tables indicate major precautions for most medications. For some people, the risk of using a medication is higher than any benefit that might occur; for them, the medication is "contraindicated."

The following precautions are not listed individually in the tables because they apply to many or all medications.

- Many medications may be potentially risky during pregnancy.
- Many medications may be passed on to infants through breast milk.
- The effect of medications must be periodically monitored by appropriate examinations or tests.
- The way a medication is taken (for example, with or without food, time of day) should be adhered to as recommended by the doctor and pharmacist.
- Various medications can interact when taken together and thus their individual effects can increase, decrease, or change. This possibility should be checked with the doctor and pharmacist.
- Do not chew or crush long-acting (slow-release) forms of medications.

Table 1. Medications for Angina: Nitrates

Type of Medication	Generic Name	Examples of Brand Names	Uses	How Taken	Specific Side Effects	Specific Precautions
Nitrates The nitrates all have the following actions: 1. Dilate veins of the body 2. Dilate arteries of the body 3. Dilate coronary arteries The effects of these actions are: 1. Redistribution of some of the volume of blood from the chambers of your heart to the veins of the body. This decreases the amount of stretching of the heart muscle. The less stretch or stress, the less oxygen the heart uses. This is the main way that nitrates lower the heart's demand for oxygen, which is helpful in view of the reduced supply 2. Lowering of the resistance the heart encounters in pumping blood into the arteries. This decreases the work load of the heart so that its need for oxygen is reduced 3. Increase in the amount of blood that can flow through partially blocked coronary arteries. This enhances the oxygen supply to the heart muscle	Nitroglycerin	*Nitrostat* (tablets)	Shorten angina attack Prevent anticipated angina attack	Let tablet dissolve under tongue at onset of angina, while sitting. If needed, repeat dose twice, 5 minutes between doses One tablet under tongue at onset of activity predicted to cause angina	See general side effects listed below Tingling under the tongue is normal	Loses potency 3–6 months after opening container Remove cotton plug and leave out Keep container tightly closed If angina persists for 15 minutes, go to doctor or emergency room
		Nitrolingual (spray)	Shorten angina attack Prevent anticipated angina attack	1 or 2 sprays on or under tongue at onset of angina, while sitting. If needed, repeat dose twice, 5 minutes between doses 1 or 2 sprays on or under tongue at onset of activity predicted to cause angina	See general side effects listed below	Do not shake container Do not inhale If angina persists for 15 minutes, go to doctor or emergency room
		Nitrogard (buccal extended-release tablets)	Prevent angina attacks	Place tablet between upper lip and gum, or between cheek and gum. Allow to dissolve over 3–5 hours	See general side effects listed below	Do not chew or swallow
		Nitrol (ointment)	Prevent angina attacks	Spread (do not rub in) the prescribed amount of ointment in thin layer on hairless area of skin at prescribed schedule. Use applicator paper that is provided	See general side effects listed below Skin irritation	Clean off previous ointment before reapplication Rotate application sites to avoid irritation

Drug	Use	Administration	Side effects	Precautions
Nitro-Bid (capsules)	Prevent angina attacks	Swallow tablet at prescribed dose and schedule	See general side effects listed below	Do not stop taking abruptly (to avoid rebound)
Minitran *Nitro-disc* *Nitro-Dur* *Transderm-Nitro* *Deponit* (transdermal patches) *Nitro-Bid IV* *Nitrol IV* *Nitrostat IV* *Tridil*	Prevent angina attacks	Apply skin patch for prescribed duration on relatively hairless skin	See general side effects listed below; Skin irritation	Rotate application sites to avoid irritation; Avoid skin with nicks or cuts; Remove patch for 6–8 hours before replacing (to avoid tolerance)
Nitroglycerin (intravenous)	Manage heart attack	Given by vein	See general side effects listed below	
Isosorbide dinitrate — *Isordil* (tablets) *Sorbitrate* (tablets) *Dilatrate* (tablets)	Prevent angina attacks; Reduce work load of heart	Swallow tablet at prescribed schedule with full glass of water on empty stomach	See general side effects listed below	Do not stop taking abruptly (to avoid rebound)
Pentaerythrityl tetranitrate — *Peritrate* (tablets)	Prevent angina attacks	Swallow tablet at prescribed schedule with full glass of water on empty stomach	See general side effects listed below	Do not stop taking abruptly (to avoid rebound)
Erythrityl tetranitrate — *Cardilate* (tablets)	Prevent angina attacks	Swallow tablet at prescribed schedule with full glass of water on empty stomach	See general side effects listed below	Do not stop taking abruptly (to avoid rebound)

General side effects: Headache, dizziness, light-headedness, fast pulse, nausea.

General precautions: After chewing chewable tablets, hold in your mouth for 2 minutes before swallowing.

Alcohol may worsen some side effects (dizziness, light-headedness).

Some side effects (headache) generally lessen after several days of taking the medication.

A rebound effect (sudden worsening of angina or a heart attack) may occur if nitrate use is suddenly stopped. A tapered withdrawal is recommended.

The effect of nitrates diminishes if a constant amount is in the bloodstream all the time ("tolerance"). Skin patches should be removed for a period of each day.

Beta blockers (see Table 2)   Calcium channel blockers (see Table 3)

This list is not comprehensive and does not represent an endorsement of any product listed.

Table 2.   Medications for Angina: Beta Blockers

Type of Medication	Generic Name	Examples of Brand Names	Uses	How Taken	Specific Side Effects	Specific Precautions
Beta blockers The beta blockers all have the following actions: 1. Slow the heartbeat 2. Decrease blood pressure 3. Reduce the contraction strength of the heart muscle The effects of these actions are: 1. Reduction of your heart's need for oxygen by reducing the number of times it beats per minute both at rest and during exertion. This is the main way that beta blockers lower your heart's demand for oxygen, which is helpful in view of the reduced supply. 2. Lowering of the pressure your heart must pump against to push blood into the arteries. The lower the pressure, the less oxygen is required	Propranolol Metoprolol Nadolol Atenolol Acebutolol Betaxolol Labetalol Penbutolol Pindolol Timolol Carteolol (tablets, capsules)	*Inderal Lopressor Corgard Tenormin Sectral Kerlone Normodyne, Trandate Levatol Visken Blocadren Cartrol*	Prevent angina attacks Lower blood pressure Slow or convert fast heart rhythms Lower risk of second heart attack	Swallow tablet at prescribed dose and schedule	Abnormal slowing of the heartbeat Fatigue or weakness Lower sexual ability Light-headedness Restless sleep Depression	Asthma, bronchitis, emphysema: may provoke wheezing and breathlessness Claudication: may worsen circulation Heart failure: may worsen heart pumping strength and provoke shortness of breath and edema Diabetes: may lower blood glucose (sugar) or make hypoglycemic episodes (insulin reactions) harder to detect and respond to
3. Lowering of the squeezing strength of your heart's contraction. This lowers the oxygen use by the heart muscle 4. Lowering of blood pressure in people with hypertension 5. Helping normalize some types of fast or irregular heart rhythms	Intravenous: Propranolol Metoprolol Atenolol Esmolol	*Inderal Lopressor Tenormin Brevibloc*	Rapid control of high blood pressure Rapid control of fast heartbeats To continue beta blocker in hospitalized patient who cannot take medication by mouth For early treatment of heart attack, to lower chances of further damage	Administered by vein		Same as above

Nitrates (see Table 1)   Calcium channel blockers (see Table 3)   This list is not comprehensive and does not represent an endorsement of any product listed.

Table 3.   Medications for Angina: Calcium Channel Blockers

Type of Medication	Generic Name	Examples of Brand Names	Uses	How Taken	Specific Side Effects	Specific Precautions
Calcium channel blockers The calcium blockers all inhibit the ability of calcium atoms to enter heart muscle and blood vessel muscle cells. This results in the following effects (although each calcium blocker differs from the others in how much it produces each effect): 1. Reduction in the heart rate, thus reducing its demand for oxygen	Verapamil	Calan Isoptin Verelan	Prevent angina attacks Lower blood pressure Slow or normalize certain fast heart rhythms	Swallow tablet at prescribed dose and schedule	Excessive slowing of heartbeat Excessive lowering of blood pressure Congestive heart failure if heart contraction already weak Constipation	Caution in people with: Abnormally slow heartbeat Weakened heart contraction Low blood pressure Interactions with other medications
2. Lowering of the squeezing strength of the heart's contraction. This lowers the oxygen use by the heart muscle	Verapamil (intravenous)	Calan Isoptin	Urgent control of certain rapid heart rhythms	Given by vein	Same as above	Same as above
3. Decreasing of blood pressure and the resistance to blood flow through the arteries. This makes the heart's task of pumping blood easier and reduces its need for oxygen	Nifedipine	Procardia Adalat	Prevent angina attacks Lower blood pressure	Swallow tablet at prescribed dose and schedule	Excessive lowering of blood pressure Headache Leg edema Flushing sensation	Caution if blood pressure is low Interactions with other medications
4. Dilation of coronary arteries so that blood flow is enhanced. This increases the amount of oxygen delivered to heart muscle	Nicardipine	Cardene	Prevent angina attacks Lower blood pressure	Swallow tablet at prescribed dose and schedule	Excessive lowering of blood pressure Headache Leg edema Flushing sensation	Caution if blood pressure is low Interactions with other medications
	Diltiazem	Cardizem	Prevent angina attacks Lower blood pressure	Swallow tablet at prescribed dose and schedule	Excessive lowering of blood pressure Excessive slowing of heartbeat Rash	Caution if blood pressure is low Interactions with other medications
5. Helping normalize some types of fast or irregular heart rhythms	Isradipine	DynaCirc	Prevent angina attacks Lower blood pressure	Swallow tablet at prescribed dose and schedule	Excessive lowering of blood pressure Headache Leg edema Flushing sensation	Caution if blood pressure is low Interactions with other medications

Table 3. Medications for Angina: Calcium Channel Blockers (Continued)

Type of Medication	Generic Name	Examples of Brand Names	Uses	How Taken	Specific Side Effects	Specific Precautions
	Felodipine	*Plendil*	Prevent angina attacks Lower blood pressure	Swallow tablet at prescribed dose and schedule	Excessive lowering of blood pressure Headache Flushing sensation Fast heartbeat Leg edema	Caution if blood pressure is low Interactions with other medications
	Bepridil	*Vascor*	Prevent angina attacks	Swallow tablet at prescribed dose and schedule	Excessive lowering of blood pressure Headache Nervousness, tremor Nausea Rhythm problems	Caution if blood pressure is low

Nitrates (see Table 1)   Beta blockers (see Table 2)

This list is not comprehensive and does not represent an endorsement of any product listed.

Table 4. Medications for Heart Attack

Type of Medication	Generic Name	Examples of Brand Names	Uses	How Taken	Specific Side Effects	Specific Precautions
Thrombolytics Thrombolytic agents are medications that promote the dissolving of clots. They are used to restore blood flow through vessels that are obstructed by a blood clot (thrombus)	Urokinase	*Abbokinase*	Dissolve clots in arteries to the lung (pulmonary embolism) Dissolve clots in coronary arteries during heart attack	Given by vein	Bleeding, including internal bleeding, bleeding into brain, bleeding from sites of injury or incisions	Avoid if recent injury or operation, bleeding tendency, severe high blood pressure
	Tissue plasminogen activator (tPA; alteplase)	*Activase*	Same as above	Given by vein	Same as above	Same as above
	Streptokinase	*Kabikinase* *Streptase*	Same as above	Given by vein	Same as above, and rare allergic reactions	Same as above, and avoid if previously received streptokinase or anistreplase
	Anistreplase	*Eminase*	Same as above	Given by vein	Same as above, and rare allergic reactions	Same as above, and avoid if previously received streptokinase or anistreplase

Nitrates (see Table 1)   Beta blockers (see Table 2)

This list is not comprehensive and does not represent an endorsement of any product listed.

Table 5. Lipid-Lowering Medications

Type of Medication	Generic Name	Examples of Brand Names	Uses	How Taken	Specific Side Effects	Specific Precautions
Bile acid sequestrants These medications chemically bind to bile acids in the intestine. Bile acids are made by the body from cholesterol. They normally pass from the liver into the intestine, but a portion return into the bloodstream through the intestinal wall. These medications do not permit them to return, so more cholesterol is used to make more bile acids, which in turn are also excreted. Eventually, the body's pool of cholesterol decreases	Cholestyramine	Questran (powder)	Lower cholesterol	Mix powder with beverage (4–6 oz)—it will not actually dissolve—and drink all the liquid. Mix with other liquid foods if desired (soup, cereal, fruit)	Constipation Abdominal pain and upset	Avoid taking at same time as other medications Take other medications 1 hour before or 6 hours after taking this medication Double-check possibility of interactions with other medications. Other cardiovascular medications that may be affected: digitalis, anticoagulants, propranolol, thiazide, diuretics
		Cholybar (chewable bar)	Lower cholesterol	Eat it like a candy bar—chew thoroughly	Constipation Abdominal pain and upset	
	Colestipol	Colestid (granules)	Lower cholesterol	Mix powder with beverage (4–6 oz)—it will not actually dissolve—and drink all the liquid. Mix with other liquid foods if desired (soup, cereal, fruit)	Constipation Abdominal pain and upset	Do not take as dry powder
Gemfibrozil This medication reduces triglyceride and VLDL cholesterol, and raises HDL cholesterol. The way it does this is not well understood	Gemfibrozil	Lopid	Lower triglycerides Raise HDL cholesterol	Swallow tablet at prescribed dose and schedule	Stomach upset Nausea, diarrhea Rash Muscle pain, weakness Liver function problems Dizziness Blurred vision	Do not take lovastatin while taking this medication. The risk of muscle inflammation increases
HMG-CoA reductase inhibitor This medication enhances your body's ability to rid itself of cholesterol	Lovastatin Pravastatin Simvastatin	Mevacor Pravachol Zocor	Lower LDL cholesterol Lower triglycerides Raise HDL cholesterol (slightly)	Swallow tablet at prescribed dose and schedule	Blurred vision Muscle pain, weakness Stomach upset Liver function problems Insomnia Headache	Do not take gemfibrozil or nicotinic acid (niacin) while taking this medication. The risk of muscle inflammation increases Other medications that may interact include

Medication	Brand names	Purpose	How to take	Side effects	Special instructions
(continued from previous page)					cyclosporine, other immunosuppressants, warfarin, clofibrate. Blood tests for liver function should be performed every 4–6 weeks for first year. Annual eye examination may be advisable
Niacin (nicotinic acid) — This medication reduces your body's ability to manufacture VLDL cholesterol	Nia-Bid, Niacels, Nicobid, Nicolar, Slo-Niacin, Nicotinex (elixir)	Lower LDL cholesterol, Lower triglycerides, Raise HDL cholesterol	Swallow tablet (or elixir) at prescribed dose and schedule. Do not break or crush long-acting forms	Flushing, warm feeling, Headache, Stomach upset, Liver function problems, Itching	Side effects can be minimized by starting at low doses, taking with food, and building up to recommended dose. Persistent flushing can be reduced by taking 1 aspirin one-half hour before dose. Blood tests for liver function should be performed occasionally
Clofibrate — This medication reduces triglycerides and, to a lesser extent, cholesterol (when triglycerides are also high), but the way it works is not understood	Atromid-S	Lower triglycerides, Lower cholesterol	Swallow tablet at prescribed dose and schedule	Gallstones, Kidney problems, Stomach upset, Muscle pain, weakness, Pancreatitis, Liver function problems	Periodic blood tests for liver function, muscle inflammation (creatine kinase), and blood count are advisable
Probucol — This medication reduces cholesterol more than triglycerides by unknown mechanisms	Lorelco	Lower cholesterol, Lower triglycerides	Swallow tablet at prescribed dose and schedule	Rhythm disorders, Stomach upset, diarrhea	Periodic electrocardiogram to detect rhythm abnormalities. Take with meals
Dextrothyroxine — This medication increases your body's ability to break down and remove cholesterol, but the mechanism is unclear	Choloxin	Lower cholesterol	Swallow tablet at prescribed dose and schedule	Heart attack, Angina, Hyperactive thyroid	Can interact with other medications, especially digitalis and anticoagulants. Avoid if heart disease is already present

Dietary measures should be attempted first except in severe cases.
Continue to follow dietary recommendations while taking medications.
For all medications, lipid values should be checked within 3 months to determine the degree of success and to decide whether a change in dose or medication is needed.

This list is not comprehensive and does not represent an endorsement of any product listed.

Table 6. Medications for High Blood Pressure

Type of Medication	Generic Name	Examples of Brand Names	Uses	How Taken	Specific Side Effects	Specific Precautions
Centrally acting agents These medications affect control centers in the brain which decrease blood pressure	Methyldopa Guanfacine Guanabenz Clonidine	*Aldomet* *Tenex* *Wytensin* *Catapres*	Decrease blood pressure	Swallow tablet at prescribed dose and schedule	Fluid retention (edema) Fever Insomnia Low blood pressure Dizziness Liver function or blood cell count abnormalities Dry mouth	May need to stand slowly from lying position to avoid sudden blood pressure drop and faintness Do not stop taking abruptly (sudden excess rebound in high blood pressure) Double-check possibility of interactions with other medications
	Clonidine (skin patch)	*Catapres-TTS*		Apply skin patch at prescribed schedule	Drowsiness Itching (skin patch)	
Direct-acting vasodilators These medications cause the muscle in the walls of blood vessels to relax	Hydralazine	*Apresoline*	Decrease blood pressure Reduce work load of heart	Swallow tablet at prescribed dose and schedule	Low blood pressure Dizziness Lupus syndrome (blisters, chest pain, joint pain, weakness) Diarrhea Headache	May need to stand slowly from lying position to avoid sudden blood pressure drop and faintness
	Minoxidil	*Loniten*	Decrease blood pressure	Swallow tablet at prescribed dose and schedule	Fast heartbeat Flushing Fluid retention (edema) Excessive hair growth	Check resting heart rate periodically Check weight (to assess fluid gain)
Peripherally acting agents These medications exert their effects on the nerves of the body which are involved in blood pressure regulation	Guanadrel Guanethidine Mecamylamine Prazosin Rauwolfia alkaloids Terazosin Doxazosin	*Hylorel* *Ismelin* *Inversine* *Minipress* *Harmonyl,* *Raudixin,* *Rauzide,* *Serpasil* *Hytrin* *Cardura*	Decrease blood pressure	Swallow tablet at prescribed dose and schedule	Fluid retention (edema) Low blood pressure Dizziness Drowsiness Difficulty ejaculating Mental depression Stomach and bowel disturbances	Double-check possibility of interactions with medications May need to stand slowly from lying position to avoid sudden blood pressure drop and faintness

Beta blockers (see Table 2)   Calcium blockers (see Table 3)   Diuretics (see Table 7)   Angiotensin converting enzyme inhibitors (see Table 7)
This list is not comprehensive and does not represent an endorsement of any product listed.

Table 7. Medications for Heart Failure

Type of Medication	Generic Name	Examples of Brand Names	Uses	How Taken	Specific Side Effects	Specific Precautions
Angiotensin converting enzyme inhibitors (ACE inhibitors) These medications dilate arteries and decrease resistance to the flow of blood being pumped from the heart. The result is lower blood pressure and easier pumping for the heart	Captopril	Capoten	Decrease blood pressure Reduce work load of heart	Swallow tablet at prescribed dose and schedule	Low blood pressure Rash Elevated potassium Persistent dry cough Abnormal sense of taste Protein in urine Stomach upset	Avoid taking simultaneously with potassium-sparing diuretics (below) Use with caution in diabetes or with kidney problems
	Enalapril	Vasotec				
	Lisinopril	Zestril, Prinivil				
	Benazepril Fosinopril Ramipril	Lotensin Monopril Altace				
Diuretics These medications promote the removal of water by the kidneys. This decreases blood pressure and decreases edema	Chlorthalidone	Hygroton, Thalitone	Milder diuretics for: Decreasing blood pressure Gentle fluid reduction	Swallow tablet at prescribed dose and schedule	Low potassium High calcium Low sodium Elevated blood glucose (sugar) Risk of gout Stomach upset Pancreatitis	Check potassium, sodium, calcium, glucose periodically
	Chlorothiazide Hydrochloro-thiazide	Diuril Esidrix, HydroDIURIL, Oretic				
	Methyclothi-azide Metolazone	Aquatensen, Enduron Diulo, Zaroxolyn				
	Amiloride Spironolactone Triamterene	Midamor Aldactone Dyrenium	As above, but without loss of potassium in the urine ("potassium-sparing")	Swallow tablet at prescribed dose and schedule	Male breast enlargement (spironolactone) Elevated potassium Stomach upset	Check potassium, sodium, calcium, glucose periodically Avoid simultaneous use of ACE inhibitors (may increase potassium markedly)
"Combination" medications						
Hydrochloro-thiazide + Amiloride + Spirono-lactone + Triamterene		Moduretic Aldactazide Dyazide, Maxzide	As above, but with reduced loss of potassium in the urine	Swallow tablet as prescribed dose and schedule	Male breast enlargement (spironolactone) Variable potassium Stomach upset	Check potassium, sodium, calcium, glucose periodically Avoid simultaneous use of ACE inhibitors (may increase potassium markedly)

Table 7.   Medications for Heart Failure (Continued)

Type of Medication	Generic Name	Examples of Brand Names	Uses	How Taken	Specific Side Effects	Specific Precautions
	Bumetanide Ethacrynic acid Furosemide (tablet or intravenous)	*Bumex* *Edecrin* *Lasix*	Potent diuretics for vigorous reduction of excess fluid	Swallow tablet at prescribed dose and schedule Administer by vein	Excess fluid output Low blood pressure Low potassium Low calcium Low sodium Elevated blood glucose (sugar) Risk of gout Stomach upset Decreased hearing Muscle cramps	Double-check possibility of interactions with other medications Check potassium, sodium, calcium, glucose periodically
Inotropic agents These medications increase the squeezing strength of the heart muscle. The effect is to increase the amount of blood the heart is able to pump through the circulation	Digitalis Digoxin Digitoxin Digoxin (intrave- nous)	*Lanoxin, Lanoxicaps Crystodigin Lanoxin*	Increase pumping strength of heart Help control certain rhythm disorders	Swallow tablet at prescribed dose and schedule Administer by vein	Stomach upset Loss of appetite Visual disturbance Slow or irregular heartbeat	Avoid low potassium level—promotes side effects Check for drug interactions, particularly drugs that can cause digitalis level to become too high, especially verapamil, quinidine
	Dopamine (intravenous) Dobutamine (intravenous) Amrinone (intravenous)	*Intropin* *Dobutrex* *Inocor*	Increase pumping strength of heart	Administer by vein	Rhythm disturbances Nausea Headache Chest pain Cold hands and feet	

Direct-acting vasodilators (see Table 6)   Nitrates (see Table 1)

This list is not comprehensive and does not represent an endorsement of any product listed.

Table 8. Medications for Rhythm Disorders

Type of Medication	Generic Name	Examples of Brand Names	Uses	How Taken	Specific Side Effects	Specific Precautions
Antiarrhythmic — Medications for fast or irregular heartbeats—alter the way in which electrical currents flow through the conduction system and heart muscle. The change in the electrical characteristics of the heart may reduce the ability of a heart rhythm abnormality to begin or continue	Quinidine	Cardioquin, Cin-Quin, Duraquin, Quinaglute, Quinalan, Quinidex, Quinora	Help control various rhythm disorders	Swallow pill as prescribed and scheduled, or administer by vein	Diarrhea, Dizziness, Stomach upset, Ringing in ears, Passing out	Avoid if known sensitivity to quinine; Digoxin dose will need to be adjusted because quinidine causes digoxin levels in blood to rise
	Procainamide (tablet, capsule, intravenous)	Procan SR, Pronestyl, Pronestyl-SR			Lupus syndrome (blisters, chest pain, joint pain, weakness)	Avoid if known sensitivity to procaine
	Disopyramide	Norpace, Norpace CR			Blurry vision, Urinary obstruction (men), Dry mouth, Congestive heart failure	Elderly patients may be more prone to side effects; Caution if milk sensitivity—tablets contain lactose (milk sugar)
	Lidocaine (intravenous)	Xylocaine			Confusion, Seizures	
	Phenytoin	Dilantin			Overgrowth of gums, Drowsiness	
	Mexiletine	Mexitil			Stomach upset, Trembling, unsteadiness	
	Tocainide	Tonocard			Stomach upset, Trembling, unsteadiness, Blood cell abnormalities	
	Flecainide	Tambocor			Congestive heart failure, Dizziness, visual disturbance	Avoid after recent heart attack; Avoid in heart failure

Table 8. Medications for Rhythm Disorders (Continued)

Type of Medication	Generic Name	Examples of Brand Names	Uses	How Taken	Specific Side Effects	Specific Precautions
	Moricizine	Ethmozine			Stomach upset Dizziness, headache	
	Propafenone	Rhythmol			Bitter taste Stomach upset Weakness Dizziness	
	Bretylium (intravenous)	Bretylol			Low blood pressure	
	Amiodarone	Cordarone			Bluish skin discoloration Overactive or underactive thyroid Lung scarring (fibrosis) Nerve damage Spots in corneas of eyes Liver abnormalities Stomach upset	Digoxin dose will need to be adjusted because amiodarone causes digoxin levels in blood to rise Periodically have blood tests and chest X-ray
	Adenosine (intravenous)	Adenocard	For rapid treatment of fast heartbeats originating from the upper parts of the heart (atria and atrioventricular node)	Rapidly injected into a vein	Chest heaviness Flushing Nausea Headache Shortness of breath/ asthma Slow heartbeat Dizziness (All side effects are very brief)	Very short-acting medication Effects enhanced by dipyridamole (see Table 9) Effects reduced by caffeine and certain asthma medications (theophyllines)

	Medication	Brand name	Use	How given	Side effects	Cautions
Medications for slow heartbeats—act by affecting the nervous system's control of heart rate	Atropine (intravenous)		For temporary acceleration of certain slow heartbeats	Administered by vein	Rapid heartbeat, Mouth dryness, Blurred vision, Difficulty urinating	Avoid in glaucoma, urinary obstruction
	Isoproterenol (intravenous)	Isuprel	For temporary acceleration of certain slow heartbeats	Administered by vein	Rapid heartbeat, Blood pressure swings	Avoid in angina

Many antiarrhythmic medications can potentially cause worse rhythm disorders; careful monitoring is necessary.
Beta blockers (see Table 2)   Calcium channel blockers (see Table 3)
This list is not comprehensive and does not represent an endorsement of any product listed.

Table 9. Medications for Vascular Problems

Type of Medication	Generic Name	Examples of Brand Names	Uses	How Taken	Specific Side Effects	Specific Precautions
Anticoagulants These medications reduce the ability of the blood to clot. They act by reducing proteins involved in blood clotting (coagulation) or changing the way they function	Warfarin Dicumarol	*Coumadin, Panwarfin*	Prevent blood clotting in high-risk situations such as: Mechanical heart valves Dilated cardio-myopathy Atrial fibrillation Previous blood clot problems	Swallow tablet at prescribed dose and schedule	Bleeding, such as: Internal bleeding into gastro-intestinal tract Excess bleeding after cuts Increased nose or gum bleeds Bleeding into joints or muscle Blood in urine Easy bruising Bluish discoloration of toes	Use with caution in liver disease Numerous medications can affect activity of anticoagulants—check with doctor Anticoagulant effect must be checked regularly with prothrombin time blood test so that dose can be adjusted if necessary
	Heparin		Prevent blood clotting in high-risk situations, such as: All of above In certain hospitalized, injured, or bed-bound patients In heart attack or unstable angina After thrombolytic therapy Pulmonary embolism Compared with warfarin, begins acting faster when medication is started, and effect ends faster when medication is stopped. Often	Administer by vein or by injection under the skin	Bleeding, such as: Internal bleeding into gastro-intestinal tract Excess bleeding after cuts Increased nose or gum bleeds Bleeding into joints or muscle Blood in urine Easy bruising Abnormal reduction of blood platelets	Anticoagulant effect must be checked frequently with blood test so dose can be adjusted if necessary

Category	Generic	Brand	Purpose	How to take	Side effects	Considerations
Antiplatelet medications These medications inhibit the normal function of platelets (blood cells involved in clotting)	Aspirin		used in place of warfarin, or while beginning warfarin, in hospitalized patients Reduce risk of blood clots, which might contribute to heart attack, stroke, unstable angina	Swallow tablet at prescribed dose and schedule One aspirin (325 mg) or one baby aspirin (81 mg) daily is generally enough for antiplatelet effects	Stomach irritation Increased chance of bleeding or bruising	Generally avoid using with an anticoagulant
	Dipyridamole	*Persantine*	Reduce risk of blood clots, which might contribute to heart attack, stroke, unstable angina	Swallow tablet at prescribed dose and schedule Usually not used alone; usually recommended with aspirin or anticoagulant	Upset stomach Increased chest pain Dizziness	
Hemorrheologic This type of medication is intended to affect the way blood flows by decreasing its viscosity ("thickness") and by making red blood cells more flexible. The effect is to make the blood flow through blocked and narrowed vessels more easily	Pentoxifylline	*Trental*	Augment blood flow in blood vessels of the limbs with atherosclerotic blockages	Swallow tablet at prescribed dose and schedule	Irregular heartbeat Stomach upset	Caution if known sensitivity to caffeine or theophylline medications

This list is not comprehensive and does not represent an endorsement of any product listed.

REHABILITATION FROM HEART DISEASE OR A HEART OPERATION

If you have had a heart attack or a heart operation, you no doubt have many questions. You probably want to do everything possible to enhance your recovery. Cardiac rehabilitation helps people who have had a heart attack or heart operation to lead active, productive lives—mentally, physically, and socially. A rehabilitation team helps you:

- Adjust physically and emotionally to your situation
- Understand your condition
- Learn ways to reduce your symptoms or limitations
- Improve your capacity for physical exercise
- Optimize a heart-healthy life-style to reduce cardiovascular risk factors and the chance of further problems.

A heart attack, other heart condition, or heart operation does not have to leave you weak, anxious, or withdrawn. Each year more than 100,000 people take part in cardiac rehabilitation programs. Going through the rehabilitation process can help restore your strength and vigor and give you the confidence to resume an active life-style. Many people come out of cardiac rehabilitation with a more healthy, happy life-style than they had before their cardiac event.

Most people with heart disease can benefit from some or all aspects of rehabilitation. Included in this group are people who have had heart attacks, a heart operation (including heart transplantation), and percutaneous translu-minal coronary angioplasty (PTCA, balloon dilation) and people with angina pectoris, silent ischemia, cardiomyopathy, or valvular heart disease.

Because individual circumstances vary, rehabilitation programs have to be tailored to each individual. What is appropriate for one person may not be appropriate for another. For example, you may have had a mild heart attack that has left you more psychologically than physically disabled. Or you may have had an extensive bypass operation that will require a longer physical recovery. The recommendations from your own doctor are crucial in making decisions about your own rehabilitation goals.

Recovery from a heart attack or other cardiac event may require various rehabilitation strategies. A diverse group of professionals are available to help you progress. This group brings together the expertise needed to help answer many of the questions that you may have about your heart condition and overall health, medications, diet, exercise, and sexual activity, especially during the early stages of your rehabilitation. The components of the program include supervised exercise and education and counseling about controlling your risk factors for heart disease.

Rehabilitation begins as soon as you are in stable medical condition after the cardiac event. Individual and group discussion and counseling sessions help you adapt psychologically to your illness. The sessions also provide information on diet, risk factors,

Members of the cardiac rehabilitation team

Member	Function
Personal doctor	Manages your general medical care
Cardiologist	Provides specialized management of your cardiovascular problem: diagnosis, medical prescriptions, treatment procedures, coordination of heart-related care
Surgeon	Does operation (if necessary), provides specialized care after surgical procedures
Nursing staff	Provides your daily care in hospital, assists with daily activities, administers medications, instructs, monitors
Inpatient cardiac rehabilitation coordinator	Organizes various rehabilitation efforts, leads discussions by team about your specific goals and outcomes
Physiatrist	Oversees physical rehabilitation, provides therapy prescriptions and medical prescriptions during hospitalization
Physical therapist	Instructs and assists you in activities to regain and maintain physical and cardiovascular fitness during hospitalization
Occupational therapist	Instructs and assists you in adjusting to daily life and how to compensate for any limitations that may be present
Psychiatrist	Provides specialized management of significant emotional difficulties that may arise, discussion, prescriptions for appropriate medications if needed
Psychologist	Provides ongoing counseling and evaluation of emotional or psychological problems if needed
Exercise physiologist	Analyzes your body's exercise capabilities or limitations, makes recommendations for improving or adapting function of heart and body during outpatient rehabilitation
Outpatient cardiac rehabilitation nurse	Oversees ongoing rehabilitation efforts after hospitalization, monitors progress, confers with cardiologist and exercise physiologist
Exercise specialist	Teaches specific exercises and conducts exercise sessions with patients individually or in groups
Registered dietitian	Analyzes nutritional needs, develops and instructs you in food selection and preparation to meet goals of reducing cholesterol level and losing weight
Chaplain	Provides support for your spiritual needs in hospital
Pharmacist	Reviews concerns about medications, such as interactions and side effects
Social worker	Assists and oversees special needs such as arranging for nursing facilities or financial assistance options if needed
Smoking cessation counselor	Makes recommendations and provides support for stopping smoking if needed

medications, physical activity, and any concerns you may have.

The objective of rehabilitation efforts is to develop a plan of action that meets your *individual* needs. This book cannot provide recommendations that meet all of your specific objectives. But it is useful as a description of how a general plan might work.

The Rehabilitation Plan

In general, programs usually involve a minimum of 6 months of rehabilitation, divided into four phases: hospitalization, early recovery, late recovery, and maintenance.

PHASE 1: HOSPITALIZATION.

This phase usually lasts throughout the hospitalization after your heart attack, operation, or other illness. Consequently, it is of fairly short duration. During your hospitalization, you begin nonstrenuous activities such as sitting up in bed and simple range-of-motion exercises. Initially, the range-of-motion exercises are passive, meaning that the therapist will move your limbs for you, but you quickly progress to active exercises. The goal of these activities is to maintain muscle tone and joint flexibility, even though you are restricted in your overall activity. You then progress to walking and limited stair climbing. Without such efforts, up to 15 percent of muscle strength can be lost in as little as 1 week in the hospital.

Step-by-Step Progression.

The physical activity program in the hospital follows a step-by-step progression. You usually advance one step, or activity level, each day. The following activity schedule follows a 6-day plan, but your doctor may adjust the timing depending on your condition.

Day 1 Morning
Remain in bed, except to use the bedside commode (avoid straining)

You may brush your teeth or dentures; the nurse will assist you as necessary

You may wash your face and hands, but the nurse will assist you with your sponge bath

You may feed yourself with your elbows supported on the tray table; the nurse will set up your tray

A physical therapist will exercise your arms and legs for you

You will need adequate rest; therefore, it will be important for you to observe the rest period

Afternoon
You may sit in the chair up to 15 to 30 minutes, depending on your tolerance

Your educational program will begin

Day 2 Morning
You may sit in the chair up to 60 minutes

You may divide your time in the chair as you choose

You may begin to exercise with the assistance of a physical therapist

Afternoon
You may sit in the chair up to 90 minutes

Day 3   Morning

You may sit in the chair up to 120 minutes; this period will include class time

You may walk in the room with professional assistance

You may have bathroom privileges and take a wheelchair shower

You may attend classes and discussion groups

Afternoon

You may walk around the nurses' station with professional supervision

You may sit in the chair as much as you like and can tolerate

Day 4   You may be up in the room and walk around the nurses' station as much as you like

You are encouraged to dress in street clothes

You may take a standing shower with the assistance of a nurse

Day 5   You may continue walking around the nurses' station as much as you like

You may climb stairs with professional assistance

Day 6   Your home-going instructions will be finalized

PHASE 2: EARLY RECOVERY.

The next 2- to 12-week phase of your rehabilitation begins when you go home from the hospital. During this phase, you gradually assume self-care activities, increase your general level of activity under supervision, and, in-stead of the physical therapist moving your arms and legs, you use your own strength to move your limbs to keep the joints limber. Your doctor may suggest home exercises that include walking, stationary cycling, and gentle calisthenics during the first few days.

After you leave the hospital, you may be advised to participate in medically supervised exercise at your local hospital or cardiac rehabilitation center. These programs generally encourage aerobic exercise and some muscle strengthening exercise at your individually tolerated level, which is usually determined with an exercise test. This phase of rehabilitation also continues to emphasize health and nutrition education and psychological counseling and support.

Gradually Increasing Physical Activity.   If you have had a heart attack, a typical scenario for your progression of activities after leaving the hospital may proceed as described below.

Week 1   Any light activity that can be done while sitting

Walking slowly for about 10 minutes on a level surface once or twice a day or use of a stationary cycle with minimal resistance

Light housework such as dishes, cooking, dusting, or sweeping with a broom

Personal hygiene such as shaving, showering, and dressing

Week 2   Social activity such as playing cards at home, visiting neighbors, or riding in the car

Walking at a relaxed pace for about 20 minutes on a level surface once or twice a day or use of a stationary cycle with slight resistance

Housework such as making beds, ironing, minor repair of appliances, bench work, or supervising farm work

Resume sexual intercourse

Week 3
Driving with a backup driver present

Housework such as vacuuming

Increase in social activity such as movies, church, and concerts

Walking at a moderate pace for about 30 minutes once or twice a day or continuing stationary cycling with slight resistance

Lifting a few (10 to 15) pounds

Week 4
Driving alone

Light gardening

Pitch-and-putt golfing

Social group activities such as club meetings, parties, and dancing

Grocery shopping (no heavy lifting)

Walking or stationary cycling for 30 minutes, once or twice a day

Perhaps a return to work part-time

During the next 2 to 4 weeks, you are encouraged to perform aerobic exercise (in addition to your usual daily activities) for up to 40 minutes at a moderate intensity. Doctors usually recommend exercising five to seven times per week, with three or fewer of the sessions at the rehabilitation center. Recommendations will vary for each individual.

Ideally, you should exercise in a medically supervised environment for several weeks after leaving the hospital. However, in reality, many people do not have access to these programs and must exercise on their own. Nonetheless, you must have your doctor's opinion before beginning your exercise program after a cardiac event. Your rehabilitation team will tell you what symptoms to watch for, the type of exercise permitted, types of equipment you might need, the importance of warm-up and cool-down exercises, and proper techniques for pacing yourself during exercise.

This phase is also a good time to consider joining a community support group, such as a local "coronary club," to help you learn how to better manage your heart disease.

Near the end of this phase, your doctor evaluates your overall progress to determine your readiness to return to work and other activities. Returning to the rehabilitation center for follow-up at several time points, such as at 3, 6, and 9 months after you complete phase 2, helps ensure that you continue with your good efforts.

PHASE 3: LATE RECOVERY.

You probably will have settled into your own comfortable exercise routine at home or at local exercise facilities about 6 to 12 weeks after your hospitalization. By this time you should also be making good progress with control of your other cardiovascular risk factors such as smoking, high blood pressure, high blood cholesterol, obesity, or stress.

Diet is an important aspect of the rehabilitation program. A registered dietitian (R.D.) can suggest ways to reduce fat, cholesterol, and salt, if necessary, from your diet. Alcohol and caffeine may or may not be allowed, depending on your condition. Following the dietary recommendations will also help you lose weight, if that is one of the goals in your rehabilitation program.

PHASE 4: MAINTENANCE.

This phase lasts indefinitely, and in some ways it is the most important part of your rehabilitation. At this point, you must regain your independence and work toward a lifelong commitment to the changes you started earlier in your recovery. Periodic visits with your rehabilitation team can help reinforce your "heart-healthy" life-style.

Psychological Adjustments

It is natural to react to a heart attack with panic and anxiety. You are confronted with the stress of the illness itself, unfamiliar surroundings, the threat of death, and pain and discomfort.

Even after your condition has stabilized and you have left the hospital, restrictions and alterations in previously routine activities can be stressful. Burdens may fall, at least temporarily, on your spouse or other family members. Reversals of responsibilities within a relationship are sometimes necessary. After a cardiac event, you may have to take new medications and change your life-style dramatically, including diet changes that may affect other family members. And, of course, the thought of death or a recurrence or worsening of your condition lingers in the background.

EMOTIONAL RESPONSES TO CARDIAC EVENTS.

Emotional responses to a heart attack often follow a common pattern. The spouse and family often experience these same emotions on a delayed time schedule.

Denial that a heart attack has occurred or that it may be serious is common when symptoms of a heart attack first begin. In fact, the denial may have been present long before the actual heart attack, as the person continued smoking and eating a high-fat diet despite advice from many sources and despite experiencing fatigue, shortness of breath, and chest discomfort signaling that something was wrong with the heart.

Shock and *fear* usually follow when the problem can no longer be denied. *Anger* is common and is often directed at medical personnel, the spouse, and oneself. Anger may take the form of "Why me?"

Within days of the event, the person may experience *depression*, which is probably related to the perceived loss of physical ability. Depression may be relatively mild and brief or severe and long-lasting, depending on the severity of the disease, the psychological makeup of the person, and the type and amount of therapy provided. Some people become depressed only after they return home, and others do not seem to experience feelings of depression. Depression may be characterized by complaints such as fatigue or nonspecific discomfort.

People may go through a *bargaining* stage where they try to get reassurance from the doctor to erase the event— "If I watch my diet closely, can I get the cholesterol out of my arteries and repair the damage to my heart?''—or from God—"Let me live through this and I'll start going to church again.''

Most people go through a stage of *excessive concern* in which they are afraid that every little muscle twitch and upset stomach is another heart attack. Unfortunately, even with full compliance with doctors' recommendations, full recovery and freedom from any future problems cannot be guaranteed. Adapting to this stage re-

Looking for the silver lining

Eventually, most people can even look at the cardiac event as a positive experience in their lives. Commonly, people report physical improvements such as weight loss and improved fitness. They have quit smoking and are eating a more healthful diet. In addition, they identify social and psychological benefits such as an improved relationship with their spouse and families, better self-image, better ability to deal with work pressures, and an awakened enthusiasm for the simple pleasures in life. In some cases, people even see a message or spiritual meaning in the cardiac event, and this gives them a sense of spiritual enlightenment or helps to resolve long-standing conflicts or doubts.

People who ultimately effectively resolve crises such as a heart attack and go on to experience personal growth adopt one or more of the following strategies:

1. Remember that there is always someone worse off than you.
2. Accept some responsibility for the event, then change that behavior to reduce the risk of future events.
3. Specifically look for the message or meaning of the event and identify the changes or experiences that have been positive.

With the help of new medications and medical procedures, in addition to changes in life-style and learning new ways to deal with stress, you can maintain or possibly improve the quality of your life after a heart attack or other cardiac event.

quires a realistic perspective and outlook.

Dealing With the Emotional Responses. Many cardiac rehabilitation programs recognize the emotional stress of heart disease and begin to help patients and their families address these issues as soon as possible. Outpatient programs, in addition to providing exercise classes, often include special group sessions at which you can discuss stress related to the event itself and also the more general stress issues that you must deal with again as you return to work and normal activities. Psychological screening may be used to help identify people who remain angry or depressed beyond a reasonable period. Many people say that learning to deal with stress more effectively was the most important change they made after a cardiac event.

Sexual Activity After a Heart Attack

It is common for people to reduce the frequency of sexual intercourse for many months after a heart attack or other cardiac event. Sexual dysfunction is also common. Some people are worried about the physical demands of sex after a cardiac event, but research indicates that this concern is unfounded.

Most people can return to sexual activity by the second week after a heart attack or heart operation. The demands placed on your heart during sexual intercourse are similar to those of taking a brisk walk, scrubbing a floor, or climbing one to two flights of stairs. In a way, sexual activity is like any other physical activity: your heart rate, breathing rate, and blood pressure increase, so you should proceed sensibly, with caution but without fear.

Just as with your other exercises, progress gradually with sex. As your confidence in the health of your heart grows, you will resume your usual sexual patterns. It is important to talk to your partner to alleviate fears and concerns. Be reassured that it is normal for your needs to have changed temporarily.

Some medications, such as beta blockers (see Table 2, page 298), can reduce sexual function, although this effect is more often due to depression or anxiety rather than the medication. Discuss reduced sexual activity with your doctor or the appropriate member of your rehabilitation team.

Talk to your doctor about any other fears and concerns, too. If you experience chest pain, extreme shortness of breath, or irregular heartbeat during sexual activity, stop. Do not try to do too much too fast.

Social Support

The importance of social support from friends and family cannot be overemphasized in terms of easing the psychological recovery after a cardiac event. Although counseling with health professionals is sometimes necessary, time heals most wounds and most people have a tendency to forget the most unpleasant parts of their ordeal.

Ways to Enhance Your Psychological Recovery After a Heart Attack

UNDERSTAND YOUR CONDITION. A heart attack occurs when a part of your heart muscle is permanently damaged from a lack of blood and oxygen. However, having one heart attack does not mean that you will have another. Look at the heart attack as a warning: you have heart disease, and you should seriously consider changing your life-style to reduce your risk of future problems.

STAY ACTIVE. Don't fall for the common myths about activity and heart disease that say you should not drive, exert yourself, or have sexual intercourse.

Follow your doctor's prescription for your individual level of activity. Exercise should be high on your list of "Things to Do." Activity affirms that you are still alive and not an invalid.

You should have the following items on your list of "Things *Not* to Do": don't smoke, don't eat too much, don't hurry, and don't worry.

GET INVOLVED. Your local coronary club is an excellent resource. Exchanging information and experiences on a regular basis with other people who are also learning to live with heart disease can help you regain your confidence and sense of well-being.

PART 6

Issues in Cardiology

If you have heart disease, you probably read or listen to any reports that suggest a new treatment or something you can do to improve your condition. Sometimes you get confusing messages, and some reports imply there is a definitive answer when there is not. There are several reasons why various topics are prominently reported in the news media: some potentially apply to a wide spectrum of individuals, some raise hopes of breakthroughs in the treatment of cardiovascular disease, and some are surrounded by controversy.

Several issues are covered in the following pages to provide a perspective from which to evaluate other reports. The first five subjects provide you with background on specific medical topics that are commonly discussed in the media and elsewhere.

The next three topics are more general in scope—they raise issues that may apply to various medical situations: Are there times when the "cure" may be worse than your illness? How can you as a patient contribute to medical progress? How should you weigh the pros and cons of undergoing any procedure or treatment?

The final topic, women and heart disease, disputes the myth that heart disease affects mainly men.

SHOULD YOU TAKE ASPIRIN?

The potential benefit that aspirin might have on cardiovascular health is based on its well-recognized ability to inhibit the activity of platelets. Platelets are one of the components of blood which contribute to clotting, and they may also have a role in the development of atherosclerosis. Aspirin reduces the tendency of blood to clot by weakening the activity of platelets. It may help reduce or prevent narrowing of blood vessels due to atherosclerosis. Aspirin might be useful in these situations:

■ Avoiding *recurrences* of conditions that are due to blood clotting or atherosclerosis (secondary prevention).

There is strong evidence that people who have already had a heart attack, stroke, transient ischemic attack (a warning sign of stroke), or unstable angina can benefit by taking medications, such as aspirin, that inhibit the activity of platelets. The risk of death among this group is reduced by 15 percent if they take aspirin, and the risk of experiencing a complication such as a nonfatal heart attack or stroke is decreased by 25 to 30 percent. Using this information, medical researchers have estimated that if 100 people with cardiovascular disease took aspirin for 2 years, one death and two major nonfatal events would be prevented. Although this does not seem like a large number, it is important when applied to the total number of people with cardiovascular disease in the world.

People who have had a coronary artery bypass operation can clearly benefit from the use of aspirin. Aspirin reduces the likelihood that the bypass grafts themselves will be blocked off by a blood clot or atherosclerosis.

Aspirin in low doses is inexpensive, generally safe, and easy to take. Most authorities highly recommend it as an effective secondary prevention measure (one that reduces future risk in people who have already had one problem).

- Preventing the *initial* occurrence of a blood clot or atherosclerosis-related complication (primary prevention).

If secondary prevention works, then why not treat everyone with aspirin and reduce the chances of anyone having a heart attack or stroke in the first place? The cardiovascular benefits of aspirin are not clear cut for people who currently have no form of heart disease. In a United States study of more than 22,000 male doctors, those who took one aspirin every other day had 44 percent fewer heart attacks than those who did not take aspirin, but they did not have fewer strokes or deaths attributable to cardiovascular diseases. A similar study of British doctors did not show fewer heart attacks with aspirin, so no definite answer (or recommendation) is available.

Whether these results apply to women is uncertain. A study of more than 80,000 female nurses suggested that women who take one to six aspirin weekly have less chance of a heart attack—but the apparent benefit was small and the study was not designed to allow a solid recommendation.

When aspirin is recommended for preventing complications of blood clot, whether it is for secondary or primary prevention, low doses are sufficient. Less than one aspirin a day substantially reduces the ability of the platelets to clot; indeed, one "baby" aspirin will suffice. One baby aspirin is equivalent to one-fourth of a regular-strength adult aspirin.

Even though there may be good reasons to take aspirin, for some people there are good reasons to avoid it— reasons that likely outweigh any benefit they might get from taking it. People who are allergic to aspirin, who already may have bleeding problems, who have stomach ulcers or irritation, or who already may be taking an anticoagulant (such as warfarin) should not take aspirin unless specifically advised to by their doctor.

- Avoiding blood clot formation in people with atrial fibrillation (see page 92), which predisposes them to abnormal clotting in the heart

People who have atrial fibrillation are at increased risk of having a stroke. One major reason for strokes in people with atrial fibrillation is that blood clots are more likely to form in the left atrium, break off, and travel to a blood vessel in the brain. Research has shown that for people with atrial fibrillation, the risk of having a stroke or other blood clot complication can be reduced by inhibiting the blood's ability to clot. If atrial fibrillation occurs along with other heart disease, the need for preventing clotting is very clear-cut. In these people, anticoagulation with warfarin is advisable.

Although one study showed that aspirin could be effective in decreasing stroke in some people with atrial fibrillation, warfarin is probably even more effective. In three major studies, warfarin (in low doses) reduced the likelihood of stroke by about 70 percent. Fortunately, taking either aspirin or low-dose warfarin does not seem to result in many bleeding problems in most people with atrial fibrillation.

In general, people who have atrial fibrillation (even if they have no evidence of other types of heart disease) should take either aspirin or warfarin. For those at low risk—young people with no evidence of other cardiovascular problems—aspirin may be sufficient. People with any evidence of other heart disease—including high blood pressure, congestive heart failure, past problems related to blood clots, reduced pumping function of the left ventricle, enlargement of the left atrium, or the presence of valve abnormalities—should receive warfarin, unless, of course, they have a condition that makes the use of warfarin dangerous, such as a tendency to bleed.

DOES FISH OIL PREVENT HEART DISEASE?

In the 1970s, scientists published an interesting observation: despite the fact that Eskimos in Greenland had a limited life span (60 years on the average), less than 4 percent of them died of coronary artery disease. Could their low rates of heart disease be related to their diet—about a pound of fish and whale meat a day? Investigators studied other populations (for example, the Japanese) and, in general, found that the more fish people eat, the less coronary artery disease they have. Some investigators suggested that eating as little as 1 ounce (on the average) of fish per day corresponded to a 50 percent reduction of coronary deaths. Although it is not certain that the fish in the diet actually was responsible for these trends, the evidence is tantalizing.

Certain fish and ocean mammals contain high concentrations of a unique type of fat—omega-3 polyunsaturated fatty acids (PUFAs). Studies in laboratories and in animals suggested that omega-3 PUFAs might have actions that could reduce atherosclerosis. They reduce triglycerides (but have variable effects on cholesterol). The dose that would be needed to reduce cholesterol levels is both excessive and expensive, and the resulting change in cholesterol is small.

Omega-3 PUFAs may weaken the activity of platelets (therefore reducing the tendency for blood clots). They also lessen the effect of experimental diets designed to produce atherosclerosis in pigs and monkeys. One study in pigs even suggested that a diet high in omega-3 PUFAs could cause atherosclerosis that was already present to disappear partially (regress). But omega-3 PUFAs in high doses tend to depress the body's immune system, and they have been associated with scarring of heart muscle in animal studies.

Because of these indications of some beneficial effects, people naturally wondered whether fish oil might prevent coronary artery disease and its complications or even reverse atherosclerosis in arteries. So far, studies are not conclusive or complete. For example, people who undergo percutaneous transluminal coronary angioplasty (PTCA; see page 270) have a risk for redevelopment of blockages in their coronary arteries. Some people who have had PTCA and taken fish oils seemed to have a reduced chance of recurrent blockage; however, studies of other people who took fish oils did not show this benefit.

To date, there is little direct evidence to support the use of fish oil capsules to prevent or treat heart or coronary artery disease. Because of expense, inconvenience, and the remote possibility of unrecognized risk associated with high doses of fish oils, their use cannot currently be recommended. However, there is compelling evidence that including fish in the diet is of benefit to cardiovascular health. Fish is lower in total fat and lower in saturated fat than most other meats. So a diet that includes fish two or three times a week (see page 158) helps to lower the amount of total and saturated fat you eat and therefore helps lower blood cholesterol levels. Whether the benefit of more fish in the diet is due to fish oils or to other substances, or whether it is simply because the fish is replacing less healthy components of the diet, remains elusive.

IS ALCOHOL GOOD FOR YOU?

It may seem surprising that drinking alcoholic beverages may have a healthful aspect, but several medical studies provide consistent information that this may be so. What is this information and, more important, what does it mean?

Several avenues of medical research suggest that small to moderate amounts of alcohol may reduce your risk of coronary artery diseases, such as heart attack. The main type of research that supports this conclusion is epidemiologic studies. This research method compares patterns of diseases in populations to determine whether certain groups of people are more prone to illness than other groups. Epidemiologic studies show that people who drink moderate amounts of alcohol have a 40 to 50 percent lower risk for the development of coronary artery disease. This result seems to hold up even when other factors that might affect coronary artery disease are taken into account, such as age and tobacco use. Indeed, observers have pointed out that the French have a lower rate of coronary artery disease than do Americans, despite relatively high consumption of fats, use of tobacco,

and a sedentary life style. An explanation that has been offered is that the French consume more alcohol per person on a regular basis, especially red wine.

Another avenue of research suggests that moderate amounts of alcohol tend to raise HDL cholesterol ("good" cholesterol); however, other studies have not consistently confirmed this potentially beneficial effect. Others point out that alcohol may increase triglyceride levels, promote weight gain, and raise blood pressure, which are not beneficial effects. Animal research supports the contention that regular intake of moderate amounts of alcohol improves the lipid profile by raising HDL cholesterol and lowering LDL cholesterol ("bad" cholesterol). "Binge drinking," however, produces an unfavorable response in the lipid profile.

What are the implications of these studies? For an answer to this question, a little perspective is necessary. Alcohol, especially when used excessively, is directly or indirectly responsible for enormous amounts of illness, death, and social problems. Few people are unaware of the burden caused by alcohol in automobile fatalities and injuries alone. Illnesses caused by alcohol include alcoholism, alcoholic liver disease, alcoholic gastritis (inflammation of the stomach lining), alcoholic polyneuropathy (nerve damage), and birth defects due to drinking during pregnancy. One form of cardiomyopathy (see page 41) is directly linked to alcohol consumption, and some heart rhythm disorders can be provoked by alcohol. Alcohol is often involved in crimes, including homicide. A recent estimate of the annual cost burden to the United States in terms of health and social consequences of excessive alcohol use was $117 billion.

With that in mind, the balance of potential benefits versus definite risks prohibits recommending the routine use of alcohol, even in modest portions, to lower the risk of coronary artery disease. It does not make good medical sense to "rob Peter to pay Paul." Small reductions in coronary risk likely would be "paid for" by increased risk of other adverse effects, especially among people who might drink excessive amounts of alcohol. Nevertheless, it is equally unjustified to recommend complete abstinence from alcohol by responsible low-level drinkers on the basis of coronary risks. Despite the impression that doctors recommend giving up all "vices" to decrease coronary risk factors, responsible alcohol use need not fall into that category.

CAN CORONARY ARTERY DISEASE GO AWAY?

The possibility that a medication can "dissolve" atherosclerotic blockages in arteries is understandably of great interest and hope for people. Likewise, if risk factors promote the *development* of atherosclerosis, then perhaps removal or treatment of risk factors (see Part 3, "Reducing Your Risk of Coronary Artery Disease," page 115) could also *reduce* atherosclerotic blockages that are already present. Is such a medicine or treatment available?

The answer contains elements of good news and bad news. The *good news* is that medical studies indicate that there are ways to cause atherosclerosis to "regress," or be reduced in its extent or severity. Not unexpectedly, most of these methods involve improving the lipid profile by lowering cholesterol (especially LDL cholesterol) and triglycerides and by raising HDL cholesterol (see page 126). Researchers have found evidence that improving cholesterol and triglyceride levels by using medication, by diet, or even (in rare cases) by special equipment that filters blood (somewhat like a kidney dialysis machine) can cause regression of atherosclerosis.

The *bad news* is that the observed reductions in the amount of artery narrowing after aggressive interventions have been small and do not occur in everyone. For example, in one study there was evidence of reduced narrowing in the coronary arteries of men with angina or previous heart attacks when they followed diet guidelines and used a medication to lower cholesterol. But this effect occurred in only about one-third of the men, and the degree of improvement was small (the average coronary artery narrowing decreased by only a tenth of a millimeter after 3 years). It is noteworthy that the treated men had considerably less progression of coronary artery disease and fewer new symptoms of heart problems.

Other studies have made similar observations: some (but not all) people at high risk for cardiovascular problems show evidence of less worsening of coronary blockages and, in some cases, slight improvement in blockages if they successfully improve their lipid profile (lower LDL cholesterol or raise HDL cholesterol) with medications. Furthermore, this improvement in the lipid profile results in fewer heart attacks or heart-related deaths and less need for coronary artery bypass or angioplasty.

The regression observed in these studies is encouraging because it does show that improving lipids imparts some benefit. The fact that *any* regression is documented shows that such an outcome is at least possible and justifies further efforts to find new ways to "undo" atherosclerosis, in both men and women. In the meantime, it is prudent to continue to focus on control of cholesterol and elimination of other risk factors (see page 119). Prevention is the best strategy, even if it results in only the slowing of the process that is blocking the coronary arteries.

DOES COFFEE AGGRAVATE HEART DISEASE?

Coffee is obviously a popular beverage, so any suggestion that it may promote coronary artery disease implies that a large number of people might be at risk. Assertions that coffee may not be healthful have been made since the turn of the century, but methodical attempts to address this issue have been made only recently. Can any conclusions be drawn from the available information?

The answer can be gleaned from the conclusions of several major studies:

■ *There is an association of coffee consumption with clinically evident coronary artery disease, which is consistent with a twofold to threefold elevation in risk among heavy (more than 5 cups a day) coffee drinkers. (This information is from a 1986 study of 1,130 male medical students followed medically for 19 to 35 years.)*

■ *Middle-aged white men who drink 6 or more cups of coffee per day may have 1.7 times the risk of death from coronary artery disease compared with those who drink less. (This information is from a 1987 study of 1,910 employees of Chicago Western Electric Company followed medically for 19 years, starting in 1958.)*

■ *Drinking 9 or more cups of coffee daily increases the risk of dying from coronary artery disease 2.2 times for men and 5.1 times for women, when compared with the risk in people who drink less than 1 cup daily. (This information is from a 1990 Norwegian study of 19,398 men and 19,166 women aged 35 to 54 years who were followed for an average of 6 years.)*

■ *There is a small increase in risk (about 1.4 times) of myocardial infarction in people who drink 4 or more cups of coffee a day compared with the risk in people who do not drink coffee.* (This information is from a 1990 study of 101,774 white and black persons admitted to northern California Kaiser Permanente hospitals between 1978 and 1986.)

■ *Increasing levels of consumption of caffeinated coffee were not associated with higher risks of cardiovascular disease. Higher consumption of decaffeinated coffee was associated with a small increase (1.6 times) in the risk of coronary artery disease.* (This information is from a 1991 study of 45,589 American men aged 40 to 75 years who were medically followed for 2 years.)

■ *Among men who smoke, there is no relationship between coffee consumption and heart attack or death from coronary artery disease. Among nonsmoking men, there is a trend toward heavy coffee drinkers having more coronary artery disease, but the difference between coffee drinkers and nondrinkers is so slight it may be just a coincidence.* (This information is from a 1991 study of 6,765 middle-aged Swedish men followed for 7 years.)

In short, medical research is not unanimous on the question of coffee's effect on coronary artery disease. Differences in the conclusions of these studies perhaps could be explained by variations in the way the studies were performed, differences among the groups of people studied (various countries, men, women, and racial differences), different types of coffee (decaffeinated or caffeinated), and different methods of coffee preparation (filtered, boiled, and so on).

Even if coffee drinking were to be conclusively linked with a higher risk of coronary artery disease, the way in which it might cause it remains elusive. Some researchers suggest that coffee drinking is simply more common in people who have other risk factors, such as smoking, fat consumption (for example, coffee drinkers may eat more cream cheese Danish than those who do not drink coffee), or inactivity. Most research has not disclosed that coffee in itself has a consistent effect on cholesterol.

Although the final word is still out, a prudent recommendation is to limit coffee intake to no more than 3 or 4 cups a day. The benefit may be limited, but because it is an easily accomplished goal for most people, it is worth aiming for.

One effect of coffee that is well recognized, especially caffeinated coffee as well as other caffeine-containing beverages (tea, cocoa, some soft drinks), is that it promotes the occurrence of some heart rhythm abnormalities, especially palpitations and supraventricular tachycardia (see page 94). If you are experiencing palpitations, a logical first step is to eliminate coffee and caffeinated substances from your diet.

SHOULD ALL PALPITATIONS BE TREATED?

A common problem that comes up in the field of cardiology and in general medical practice is how to handle "minor" problems. A good example of this dilemma is the problem of palpitations—the awareness of heartbeat irregularities caused by "flip-flops" or "skips" in the chest (see page 31). Palpitations can signal a potentially serious problem with the heartbeat or they can be a clue to significant problems with the heart muscle, valves, or coronary arteries. But the vast majority of palpitations that are not associated with other symptoms—such as lightheadedness, blacking out, shortness of breath, or chest discomfort—do not pose any problem for a person's overall health.

Nevertheless, palpitations can be an uncomfortable nuisance if they occur frequently or seem strong, and they certainly can provoke a high level of anxiety in some people. Consequently, it has always seemed reasonable to both patients and doctors that some palpitations should be treated with antiarrhythmic medications (see Table 8, page 307) in an attempt to suppress them and to reduce or eliminate symptoms. But is this a wise approach?

Symptomatic palpitations (or certain types of frequent extra beats observed on an electrocardiogram) sometimes warrant an evaluation for various types of heart disease. Also, they may require evaluation to determine that they are not the "tip of the iceberg" (that is, more serious rhythm problems are also present). But, again, most palpitations are very seldom an indication that there is a more serious underlying problem.

What about situations in which an underlying problem is searched for and not found and yet the palpitations continue to be bothersome? Several factors must be weighed in deciding the best way to approach this perplexing problem. How bad are the symptoms—barely noticeable, a nui-

sance, or virtually disabling? What are the chances that the rhythm abnormality will become more serious or symptomatic in the future—slight (there is no such thing as "no chance" in medicine) or highly probable? What is the likelihood of a medication helping the symptoms—low or high? Most important, what is the chance that a medication will create new problems—a side effect or even worsening of the heart rhythm?

Traditionally, doctors attempted treatment even if the symptoms were relatively minor, even if they were relatively unlikely to get worse, and even if the medication might not be very effective. The rationale for doing so could be summed up by the following philosophy: "It can't hurt to try." However, new information about the final consideration—the possibility of side effects—has raised major questions about that approach. As it turns out, in some people it *can* hurt to try.

This concern was raised by the results of a medical study examining the effects of various antiarrhythmic medications on patients with certain types of rhythm abnormalities occurring after a heart attack. The study was called the Cardiac Arrhythmia Suppression Trial (CAST); it was intended to discover whether reduction of extra beats after a heart attack would promote long-term survival and which of several medications might be best at accomplishing that.

This study included patients who had had a heart attack and who had extra beats in the ventricle which could be reduced by treatment with an antiarrhythmic medication. These patients were then randomly assigned either to continue receiving one of three antiarrhythmic medications or to receive no antiarrhythmic medications. The results: in less than 1 year, nearly three times as many patients who received medication died of severe heart rhythm abnormalities compared with those who did not receive a medication. And *more than three times as many* died of heart problems not caused by rhythm abnormalities as those who received no rhythm medication. Indeed, as this trend became apparent, the study was discontinued so that no further patients would receive the risky treatment.

The results of the CAST study do not mean that antiarrhythmic medications do not have a useful role. These types of medications *have* been shown to be effective in treating certain rhythm disorders. The results *do* mean that the medications must be used very cautiously and only when they are clearly required. General guidelines for their use are:

- If a heart rhythm abnormality is benign (that is, if your risk of future problems is *not* predictably increased) and does *not* produce symptoms, DO NOT USE MEDICATIONS.

- If a heart rhythm abnormality is benign but causes palpitations, TRY TO TOLERATE THE PALPITATIONS TO AVOID THE RISK OF MEDICATIONS.

- If palpitations cannot be tolerated, USE MEDICATIONS WITH THE LOWEST POSSIBLE RISK. Fortunately, low-risk medications, such as beta blockers (see Table 2, page 298), are often effective.

- If a heart rhythm abnormality is "prognostically significant" (that is, it may be a clue that future problems may develop) or malignant (there is a high risk of dangerous developments in the near future), USE THE MOST EFFECTIVE MEDICATION (OR AN IMPLANTABLE CARDIOVERTER-DEFIBRILLATOR) BASED ON APPROPRIATE TESTING.

SHOULD YOU PARTICIPATE IN MEDICAL RESEARCH?

Medical knowledge is continually evolving and expanding. The development of new medications, medical devices, operations, and procedures comes from years of testing and refining. Of course, many steps in the development of any new treatment for heart disease focus on assuring that the treatment provides benefits without undue risk and that it is an improvement on existing approaches. How does the process of providing these assurances occur?

The development of medications and medical devices is regulated by the U.S. Food and Drug Administration (FDA). The FDA requires several phases of investigation before a new treatment is certified as being safe and effective. The ultimate test is whether it produces the desired effect in people who have the disease for which treatment is being sought.

The question of whether a new medication (or device) is safe and effective requires a lengthy, thorough investigation. Simply providing the treatment to patients with the disease and observing what happens rarely provides useful information. Instead, studies must be designed to give information that is so "solid" that the FDA—as well as doctors and their patients—can be as confident as possible that the medication is safe and effective. They must also know what to expect in terms of possible side effects.

Someone must be among the first to take the new medication or use the new medical device, once preliminary tests show that there is reason to believe that it *might* be effective. People who are willing to be these early recipients of a medical treatment participate in a clinical study. Clinical studies are monitored by the scientists conducting the research, in addition to a special committee (called an institutional review board, or IRB) that is composed of scientists from many fields and representatives from the community. This committee exists by law, and *no* experiment involving humans can be done without its approval. The IRB is an advocate for human research subjects.

Why would anyone participate in a clinical study? After all, there is no assurance that the experimental treatment is effective—that is why it is being studied. Furthermore, many studies are designed so that some participants in the study may not even get the experimental treatment. They might actually receive a placebo (inactive substance) instead.

There are several reasons why a person might choose to be a "study subject." One reason is that some people get tremendous satisfaction in helping advance medical science. These people believe, "If it can help someone else in the future, I'd like to get involved." Another reason is that for some illnesses there are no currently effective treatments; the study may offer the hope that the new medication will be effective and directly help the patient. Similarly, some patients simply may not benefit from medications

that are already available, and their goal is to see if a new variety of medication may possibly help them. Yet another aim for a study patient may be financial; most clinical studies provide the study medication, many tests, and examinations at no charge—consequently, the patient can receive closely monitored medical care at minimal cost.

Doctors, patients, the manufacturers of new products, and the FDA must all cooperate in assessing the effect of new types of treatment. Several types of information need to be gathered to determine whether a new treatment is effective. First, the types of patient in whom the treatment is to be tested must be carefully defined, so "inclusion" and "exclusion" criteria are specified. For example, to participate in a study of a medication intended to treat congestive heart failure, you might be eligible only if your ejection fraction is less than 35 percent (see page 6). This criterion assures that only people with diminished pumping function are included in the study. Even if you had the disease being studied, you might be excluded if you had another major illness. This criterion assures that other diseases will not interfere with the evaluation of the medication. For example, little could be learned about the effect of a medication for congestive heart failure in a study participant who was experiencing most of his or her symptoms from cancer or who may not survive to the end of the study.

Second, each study must have a method to measure or determine whether the treatment is altering the illness. A new treatment for congestive heart failure would need to assess the effect of the medication on the pumping function of the heart, on the ability of the patient to exert himself or herself, or on the length of life of the patient.

Finally, some type of comparison must be done to determine whether the course of an illness when the medication is given is different from the course when the medication is not given. Such comparisons can take several forms. One common form is to compare groups who receive the treatment with those who do not. In this type of study, individuals are randomly assigned to either receive or not receive the treatment: neither the doctor nor the manufacturer can determine who gets the treatment—it is a matter of chance only. The goal is to avoid any possibility of subtly influencing the outcome by tending to put "favorable" patients in the treatment group and "sicker" patients in the nontreatment ("control") group.

Another form of comparison study is to compare how patients do while they receive treatment with how they do while they are not receiving the treatment. In this type of study, participants "cross over" from treatment to nontreatment (or vice versa) after a period of time. The order of the treatment-nontreatment sequence is generally randomly determined, again to avoid introducing any unintentional bias into the results.

Most comparison forms of study use a "placebo-controlled" format. In this type, patients who do not receive the actual medication (because they were randomized to "control") instead receive an inactive "medication" that looks just like the real medication but contains only sugar or some other inactive ingredient. Commonly, studies are "double-blind," meaning that neither the doctor nor the patient knows who is receiving the active medication or the placebo—at least until the study is finished, and then the code identifying the medication is revealed. In a "randomized, double-blind, placebo-controlled" study, the study is done and the results analyzed by investigators who do not have access to the code. The code is revealed only after the results are finalized. (Many studies have a "data monitoring and safety committee" that knows the results as they become available from the investigators. If this monitoring committee sees that one group is doing far worse than the other, they may stop the study early to prevent further risk for members of the group experiencing poor results.) Some studies are "single-blind"—only the patient is unaware of what he or she is receiving.

The purpose of placebo-control and "blinding" is to assure even further that any effects observed in the actively treated patients are *really* due to the medication and not due to biases of the researchers or the subjects. There is a well-recognized tendency for some people who think they are receiving a treatment to improve (the "placebo effect"), both subjectively in terms of symptoms and also, surprisingly, in ways that you would think they do not have control over. In a sense, placebo-controlled studies subtract the extent of changes seen in the placebo group from the extent of changes in the medication group to get a "true" assessment of the actual effects of the medication.

Doctors and patients are sometimes reluctant to participate in a study in which the patient (who, after all, has a problem that needs treatment) might receive a placebo. If the patient received the placebo, wouldn't he or she be deprived of a new and effective form of treatment? The answer is: no one knows—that is the whole point of the study. Reread the section Should All Palpitations Be Treated? (page 328) and decide whether the treated or "untreated" group was at an advantage. Furthermore, in most studies, conventional treatment is continued, even in the control group, so the patients are not deprived of the best known treatment available.

If you have the opportunity to participate in a study, read the consent form carefully. Know what is expected of you and what you should expect from participation in the study. Key elements of the consent form are a description of the study and why it is being done, what the sequence of events will be and what tests will be done, what alternative noninvestigational treatments are available, the risks of participating in the study, whether there are costs associated with being in the study, what will be done if complications occur, and who to get in touch with about any questions that might arise. Signing the consent form is a requirement for participating, but it is not a contract—the consent form should specify that you can withdraw from the study and that there will be no penalty whatsoever.

Once a study is completed, the data are reviewed by the FDA so that it can determine whether the treatment should be approved, studied further, or rejected. Often the data are also published in a medical journal. Articles in reputable medical journals are carefully reviewed for accuracy and sound reasoning by other doctors and scientists ("peer review")—this is further assurance that the information is reliable.

Some "new" medications or treatments gain publicity through the general media without ever having been subjected to carefully designed studies or peer-reviewed publication. An example is chelation therapy—the use of agents that bind to calcium and, according to proponents, open blood vessels obstructed by atherosclerosis. Almost invariably, these treatments must be regarded skeptically—they are at best unproven. The claims regarding the treatment are almost exclusively made by those who stand to profit directly by its use. Treatments that provide any benefit, even small, are able to prove it by careful testing and critical review.

WEIGHING THE PROS AND CONS OF MEDICAL OPTIONS

Most decisions in medicine, whether choosing a test to evaluate a problem, interpreting the test result, or selecting a treatment, involve weighing the pros and cons. One form of decision weighs the factors "risk" and "benefit." Another type, which is becoming increasingly important as society becomes more concerned about the costs of health care, weighs "cost" and "benefit." Each of these decisions involves probability: What is the probability that the benefit to the patient will outweigh the chance of harm? What is the likelihood that the benefit will justify the cost (that is, expense, inconvenience, discomfort, or risk)?

These complex decisions are some

of the toughest issues facing modern medicine, including escalating health care costs, malpractice lawsuits, and ethical dilemmas such as how best to care for terminally ill people. But they are also involved in the day-to-day practice of medicine. For example, everyone wants to know the chances of a complication occurring during the course of coronary artery catheterization. An expanded version of this question is, What are the *odds* that a complication will occur as a result of this procedure, how major might the complication be (*stakes*), and are the magnitude and likelihood of *benefit*

worth the *risk* (odds and stakes together are the risk)? Answers to these questions require knowing the following:

- the types of complications that could occur
- the chances of each complication occurring
- the goals of the procedure
- the chances of successfully achieving these goals

All of these components should be addressed in your discussions with your doctor.

Let us consider the decision of whether to do coronary artery catheterization.

Factors that affect your risks and benefits

- **The chance that the test will give useful information:** Do the symptoms, examination, and tests already done point to a problem that requires catheterization to solve?
- **The stability of the patient:** Is the catheterization being done on a scheduled basis or in the midst of a heart attack?
- **The existence of other problems:** Does the patient also have evidence of severe narrowing of the carotid arteries (to the brain) which could cause a stroke if the blood pressure temporarily decreased during the catheterization?
- **The general medical status of the patient:** Is he or she robust or frail?
- **The severity of the problem being investigated** (this may not be known ahead of time): Is there severe blockage of all the coronary arteries, or minimal blockage in one?
- **The skill and experience of the medical team:** Does the team do thousands of catheterizations each year, or dozens?
- **The availability of support services:** If a complication develops, are there ways to deal with it effectively (that is, coronary artery bypass), if necessary?

Reasons to do coronary catheterization (benefits)	Reasons to avoid coronary catheterization (risks and costs)
Determine whether coronary blockage is present Determine the severity of coronary blockage Determine the location of the coronary blockage Determine whether bypass operation or balloon angioplasty can be done	Small chance of serious complication Other tests may give much information Minor discomfort Expense

Remember, not all of the risks facing a patient are caused by the coronary catheterization. There is also a risk of missing out on an effective treatment if the coronary catheterization is not done. The risk of dying during a coronary catheterization is very small—less than 1 chance in 1,000. The risk of dying due to a blockage of the left main coronary artery is about 1 chance in 10 *every* year, unless a coronary bypass is done. Unfortunately, if a person with left main coronary blockage does not have a coronary catheterization, the blockage will not be discovered and an operation will not be done. The highest risk is obviously in *not* doing the catheterization. So it is important to have a clear idea of the possible risks and possible benefits of all courses of action before a procedure is done.

Another major component of the question cannot be easily quantified. Look at the question again, but with a different emphasis: What are the odds that a complication will occur as a result of this procedure, how major might the complication be (stakes), and are the magnitude and likelihood of benefit *worth* the risk? Determining the worth or value of a medical test or procedure (again, in terms of expense, inconvenience, discomfort, and risk) requires input from several sources: the patient, the people who care most for the patient (such as friends and family), and society's values. Many major hospitals have chaplains who are trained to help people reflect on and clarify values. The doctor may contribute, but more as a member of society than as an "expert."

Is there value in trying everything possible, even expensive and uncomfortable procedures, to extend the life

Examples of possible options for resuscitation

- **Do not resuscitate:** If the patient experiences a fatal heart rhythm, no action will be taken to reverse the problem.
- **Medical resuscitation only:** If a fatal heart rhythm or other abnormality develops, medications may be given (by vein) in the hope they may convert the rhythm to normal. But if they do not succeed, no further action will be taken.
- **Do not intubate:** If a fatal heart rhythm or other complication develops, medications and defibrillation can be used, but a breathing tube and ventilator should not be used. If the patient cannot breathe on his or her own, no further action will be taken. This might be specified if the patient's condition makes it unlikely that he or she will ever breathe independently again. If breathing capability is likely to require only brief and temporary assistance, then this option is unwise.

of an elderly and terminally ill person, or is there more value in promoting that person's comfort and dignity by "supportive" care? There is no single correct answer. Only candid discussions among the patient, family, and doctor can result in the appropriate medical care under the circumstances.

Diseases of the heart are often matters of life and death. Decisions about the evaluation and treatment of heart disease, therefore, are often life and death decisions. Although most of the efforts of doctors and patients are directed to saving and enhancing life, there may be a time when the decision to limit these efforts is best. This may mean giving instructions that in the event of a cardiac arrest (sudden cardiac death; see page 96) no resuscitation or only limited resuscitation should be undertaken. Most doctors of very ill hospitalized patients will seek the patient's and family's guidance on these issues; if not, the patient or family should bring up the subject. Ideally, families should discuss these serious matters before they occur. Having a "living will" (also called an "advance directive") is one option that can provide guidelines beforehand, and it should be considered by everyone regardless of their age.

By law (the Patient Self-Determination Act), whenever you are admitted to a hospital, you will be asked whether you have an advance directive. It would be wise to have thought about it before the need arises to declare this. An important component of your advance directive is to specify who should make decisions for you if you are incapacitated.

WOMEN AND HEART DISEASE

Being male is one of the risk factors for heart disease. It is not surprising, then, that many women worry about the development of heart disease in their husbands, their fathers, and other men in their lives. But heart disease is also the number one killer of women. In fact, almost 500,000 women die from some form of heart and blood vessel disease each year—twice the number of deaths from all forms of cancer.

The 240,000 women who die of heart attack each year represent close to half the 500,000 heart attack deaths in the United States. Despite the legitimate concern about, for example, breast cancer in women, breast cancer kills about 42,800 women, or only one-sixth the number of women who die of heart attack each year. These statistics show that the belief that heart disease is a man's problem is a dangerous misconception.

The myth that heart disease does not affect women is dangerous because it can cause women to neglect reducing their risk factors for heart disease. Furthermore, women may ignore symptoms that should send them for urgent medical evaluation. Women who have heart attacks are twice as likely to die as men within the first few weeks, but

women (or their doctors) may tend to misinterpret or discount symptoms suggesting heart attack.

Have Women Been Undertreated?

Women themselves often downplay or underestimate the severity of symptoms of heart disease or attribute the symptoms to another cause. Now, evidence shows that when women do enter the medical system, they may be managed less aggressively than men.

DIAGNOSIS. Women undergo fewer diagnostic procedures. One explanation for this difference is that some diagnostic tests are less accurate in women. For example, some types of exercise tests may show more "false-positive" results in women, and doctors are reluctant to use a test unless it has a high degree of accuracy.

TREATMENT. The use of some types of treatment for heart disease among men and women seems to differ. For example, figures show that four times as many men as women have coronary artery bypass operation.

RESULTS OF TREATMENT. Women also tend to have worse outcomes than men after procedures such as coronary artery bypass operation or balloon angioplasty. Part of the reason for this difference is that women tend to be older and sicker when the procedures are done. Another part of the reason is that women's coronary arteries are often smaller and so the procedures are more difficult to perform. But women also seem to have worse survival rates after having heart attacks, even when they are treated exactly like men with the most effective clot-dissolving medications available.

Yet the perception remains that heart disease does not affect women. Why don't women take this deadly disease more seriously? One reason is that women are not affected by heart disease as *early* as men are. Heart disease usually shows up in women almost 10 years later than it does in men. However, after age 50 years, it is the leading cause of death in women; by age 65 years, women's risk is almost equal to that of men's. One in three women aged 65 years or older has some form of heart disease.

Another reason is that most studies of heart disease have used men as subjects. For example, the Physicians' Health Study used only male physicians as subjects and showed that aspirin could help decrease the risk of heart attack in men. The Multiple Risk Factor Intervention Trial, which provided much information about risk factors, also studied only men. It is not clear whether findings that apply to men apply equally to women.

The Framingham Study, a large ongoing study of residents of Framingham, Massachusetts, includes 2,873 women in its study population, and it has provided valuable information

concerning the prevalence of and risk factors for heart disease in both men and women. However, there are still many unanswered questions, and much more research is needed. Fortunately, the need for more research involving women is being encouraged by the National Institutes of Health, the government agency that funds many important studies.

Until results are available to show whether and how prevention, diagnosis, and treatment of heart disease differ for men and women, women should use the information available today to assess their individual risks with their doctor. Guided by this information, you and your doctor can determine the best way to reduce your individual risk.

Factors That Remove Women's "Gender Protection"

Although heart disease develops later in life in women than in men, women are not immune to the influences that smoking, diabetes, high blood pressure, obesity, high blood cholesterol level, lack of exercise, and stress have on heart disease. (See Part 3, "Reducing Your Risk of Coronary Artery Disease," page 115, for a more detailed discussion of risk factors.) Of course, some risk factors are worse than others. In fact, smoking and diabetes may remove women's "gender protection" altogether.

SMOKING. For women, smoking is the greatest risk factor for heart attack. Women who smoke have two to six times the risk of having a heart attack as women who do not smoke. If you smoke and have a heart attack, you are more likely to die from it. Women smokers are also two to four times as likely to die suddenly of heart disease. Smoking seems to promote a more dangerous distribution of body fat (apple-shaped) (see page 139). The combination of smoking and the use of birth control pills dramatically increases the risk of a heart attack. Smokers, including women smokers, generally have lower levels of protective HDL cholesterol than nonsmokers.

These are frightening statistics in view of the fact that teenaged girls are the only group in our population that is increasing its use of cigarettes. On the positive side, a woman who quits smoking reduces her risk to a level that is almost as low as that of a nonsmoker in 2 or 3 years.

DIABETES. Diabetes mellitus is a disease in which too much sugar (called glucose) remains in the bloodstream rather than being transferred into cells throughout the body. Both type I and type II diabetes are associated with a higher risk of cardiovascular disease (see pages 140–142). Women with diabetes have rates of cardiovascular disease that are two to five times higher than in women without diabetes. For men, diabetes is not such a strong predictor of heart-related complications.

Special Issues Concerning Women

Research is starting to reveal how factors such as age, menopause, estrogen replacement therapy, and use of birth control pills affect your risk of heart disease. Some studies suggest that certain risk factors such as blood cholesterol levels may have different implications for women than they have for men.

AGE AND MENOPAUSE. One major difference between men and women is the age at which their risk of heart disease starts to climb. Women's risk of heart disease remains relatively low compared with men's until menopause, when the risk of heart attack increases gradually until it almost equals men's risk by age 65 years.

The reasons for this increase in risk are complex and not entirely understood. The female hormone estrogen may exert a protective effect. Estrogen tends to raise a woman's HDL ("good") cholesterol level and lower her LDL ("bad") cholesterol. Even if a woman's total cholesterol level is relatively high, she is likely to have a higher level of the protective HDL than a man with a similar total cholesterol level. However, after menopause, estrogen production is drastically reduced and its potentially beneficial effects are lost.

ESTROGEN REPLACEMENT THERAPY. If estrogen provides some protection from heart disease for younger women, why not replace the sharp decrease in estrogen after menopause? Estrogen replacement therapy was first used in the 1960s to relieve distressful symptoms such as hot flashes and vaginal dryness that accompany menopause in some women. Studies showed that supplemental estrogen seems to protect women against heart disease, but high doses also increase the risk of endometrial cancer (cancer in the lining of the uterus). The addition of the hormone progestin seems to cancel that risk, and it may even protect against endometrial cancer. Unfortunately, it may also partly cancel the protective effect of estrogen against heart disease.

So far, no conclusive evidence for or against estrogen replacement therapy for the prevention of heart disease is available, because studies have used subjects with different ages, health status, and risk factors. In addition, the dosages used today are much lower than they were in the past.

A study of groups of women aged 40 to 59 years in Rochester, Minnesota, indicated that the use of estrogen could reduce heart disease. However, estrogen could not counterbalance the bad effect of smoking. Most researchers agree that the risk of heart disease can be reduced by more than 30 percent in postmenopausal women who take replacement estrogen. This benefit seems to be due at least in part to increased HDL levels. Estrogen delivered by skin patches (transdermally) bypasses the liver and may not improve HDL levels as much.

In view of the possible risks of using estrogen replacement therapy, you should discuss your individual situation with your doctor and take your family history and risk factors for both heart disease and cancer into consideration. The American Heart Association suggests estrogen replacement therapy may not be necessary in women with no menopausal symptoms. Women with a personal or family history of uterine or breast cancer may want to avoid it. However, if you have had a hysterectomy, your risk of heart disease is real, whereas uterine cancer is not, so you may choose to take replacement estrogen to protect against heart attack.

BIRTH CONTROL PILLS. In contrast to the possible benefit of estrogen *replacement* therapy after menopause, the use of estrogen in birth control pills during the reproductive years may be associated with some increase in cardiovascular risk. Young women taking birth control pills may have a risk of heart attack up to three to four times that of women not taking them, although at that age the overall risk of heart attack still remains very small. Women who use birth control pills for more than 5 years may have a higher risk of heart attack for up to 10 years after they stop taking them. Birth control pills may slightly increase blood cholesterol level, blood pressure, and blood sugar level in some women. They also may lead to the development of blood clots. The amount of estrogen in birth control pills is less than that used previously, which probably reduces the risk substantially. Thus, the Food and Drug Administration has recommended that birth control pills can be used safely by women, even women older than 40 years, if they are otherwise healthy and do not smoke. Simultaneous risk factors tend to augment each other's effect, and the same is true for use of birth control pills: concurrent use of birth control pills and smoking multiplies the risk of heart attack up to 39 times compared with the risk in those who do not smoke *or* take oral contraceptives.

BLOOD LIPIDS. Total cholesterol level in the blood is a risk factor for coronary artery disease in women as well as in men. Women whose total cholesterol level is more than 265 mg/dl have more than twice the risk for the development of coronary artery disease as women whose level is less than 205 mg/dl. Although the association between coronary artery disease and total cholesterol is significant, women are even more susceptible to the risks of having a low HDL ("good") cholesterol level. The cardiovascular health of women also seems to be more influenced by triglyceride level than is men's. Women with a triglyceride level of more than 190 mg/dl have a greater risk, whereas men do not appear to increase their risk until the triglyceride level reaches 400 mg/dl.

BODY SIZE AND TYPE. Women tend to be smaller than men and, in turn, their hearts and coronary arteries are smaller. Some experts believe that smaller coronary arteries can become blocked by atherosclerosis more easily than larger arteries. In fact, some studies suggest that men and women of similar size have similar risks.

Smaller size makes procedures such as balloon angioplasty more difficult in women. They suffer more complications and have a lower rate of success with these procedures, although newer, appropriately sized equipment makes this less of a problem.

Although women tend to have a higher percentage of body fat than men, the fat tends to be distributed differently. Many men are shaped like apples, with fat around the waist, while many women are shaped more like pears, with fat around the hips. However, a woman may be apple-shaped, and this pattern of fat distribution tends to carry a higher risk of coronary artery disease.

The main point is that heart disease is not just a man's problem. Men and women alike should take steps to reduce their risk factors for coronary artery disease. In fact, developing a heart-healthy life-style should begin at a young age. Both men and women can play a role in preventing heart disease in future generations.

Pregnancy and Heart Disease

Heart disease in pregnant women requires careful medical management, but outcomes have changed dramatically. Women with any type of heart disease used to be told that they should not become pregnant. During the past 50 years, however, doctors have gained a better understanding of the changes that occur in a woman's body—especially her cardiovascular system—during pregnancy. Now, many women with heart disease are able to deliver healthy babies.

Pregnancy puts an extra burden on your heart. Your blood volume increases up to 50 percent by the 32nd week of pregnancy. You therefore have 6 to 8 liters (slightly more than 6 to 8 quarts) more body fluid than before you were pregnant. Your heart has to pump all that extra fluid to your body and your developing baby. To handle this increased load, your heart beats faster and also pumps out more blood with each contraction.

Different kinds of heart disease have different effects on your heart's ability to handle the stresses of pregnancy, labor, and delivery. Therefore, if you have heart disease, you should talk to your doctor before you become pregnant so that you both can evaluate your individual situation. Most women with heart disease can have a successful pregnancy, especially under the care of both an obstetrician and a cardiologist. But some heart problems (such as cyanotic congenital heart disease, pulmonary hypertension, and severe aortic stenosis) pose a high risk to both the mother and the fetus. Women with these problems are still advised to avoid pregnancy, unless the problem can be corrected first.

During prenatal counseling your doctor will be able to talk to you about possible physical risks for you and your baby during pregnancy, as well as the potential for passing on any congenital heart problems to your child. The rate of congenital heart disease is about 4 to 5 percent in children of women with significant congenital heart disease, whereas it is 1 percent in the general population. In some conditions, the chances of passing along a defect are as high as 50 percent.

Medication for various heart conditions, although necessary for the mother, may pose a potential risk for the fetus. Discuss your medication op-tions thoroughly with your doctor before you are pregnant.

Once you are pregnant, your doctor will monitor the development of your fetus and the effect of the pregnancy on your heart. Your doctor may tell you to cut back on your activities and take frequent breaks for 20 to 30 minutes in bed to give your heart a chance to rest. You should rest on your left side so your uterus does not compress your inferior vena cava, the main vein in the lower part of your body that returns blood to the heart. Other adjustments may include restricting salt in your diet and avoiding hot baths or long hot showers, which may dilate the blood vessels in your arms and legs. Dilated blood vessels are your body's response to hot temperatures, but they divert blood flow away from the fetus. It is important to have early prenatal care and ready access to a high-risk pregnancy center if you experience any problems.

Heart Drug Directory

Tables 1 through 9 appear on pages 296–311.

Name*	Table	Name*	Table
Abbokinase	4	Carteolol	2
Acebutolol	2	Cartrol	2
Activase	4	Catapres	6
Adalat	3	Catapres-TTS	6
Adenocard	8	Chlorothiazide	7
Adenosine	8	Chlorthalidone	7
Aldactazide	7	Cholestyramine	5
Aldactone	7	Choloxin	5
Aldomet	6	Cholybar	5
Altace	7	Cin-Quin	8
Amiloride	7	Clofibrate	5
Amiodarone	8	Clonidine	6
Amrinone	7	Colestid	5
Anistreplase	4	Colestipol	5
Apresoline	6	Cordarone	8
Aquatensen	7	Corgard	2
Aspirin	9	Coumadin	9
Atenolol	2	Crystodigin	7
Atromid-S	5	Deponit	1
Atropine	8	Dextrothyroxine	5
Benazepril	7	Dicumarol	9
Bepridil	3	Digitalis	7
Betaxolol	2	Digitoxin	7
Blocadren	2	Digoxin	7
Bretylium	8	Dilantin	8
Bretylol	8	Dilatrate	1
Brevibloc	2	Diltiazem	3
Bumetanide	7	Dipyridamole	9
Bumex	7	Disopyramide	8
Calan	3	Diulo	7
Capoten	7	Diuril	7
Captopril	7	Dobutamine	7
Cardene	3	Dobutrex	7
Cardilate	1	Dopamine	7
Cardioquin	8	Doxazosin	6
Cardizem	3	Duraquin	8
Cardura	6	Dyazide	7

Name*	Table	Name*	Table
DynaCirc	3	*Lanoxicaps*	7
Dyrenium	7	*Lanoxin*	7
Edecrin	7	*Lasix*	7
Eminase	4	*Levatol*	2
Enalapril	7	Lidocaine	8
Enduron	7	Lisinopril	7
Erythrityl		*Loniten*	6
tetranitrate	1	*Lopid*	5
Esidrix	7	*Lopressor*	2
Esmolol	2	*Lorelco*	5
Ethacrynic acid	7	*Lotensin*	7
Ethmozine	8	Lovastatin	5
Felodipine	3	*Maxzide*	7
Flecainide	8	Mecamylamine	6
Fosinopril	7	Methyclothiazide	7
Furosemide	7	Methyldopa	6
Gemfibrozil	5	Metolazone	7
Guanabenz	6	Metoprolol	2
Guanadrel	6	*Mevacor*	5
Guanethidine	6	Mexiletine	8
Guanfacine	6	*Mexitil*	8
Harmonyl	6	*Midamor*	7
Heparin	9	*Minipress*	6
Hydralazine	6	*Minitran*	1
Hydrochlorothiazide	7	Minoxidil	6
HydroDIURIL	7	*Moduretic*	7
Hygroton	7	*Monopril*	7
Hylorel	6	Moricizine	8
Hytrin	6	Nadolol	2
Inderal	2	*Nia-Bid*	5
Inocor	7	*Niacels*	5
Intropin	7	Niacin	5
Inversine	6	Nicardipine	3
Ismelin	6	*Nicobid*	5
Isoproterenol	8	*Nicolar*	5
Isoptin	3	*Nicotinex*	5
Isordil	1	Nifedipine	3
Isosorbide dinitrate	1	*Nitro-Bid*	1
Isradipine	3	*Nitro-disc*	1
Isuprel	8	*Nitro-Dur*	1
Kabikinase	4	*Nitrogard*	1
Kerlone	2	Nitroglycerin	1
Labetalol	2	*Nitrol*	1

Tables 1 through 9 appear on pages 296–311.

Name*	Table	Name*	Table
Nitrolingual	1	Rauzide	6
Nitrostat	1	Rhythmol	8
Normodyne	2	Sectral	2
Norpace	8	Serpasil	6
Norpace CR	8	Simvastatin	5
Oretic	7	Slo-Niacin	5
Panwarfin	9	Sorbitrate	1
Penbutolol	2	Spironolactone	7
Pentaerythrityl		Streptase	4
tetranitrate	1	Streptokinase	4
Pentoxifylline	9	Tambocor	8
Peritrate	1	Tenex	6
Persantine	9	Tenormin	2
Phenytoin	8	Terazosin	6
Pindolol	2	Thalitone	7
Plendil	3	Timolol	2
Pravachol	5	Tissue plasminogen	
Pravastatin	5	activator	4
Prazosin	6	Tocainide	8
Prinivil	7	Tonocard	8
Probucol	5	Trandate	2
Procainamide	8	Transderm-Nitro	1
Procan SR	8	Trental	9
Procardia	3	Triamterene	7
Pronestyl	8	Urokinase	4
Pronestyl-SR	8	Vascor	3
Propafenone	8	Vasotec	7
Propranolol	2	Verapamil	3
Questran	5	Verelan	3
Quinaglute	8	Visken	2
Quinalan	8	Warfarin	9
Quinidex	8	Wytensin	6
Quinidine	8	Xylocaine	8
Quinora	8	Zaroxolyn	7
Ramipril	7	Zestril	7
Raudixin	6	Zocor	5
Rauwolfia alkaloids	6		

*Generic names are in regular type, and *brand names are in italic type.*

Tables 1 through 9 appear on pages 296–311.

Glossary

Abdominal aorta (ab-DOM-ih-nal ay-OR-tah): portion of the aorta in the abdomen

Ablation (ah-BLAY-shun): elimination or removal

Adventitia (ad-ven-TISH-ah): outer layer in the wall of an artery

Alveoli (al-VEE-o-li): air sacs in the lungs where oxygen and carbon dioxide are exchanged

Amaurosis fugax (am-ah-ROW-sis FU-jax): temporary visual defect, usually in one eye, caused by inadequate blood flow to the eye

Amyloidosis (am-i-loy-DOE-sis): rare condition in which certain blood cells produce excessive protein deposits in the tissues. If the deposits are in the heart, heart failure can result

Aneurysm (AN-yu-riz-em): bulge in a blood vessel

Angina pectoris (AN-jin-ah PEK-ta-ris): chest pain or discomfort caused by too little blood flow in the coronary arteries to meet the oxygen needs of the heart muscle

Angiogram (AN-jee-o-gram): X-ray picture of any arteries or veins

Angiography (an-jee-AHG-ra-fee): method for taking X-ray pictures of the coronary arteries

Angioplasty (AN-jee-o-plas-tee): method for dilating narrowed or blocked part of an artery with a catheter

Annulus (AN-yu-lus): the ring around a heart valve where the valve leaflet merges with the heart muscle

Antianginal (AN-ti-AN-jih-nal): preventing or treating angina

Antiarrhythmic (AN-ti-ah-RITH-mik): preventing or alleviating arrhythmias

Anticoagulant (AN-ti-co-AG-u-lant): medication that keeps blood from clotting; "blood thinner"

Aorta (ay-OR-tah): the artery carrying oxygen-containing blood from the left ventricle of your heart to all parts of the body

Aortic (ay-OR-tik) **valve:** valve between the left ventricle and the aorta

Apoproteins (ap-oh-PROE-teens): proteins that combine with lipids to make them dissolve in blood

Arrhythmia (ah-RITH-mee-ah): abnormal heartbeat

Arteriogram (ar-TEER-e-o-gram): angiogram of arteries; a coronary arteriogram is an angiogram of the coronary arteries

Arteriole (ar-TEER-ee-ole): smaller branch of an artery

Arteritis (art-ah-WRITE-us): inflammation of arteries

Artery: blood vessel that transports blood from the heart to the body or lungs

Ascending aorta (ah-SEN-ding ay-OR-tah): the first part of the aorta that emerges from the left ventricle

Atherectomy (a-ther-EK-toh-mee): method for shaving or removing plaque from inside arteries with a specially designed catheter

Atherosclerosis (ath-e-roe-skleh-ROE-sis): fatty deposits in and on artery walls, producing narrowing; "hardening of the arteries"

Atrial septal defect: see *Septal defect*

Atrioventricular (ay-tree-o-ven-TRIK-yu-lar): between the atria and ventricles

Atrioventricular block: block of the electrical signal between the atria and ventricles; can vary in severity from first, second, or third degree (complete heart block)

Atrioventricular node; also called AV node: cluster of cells between the atria and ventricles that slows the electrical current of the heart rhythm as it passes through to the ventricles

Atrium (AY-tree-um): one of two small upper receiving chambers of the heart; plural form is "atria"

Bicuspid (by-CUS-pid): having two cusps

Biopsy (BY-op-see): method of taking a small sample of tissue for examination

Blalock-Taussig (BLAY-lok TAW-sig) **procedure:** a palliative operation that partially improves the condition of some patients with cyanotic heart disease

Bradycardia (bray-de-KAR-dee-ah): slow heartbeat

Bruit (BREW-ee): sound of blood flowing through a narrowed vessel

Bundle-branch block: condition in which portions of the heart's conduction system become defective and are unable to conduct the electrical signal normally (can be right or left bundle-branch block)

Bypass: see *Cardiopulmonary bypass* and *Coronary artery bypass graft*

Capillaries (KAP-ih-ler-ees): smallest blood vessels connecting arteries and veins where oxygen and nutrients are exchanged for waste products

Cardiac arrest: condition in which the heart stops beating and breathing ceases abruptly

Cardiac cycle: period from the beginning of one heartbeat to the beginning of the next

Cardiac output: the amount of blood the heart pumps through the circulatory system in 1 minute (stroke volume multiplied by heart rate)

Cardiomyopathy (kar-dee-oh-my-OP-ah-thee): diseases of the muscle of the heart (myocardium)

Cardiopulmonary bypass (kar-dee-oh-PUL-mah-ner-ee BY-pass): method by which a machine takes over the function of the heart and lungs so the heart can be stopped for surgery

Cardiopulmonary resuscitation (kar-dee-oh-PUL-mah-ner-ee ree-SUS-ih-TAY-shun): use of rescue breathing and chest compressions to supply oxygen and blood to a person whose heartbeat and breathing have stopped

Cardioversion (KAR-dee-o-VER-zhun): electrical shock applied to the chest to convert an abnormal heartbeat to normal

Carotid (ka-RAH-tid) **arteries:** main arteries supplying the head

Catheter (KATH-et-er): long, thin, flexible, hollow tube inserted into the body

Catheterization (kath-et-er-ih-ZA-shun): any procedure in which a catheter is inserted into the body; it can be used to assess the condition of coronary arteries, valves, and heart muscle and to open blocked arteries and reshape heart valves

CCU: cardiac (or coronary, in some hospitals) care unit

Cerebral embolism (seh-REE-bral EM-boe-lis-m): a clot that travels through blood vessels from the site where it formed and blocks blood flow in the brain

Cerebral hemorrhage (seh-REE-bral HEH-mor-ij): bleeding into the brain

Cheyne-Stokes (CHAIN stokes) **respiration:** alternating periods of slow breathing with pauses and periods of rapid, deep breathing

Cholesterol (ko-LES-ter-ol): a type of lipid (fat) used by your body to build cells and certain hormones; also one of the fats found in foods derived from animal sources

Chordae tendineae (KOR-dee ten-DIN-eeah): strong chords that stretch from the tricuspid and mitral valve edges to the heart muscle and restrict how far the valve leaflets swing when they close

Claudication (claw-dih-KAY-shun): limb pain or tiredness due to inadequate oxygen supply to the muscles; caused by narrowed arteries

Coarctation (co-ark-TAY-shun) **of the aorta:** congenital constriction or narrowing of the aorta that impedes blood flow from the heart to the lower part of the body and increases blood pressure

Collateral (ko-LAT-er-al) **vessels:** small branches of blood vessels that develop to bypass narrowed or blocked sections

Compensatory (com-PEN-sah-tor-ee) **pause:** after a premature contraction, the heart waits a little longer before it beats

Computed tomography (toh-MOG-ra-fee); also called CT or CAT scan: X-ray technique that uses a computer to construct a cross-section image of the body

Conduction system: special muscle fibers that conduct electrical impulses throughout the muscle of the heart

Congenital heart defect: defect in the heart which is present at birth

Congestive heart failure (also called heart failure): condition caused when the heart is unable to pump enough blood to meet the needs of the body; also characterized by fluid collecting in various parts of the body (such as legs, lungs, liver)

Coronary arteries: arteries supplying blood to the heart muscle itself

Coronary artery bypass graft (CABG) operation: an operation that reroutes the blood supply by bypassing blocked coronary arteries

Coronary artery disease: blockage of one or more of the coronary arteries

Coronary sinus: the main coronary vein that drains blood into the right atrium from the smaller coronary veins

Coronary veins: veins returning blood from the heart muscle to the coronary sinus

CPR: cardiopulmonary resuscitation

Cusp: a heart valve leaflet

Cyanosis (sigh-ah-NO-sis): bluish coloring of skin, nails, lips, or tongue due to lack of oxygen-containing blood

Cyanotic heart disease: birth defects of the heart which permit oxygen-depleted (blue) blood to circulate to the body without passing through the lungs

Deep vein thrombosis: a blood clot in the deep vein of the calf

Defibrillation (dee-fih-brih-LAY-shun): electrical shock applied to the chest to stop fibrillation

Defibrillator (dee-FIH-brih-lay-tor): machine used to deliver an electrical shock to the chest to stop fibrillation; it may be internal (implanted) or external

Deoxygenated (dee-OX-ee-jen-ay-ted): without much oxygen

Diabetes (die-a-BEE-teez): a disease in which too much sugar (called glucose) remains in the bloodstream rather than being transferred into the cells throughout the body

Diastole (die-ASS-toe-lee): period of the cardiac cycle when the heart relaxes to allow blood to flow in

Dilated (DIE-lay-ted): enlarged

Dissection (di-SEK-shun): separation of the inner layers of a blood vessel from the outer layers

Diuretic (die-ur-EH-tik): "water pill"; promotes urine production

Doppler ultrasound: technique used to characterize blood flow in the heart or blood vessels in which ultrasound waves are reflected off blood cells as they move in the bloodstream

Duplex scanning (DU-pleks scanning): ultrasound test showing blood flow and blood vessel structure; used to detect blockages and various other circulatory problems in the arteries or veins

Dyspnea (DISP-nee-a): shortness of breath

Ebstein's anomaly (EB-stinz ah-NOH-ma-lee): congenital heart disease characterized by abnormally developed tricuspid valve leaflets

Echocardiography (EH-ko-kar-dee-OG-ra-fee): use of ultrasound to "look" directly at the heart without penetrating the skin

Edema (eh-DEEM-a): swelling caused by leakage of fluid from the bloodstream into the surrounding tissue

Effusion (eh-FEW-zhun): fluid accumulation

Eisenmenger's (EYE-sen-men-gerz) **complex:** condition that occurs when a congenital heart defect leads to an increase in blood flow to the lungs and to irreversible high blood pressure in the lungs

Ejection fraction: the portion of blood that is pumped out of a filled ventricle (normal is 50 percent or more)

Electrocardiogram (ee-lek-troe-KAR-dee-o-gram): recording of the electrical activity of the heart

Electrophysiology (ee-lek-troe-fiz-ee-OL-o-jee) **studies:** a type of catheterization in which electrode catheters rather than hollow catheter tubes are inserted through blood vessels into the heart to sense electrical impulses and also to pace the heart

Embolism (EM-boe-liz-em): the blocking of a blood vessel by a blood clot that has formed in one place but traveled to another point in the circulation and lodged

Endarterectomy (end-ar-ter-EK-toh-mee): surgical removal of material (such as atherosclerosis) from an artery

Endocarditis (en-doe-kard-EYE-tis): inflammation of the membrane that lines the chambers and valves of the heart, usually caused by an infection of the valve

Endocardium (en-doe-CARD-ee-um): smooth membrane covering the inside surfaces of the heart

Endothelium (en-doe-THEE-lee-um): a layer of cells on the inner surface of the blood vessels

Endotracheal (en-doe-TRAY-kee-al) **tube:** tube inserted into the trachea (windpipe) to allow assisted breathing with a ventilator

Epicardium (eh-pih-KAR-dee-um): thin membrane covering the outside surface of the heart muscle

Erythema (eer-eh-THEE-mah): abnormal reddish coloring of the skin

Estrogen (ES-troe-jen): female hormone that may protect women against heart disease

Extrasystole (ex-tra-SIS-toe-lee): premature heartbeat

Familial hypercholesterolemia (fah-MIL-yul hy-per-koe-les-ter-ol-EE-mee-ah): a genetic predisposition to have dangerously high cholesterol levels

Fatty acids; also called "fats": substances that occur in several forms in the foods you eat; different fatty acids have different effects on lipid profiles

Fibrillation (fih-brih-LAY-shun): rapid and uncoordinated beating of chambers of the heart

Fluoroscopy (flur-OS-ko-pee): use of X-rays to see motion, as opposed to still X-ray films

Flutter: rapid, ineffective beating of a heart chamber, but more coordinated than fibrillation

Gangrene (GAN-green): death of tissue due to loss of blood supply

Gynecoid (GUYN-eh-koid) **fat distribution:** body shape that is fairly thin in the upper body with fat accumulated in the hips and thighs; more typical of females

HDL cholesterol (high-density lipoprotein [lih-poe-PROE-teen] **cholesterol):** a combination of about 50 percent apoproteins and 20 percent cholesterol; it tends to help remove excess cholesterol from blood

Heart block: see *Atrioventricular block*

Heart failure: see *Congestive heart failure*

Heart-lung machine: machine that oxygenates and circulates blood during open-heart surgery; see also *Cardiopulmonary bypass*

Heimlich (HIME-lik) **maneuver:** abdominal thrusts applied manually below the diaphragm to dislodge an object blocking the windpipe

Hemochromatosis (hee-mo-kro-mah-TOE-sis): a defect in iron metabolism that permits iron to build up in the body

Hemorrhage (HEH-mor-ij): heavy bleeding

His-Purkinje (his pur-KIN-jee) **system:** system of branching pathways of specialized electricity-conducting tissue in the ventricles

HOCM: hypertrophic obstructive cardiomyopathy; overgrowth of heart muscle that creates a bulge into the ventricle, impeding blood flow

Holter (HOLE-ter) **monitor:** a portable device that records an electrocardiogram on tape or computer chip

"Hot reactor": a person whose body responds dramatically to stress

Hyperglycemia (hy-per-gly-SEE-mee-ah): high blood levels of glucose

Hypertension: high blood pressure

Hypertrophic (hy-per-TROE-fik) **cardiomyopathy:** overgrowth of heart muscle that impedes blood flow into and out of the heart

Hyperventilation (hy-per-ven-tih-LAY-shun): repetitive sighing type of rapid breathing and a sense that you cannot breathe deeply enough

IHSS: idiopathic hypertrophic subaortic stenosis; another term for HOCM

Immunosuppressive (ih-mu-no-suh-PREH-siv) **medications:** drugs that suppress the immune system to minimize the chances that it will reject a new transplanted organ (heart)

Impedance plethysmography (im-PEED-ens ple-thiz-MOG-ra-fee): a test to evaluate blood flow through leg veins

Infarct (IN-farkt): area of permanently damaged tissue (scar) caused by inadequate oxygen supply

Inferior vena cava (VEE-nah CAY-vah): large vein returning blood from your legs and abdomen to your heart

Inotropic (ine-o-TRO-pik) **medications:** medications that increase the strength of the heart's contraction

Intima (IN-tim-a): inner layer in the wall of an artery

Ischemia (is-KEE-mee-a): insufficient amount of blood and oxygen reaching the tissues

Jugular (JUG-yu-lar) **veins:** veins that carry blood back from the head to the heart

Korotkoff (ko-ROT-kof) **sounds:** sounds made by the pulse that are heard when a blood pressure is taken

LDL cholesterol (low-density lipoprotein [lie-poe-PROE-teen] **cholesterol):** a combination of about 25 percent apoproteins and 45 percent cholesterol; it provides cholesterol for necessary body functions, but in excessive amounts it tends to accumulate in artery walls

Left heart failure: blood flow to the body is decreased and fluid accumulates in the lungs; see also *Congestive heart failure*

Lipid profile: measurement of various lipids in the bloodstream

Lipids (LIH-pids): general term referring to fats circulating in the bloodstream

Lipoproteins (lih-poe-PROE-teens): lipids combined with apoproteins

Lumen (LUE-men): the channel within blood vessels in which blood flows

Lung scanning: a test designed to assess the circulation through the lungs

Magnetic resonance (REZ-n-ens) **imaging; also called MRI:** uses magnetic fields and radio waves to construct images of internal body structures

Media: middle muscular layer in the wall of an artery

Mitral (MY-tral) **valve:** valve between the left atrium and left ventricle

Mitral valve prolapse (MY-tral valve PRO-laps): bulging of the leaflets of the mitral valve into the left atrium during the heart's contraction; also called "click murmur syndrome"

mm Hg: millimeters of mercury; unit for measuring blood pressure

Murmur: sounds made by turbulent blood moving through the chambers and valves of the heart or through the blood vessels near the heart, usually signifying an abnormality of blood flow caused by a structural defect in the heart or valves

Myocardial infarction (my-o-KAR-dee-al in-FARK-shun): heart attack; an area of heart tissue dies because its blood supply is blocked

Myocarditis (my-o-kard-EYE-tis): inflammation of the heart muscle

Myocardium (my-o-KAR-dee-um): heart muscle

Necrosis (neh-KROE-sis): death of areas of tissue

Nuclear (NU-klee-ar) **heart scanning:** test used to show features of heart function and blood flow; it involves injection of radioactive material ("tracers") into the bloodstream

Occlusion (oh-KLU-zhun): total blockage of a blood vessel

Oculoplethysmography (OPG) (AH-ku-loe-ple-thiz-MOG-ra-fee): test used to measure eye pressure; it indirectly helps to determine whether a carotid artery is blocked

Open heart surgery: opening the heart to operate on its structures; see also *Cardiopulmonary bypass*

Orthopnea (or-THOP-nee-a): difficulty breathing except in an upright position (*ortho* means "straight" or "upright")

Orthostatic hypotension (or-thoe-STAT-ik hy-poe-TEN-shun): low blood pressure upon standing that may lead to light-headedness or passing out

Pacemaker: device that delivers electrical stimulus to the heart, which causes it to contract

Palliative (PAL-e-at-iv): treatment, such as an operation, that does not cure a problem but makes adjustments to improve the situation

Pallor (PAL-er): paleness

Palpation (pal-PAY-shun): examining by touch

Palpitations (pal-pi-TAY-shuns): uncomfortable sensations of your heartbeat in your chest

Paroxysmal nocturnal dyspnea (par-ox-SIZ-mal nok-TUR-nal DISP-nee-a): shortness of breath developing at night which causes awakening and gasping for air

Percutaneous transluminal coronary angioplasty (per-kew-TAY-nee-us trans-LUE-mih-nal KO-ro-NAIR-ee AN-jee-o-plas-tee); PTCA: the use of catheters to reopen obstructed coronary arteries

Perfusion (pur-FEW-zhun) **scanning:** a test that produces an image of the heart muscle with radioactive tracers. It can show areas of the heart muscle that do not receive adequate blood flow

Pericardiectomy (pair-ih-kar-dee-EK-tah-mee): removal of the pericardium

Pericardiocentesis (pair-ih-kar-dee-o-sen-TEE-sis): withdrawing excess fluid (pericardial effusion) from the pericardium through a needle

Pericarditis (pair-ih-kard-EYE-tis): inflammation of the pericardium

Pericardium (pair-ih-KAR-dee-um): the sac or membrane surrounding the heart

Placebo (plah-SEE-boe): inactive substance

Plaque (plak): material that builds up inside an artery which can reduce or block blood flow; see also *Atherosclerosis*

Platelets (PLAYT-lets): one of the components of blood that contribute to clotting

Positron emission tomography (PA-zih-tron ee-MIH-shun toh-MAH-gra-fee); PET scanning: investigational imaging technique used for measuring blood flow and the metabolism of the tissues of the body, including the heart

Premature contraction: a heartbeat that comes too soon; see also *Extrasystole*

Presyncope (pree-SIN-ko-pee): lightheadedness

Prolapse: see *Mitral valve prolapse*

Prothrombin (proe-THROM-bin) **time test:** test that measures the activity of certain clotting factors; it is often used to determine whether a person is receiving the correct dose of the anticoagulant warfarin

Pulmonary (PUL-mah-ner-ee) **artery:** blood vessel that carries oxygen-depleted blood from the right ventricle to the lungs

Pulmonary edema (PUL-mah-ner-ee eh-DEE-mah): fluid buildup in the lungs

Pulmonary (PUL-mah-ner-ee) **valve:** valve at the opening from the right ventricle to the pulmonary artery

Pulmonary (PUL-mah-ner-ee) **vein:** blood vessel that carries newly oxygenated blood from the lungs back to the left atrium of the heart

Pulse: the rhythmic expansion of an artery, caused by contractions of the heart; it can be felt with the finger

Radionuclide ventriculography (ray-dee-o-NU-klide ven-TRIH-ku-log-ra-fee): a test used to determine the size and shape of the heart's pumping chambers, the ventricles

Rales (rayls): abnormal breathing sounds, sometimes indicating fluid in the air sacs of the lung

Raynaud's (RAY-noze) **phenomenon:** spasm of the small vessels in the fingers, especially when exposed to cold

Regurgitation (ree-gur-ji-TAY-shun): backward flow

Renal (REE-nal): relating to the kidneys

Reperfusion (ree-per-FEW-zhun): resumption of blood flow

Rheumatic (rue-MAT-ik) **fever:** inflammatory illness that sometimes follows strep throat and may damage the heart valves

Right heart failure: decreased blood flow resulting in swelling in the legs and abdominal organs, including the liver (see *Congestive heart failure*)

Sedentary (SEH-den-tare-ee): lacking exercise

Septal (SEP-tal) **defect:** hole in the wall separating the atria or in the wall separating the ventricles

Septum (SEP-tum): wall separating the left and right atria and the left and right ventricles

Shock: collapse of the circulatory system

Shunt: connection allowing abnormal blood flow between two locations

Sick sinus syndrome: failure of the sinus node to perform its normal function of regulating the heartbeat. It often results in periods of fast heartbeat and periods of slow heartbeat

Silent ischemia (is-KEE-mee-a): insufficient amounts of blood and oxygen reach portions of the heart muscle, but angina is not produced

Sinus node: the heart's natural pacemaker

Sphygmomanometer (sfyg-moe-mah-NAH-meh-ter): a device for measuring blood pressure

Stable angina (AN-jin-ah): chest pain caused by myocardial ischemia and with a predictable pattern

Stenosis (steh-NO-sis): narrowing, stiffening

Sternum (STER-num): breastbone

Stethoscope (STETH-o-scope): device for listening to heart sounds

Strain gauge plethysmography (plethiz-MOG-ra-fee): a test used to evaluate how efficiently blood is flowing through a leg artery

Strep throat: bacterial (streptococcal) infection of the throat that can lead to rheumatic fever if untreated

Stroke: a brain injury that is caused by an inadequate supply of blood to the brain

Stroke volume: the actual amount of blood pumped by the left ventricle with one contraction

Sudden cardiac death: cardiac arrest; usually caused by ventricular fibrillation

Superior vena cava (VEE-na CAE-va): large vein returning blood from your head and arms to your heart

Swan-Ganz catheter: a monitoring catheter; used to assess the cardiac output and pressures in the right heart chambers and pulmonary artery

Syncope (SIN-ko-pee): loss of consciousness due to temporary insufficient blood supply to the brain, often caused by a serious arrhythmia

Systole (SIS-toe-lee): period of contraction in the cardiac cycle when the heart squeezes or pumps

Tachycardia (TAK-ee-KAR-dee-ah): rapid heartbeat

Tachypnea (ta-KIP-nee-ah): rapid breathing

Tamponade (tam-pon-ODD): excess fluid in the pericardium prevents the heart from expanding enough during diastole to fill sufficiently

Thrills: vibrations in the chest from abnormal blood flow

Thrombolysis (throm-BOL-ih-sis): use of medication to dissolve blood clots

Thrombolytic (throm-boe-LIH-tik) **agents:** drugs that dissolve clots

Thrombophlebitis (throm-boe-fleb-I-tis): clotting of blood and inflammation in a vein, most commonly in a leg

Thrombosis (throm-BOE-sis): formation of a blood clot (thrombus) within the heart or blood vessels

Thrombus (THROM-bus): blood clot

TIA: transient ischemic attack; temporary lack of circulation to part of the brain

Transcutaneous oximetry (trans-kew-TAY-nee-us oks-IH-meh-tree): measurement of the amount of oxygen in a region of skin with a special patch taped to the skin

Transesophageal (trans-eh-SOF-ah-jeel) **echocardiography:** echocardiography in which a transducer is placed in the esophagus to gain clearer images of the heart

Transplantation: replacing a defective organ with one from a donor

Tricuspid (try-KUS-pid) **valve:** valve between the right atrium and ventricle

Triglycerides (try-GLIH-ser-ides): a type of lipid used by the body as a source of energy; elevated triglycerides contribute to atherosclerosis

Truncal (TRUN-kal) **obesity:** fat deposited in the upper body and abdomen, instead of the hips and thighs; more typical of males

Unstable angina (AN-jin-ah): new or increasing angina

Valvuloplasty (VAL-vu-lo-plas-tee): reshaping of a heart valve with surgical or catheter techniques

Variant angina (AN-jin-ah): chest pain caused by spasm of the muscle encircling the coronary arteries

Varicose veins: abnormally dilated veins

Vascular system: blood vessels; arteries and veins

Vasodilators (vay-so-DIE-lay-tors): medications that widen or dilate the arteries

Vasopressors (vay-so-PRES-ors): drugs that elevate blood pressure

Vasovagal syncope (vay-zoe-VAY-gal SIN-koe-pee): simple faint

Vein: a blood vessel that returns blood to the heart from the body or lungs

Venogram: angiogram of veins

Ventilation/perfusion scanning: see *Lung scanning*

Ventricle (VEN-trih-kel): one of two large lower pumping chambers of the heart

Ventricular septal defect: see *Septal defect*

Venule (VEEN-yule): a small vein

Vertigo (VER-tih-go): dizziness; the sense that you are spinning

Wolff-Parkinson-White syndrome: condition in which an extra electrical pathway connects the atria and ventricles; it may cause a rapid heartbeat

X-ray: form of radiation used to create a picture of internal body structures on film

Yo-yo syndrome: weight goes up and down because of intermittent dieting alternating with regaining the weight; weight cycling

INDEX